Doctors and the State

DOCTORS
and the STATE:

THE BRITISH MEDICAL PROFESSION
AND GOVERNMENT ACTION IN
PUBLIC HEALTH, 1870-1912

BY JEANNE L. BRAND

THE JOHNS HOPKINS PRESS
BALTIMORE, MARYLAND

Preface

THE PATTERNS of government action for the public health and welfare which evolved in England in the last hundred years differ markedly from those of the United States of America. England and many Western European countries have long since adopted comprehensive national medical care plans which even the liberal United States Congress of 1965 would hesitate to consider.

The earlier growth of such schemes abroad stemmed from a greater need—a wider gap between the rich and poor, which environmental opportunity and economic self-help could not bridge. Elsewhere, national health insurance plans developed out of the broader social goals of a labor vote, and the existence of smaller, more homogeneous populations with a single, central government, and not, as in the United States, a federal government whose powers are shared with the states. In some nations, notably Germany and czarist Russia, single leaders pushed through medical care or sickness insurance plans in the last century.

At a time when America is on the threshold of adopting a limited national health plan for the aged members of our society, a review of earlier patterns of preventive and social medicine, and of the role of the medical profession in such developments, may offer fresh perspectives. The years 1870 to 1912 in England and Wales are particularly appropriate for such observations. They witnessed the start of a new central authority for public health, remarkable developments in medicine and science, a shift in emphasis from environmental hygiene to personal health services, and the assumption of government responsibility for curative medicine. These years also brought fundamental changes in the social and economic conditions of the English people which led to the new society of the twentieth-century state. And from a population in 1870 of 22,457,366, there developed by 1912 a nation of 36,539,636, an increase of more than 60 per cent.

The widely publicized opposition to "state medicine" expressed by professional medical groups in many western countries often obscures the substantial contributions of physicians in the extension of government action for the health of society. In England medical men, within and without the government structure, supported much of the legislation which established public responsibility for preventive and curative medicine.

The width of the field has limited the study to topics most central to the subject. It has been necessary, for example, to exclude the whole area of reforms in the care of the mentally ill, to limit detailed observations of the development of preventive medicine to the years prior to 1900, and to consider only briefly the medical programs of the British military and colonial services. These are substantial studies in their own right. Again, in tracing primarily national developments, the work of some private medical practitioners, whose contributions were essentially regional, may be slighted. Problems of selection and emphasis necessarily enter into any study, requiring in the end arbitrary decisions, made with the hope that readers will accept the scope of a book as an author conceived it. While it has been occasionally desirable to include some international perspective on contemporary developments in preventive and curative medicine, this is primarily a study of British medicine and society.

The social historian aims for objectivity but can never wholly escape his biases. It is, therefore, only fair to acknowledge a conscious bias in favor of government action for the health of a society—a belief that the healthy and strong have a fundamental obligation toward the weak—and that a scientifically informed humanitarianism is an essential component of a civilized society. To the degree that this conviction might color an analysis of earlier societies in which it was not widely held, this study may not be wholly "objective" history. Every effort has, nevertheless, been made to view those who constitute this story in the framework of their contemporary thinking. This book does not set forth any blanket plea for central government action as the sole approach to national health. Nor does it assume that the passage of laws is sufficient to guarantee to the public universally competent and efficient medical care. But national legislation can, and has, provided baselines for the development of sound programs of preventive and curative medicine.

The original topic was formulated in seminars with the late Professor J. Bartlett Brebner at Columbia University. The major portion of the research was carried out in England under a Fulbright scholarship and Leverhulme grant at the London School of Economics and Political Science.

The study owes most to the wide erudition and kindness of Mr. H. L. Beales, formerly Reader in Economic History at the London School of Economics. Both Dr. Iago Galdston and Dr. George Rosen read a draft of the manuscript in its entirety, and I am deeply grateful for this generous gift of their time and for their comments and suggestions. Among others who offered constructive criticism of the study, at various stages, were Dr. James M. Mackintosh, Dr. Joseph S. Pegum, Dr. James Cassedy, Dr. Marcus Goldstein, and Dr. Leanore Laan. Responsibility for possible errors must, of course, rest with the author.

I am also most appreciative of the assistance of staff members of many London and United States libraries, more particularly the Royal Society of Medicine, the Wellcome Historical Medical Library, the New York Academy of Medicine, the Library of Congress, and the National Library of Medicine. Much help was obtained from staff of the British Museum, the Public Record Office, the Ministry of Housing and Local Government, and the Society of Medical Officers of Health. I am especially indebted to the National Library of Medicine and to Dr. F. N. L. Poynter, Director of the Wellcome Historical Medical Library and Museum, for the location and reproduction of contemporary illustrations for the book.

The book was completed during various periods of leave from the National Institute of Mental Health. It in no way reflects any official views of the United States Public Health Service.

JEANNE L. BRAND

Washington, D.C.
June, 1965

ABBREVIATIONS

C.B.	Companion Order of the Bath
C.B.E.	Commander Order of the British Empire
Ch.M., C.M., M.S.	Master of Surgery
D.C.L.	Doctor of Civil Laws
D.P.H.	Diploma in Public Health
F.R.C.P.	Fellow Royal College of Physicians
F.R.C.S.	Fellow Royal College of Surgeons
F.R.S.	Fellow Royal Society
K.C.B.	Knight Commander Order of the Bath
L.R.C.P.	Licentiate Royal College of Physicians
L.R.C.S.	Licentiate Royal College of Surgeons
L.S.A.	Licentiate Society of Apothecaries
M.B.	Bachelor of Medicine
M.P.	Member of Parliament
M.R.C.P.	Member Royal College of Physicians
M.R.C.S.	Member Royal College of Surgeons

Contents

List of Tables

Doctors and the State

Introduction

The growth of civilization means the growth of towns, and the growth of towns means, at present, a terrible sacrifice of human life. . . . The fact is that in creating towns, men create the materials for an immense hotbed of disease, and this effect can only be neutralized by extraordinary artificial precautions.

The Times October 8, 1868

ENGLAND led the world on both sides of the Atlantic in initiating public health legislation. It had the most urgent need to do so. The first country to industrialize, England was the first to grapple with resulting urban slums, polluted by dungheaps, open sewers, and contaminated water supplies.

In the years 1801 to 1851, the population of the principal towns and cities of England and Wales almost tripled. From 8,892,000 inhabitants at the opening of the nineteenth century, England had grown, by 1851, into a nation of 17,927,000 persons, crowded in great urban centers recurrently ravaged by epidemic disease.[1]

With the steadily expanding population came new sanitary problems and mounting urban deaths. *Laissez faire,* still the favorite nineteenth century watchword, provided no solution. But the philosophical formula of Benthamite utilitarianism, at first interpreted in support of individualism and *laissez faire,* was gradually being liberalized. A degree of scientific central administration and inspection came to be recognized as promoting "the greatest happiness for the greatest number." Increasingly, the doctrine of "utility" led in England toward an interventionist approach.

As the squalid industrial cities swelled, it became more and more clear to the English Victorian that the man of property was as susceptible to disease as his poorer neighbor. No one force overcame the barriers to public health legislation—barriers of ignorance, apathy,

1

and vested property rights. In part, the climate fostered by the humanitarian movement focused attention on the welfare of the individual. Methodism and the early nineteenth century religious revival strengthened the spirit of philanthropy and increased moral sensitivity, even while bolstering reaction against the French Revolution.

Scientific advances throughout the late eighteenth and early nineteenth centuries led to differentiating diseases, but most epidemics still ran their course unchecked. Bacterial infectivity was not widely acknowledged until late in the nineteenth century. Asiatic cholera, however, proved a powerful spur to sanitary statutes. This disease in epidemic form struck England for the first time in 1831. Other severe outbreaks followed in 1848 and 1853. Each time they inspired movements for sanitary reform, which waned with the passing of the epidemic.

With the development of vital statistics, a new tool became available for public health reformers. Prior to the establishment in 1836 of the Office of the Registrar-General of Births, Deaths and Marriages, such bills of mortality and other medical statistics as were available were almost useless for scientific purposes. The solid statistical foundation developed by Dr. William Farr (1807–1883), who was appointed Compiler of Abstracts in 1839, was an essential element in comprehending the etiology of disease. Farr became the foremost expert in vital statistics throughout the western world before his retirement from public service in 1879.*

British medical men spearheaded the developing movement for sanitary reform. When faced with epidemics, English physicians at first favored specific emergency regulations such as quarantine. As the nineteenth century wore on, physicians increasingly attempted to educate public authorities to the overwhelming demand for public health measures. Medical practitioners in growing numbers also served the state as expert advisers, and parliamentary inquiries into health matters relied increasingly upon medical testimony.

Forerunners of the nineteenth century medical reformers were men

---

* Farr studied medicine at the Shrewsbury Infirmary, 1826–1828, in Paris, 1829–1831, and at University College, London. L.S.A., 1832. An 1837 article Farr wrote on "Vital Statistics" is credited with laying the foundations for this new science. Much of Farr's subsequent work was issued in the *Reports of the Registrar-General* from 1839 to 1880. A selection of his papers, edited by Noel A. Humphreys, was published in 1885 by the Royal Sanitary Institute. Farr's many honors included an honorary M.D. from New York in 1847; F.R.S., 1855; D.C.L. from Oxford, 1857; C.B. 1880.

like John Haygarth (1740–1827), the fever specialist, Thomas Percival (1740–1804), early British medical advocate of factory legislation, John Ferriar of Manchester (1761–1815), and Sir John Pringle (1707–1782), the military sanitarian. These physicians were, above all, practical men, respected in their communities and trained in the best scientific techniques of their time. They wielded considerable influence. In Manchester, Percival and Ferriar helped to set up a voluntary board of health. Dr. James Currie (1756–1805) in Liverpool steered a similar movement. Like his contemporaries, Currie aimed at introducing preventive health measures. Working sometimes in combination with one another, sometimes in community efforts with philanthropic laymen like John Howard (1726?–1790), these men provided the initial impetus for sanitary reform.

Some of the most prominent medical reformers of the early nineteenth century associated themselves with the dynamic Edwin Chadwick (1800–1890), who by 1834 was serving as Secretary of a Commission of Inquiry into the Working of the Poor Laws. Among Chadwick's colleagues were men like Dr. Thomas Southwood Smith (1788–1861), physician to the London Fever Hospital, Dr. Neil Arnott (1788–1874), who became Physician Extraordinary to Queen Victoria, and Dr. James Kay-Shuttleworth (1804–1877), author of treatises on the moral and physical conditions of the working classes.

All the earlier sanitary investigations were dwarfed in 1842 by Chadwick's monumental report on the *Sanitary Condition of the Labouring Population of Great Britain.* Chadwick's recommendations were supported by page after page of medical testimony on the sanitary ills of the nation. His report laid the basis for much of the sanitary legislation which followed. By 1845, with the appearance of the *Report of the Health of Towns Commissioners,* which strengthened the recommendations of the Chadwick Report, the British public had awakened to some recognition of the appalling sanitary conditions in which the nation dwelt. Highlighted now was the confusion of sanitary administration (where it existed at all), the pollution of drinking water, the stagnating sewers and cesspools, and those breeding grounds for epidemics—the damp, unhealthy houses, crowded with the poor.

Goaded by the repeated cholera epidemics and by the new awareness of the country's sanitary conditions, Parliament attempted a six-year experiment and established the General Board of Health under the Public Health Act of 1848. The Board's administrators were intelligent and energetic, but the Board's role had been poorly planned, giving to a central authority powers for which the climate of opinion was as yet unprepared. This weakness, accentuated by the Board's lack of direct connection with one of the ministries and coupled with the difficult personalities of its administrators, Edwin Chadwick and Lord Shaftesbury, made the Board immensely unpopular. Its early demise in 1854 was mourned only by a few exponents of the sanitary idea. The press rejoiced. Among the Board's many influential enemies had been the Royal College of Physicians.

The First General Board of Health was, nevertheless, useful in enforcing cholera regulations and in propagandizing against dirt and uncleanliness. Outside of London some progress was made, but the Board was wholly unsuccessful in fighting vested London property interests in attempting to establish a proper drainage and water supply in the nation's capital. A second, reconstituted General Board of Health was set up on an annual basis until 1858, when its public health responsibilities were transferred to the Privy Council.

Despite the failure of the General Board of Health, sanitary reformers continued their pressures for broader central authority. The remarkable John Simon (1816–1904), who served as Medical Officer of the Privy Council from 1858 to 1871, conceived the state's role as that of a superintendent-general of health—an earnest adviser and supervisor of local sanitary administration, ready in the last resort to enforce the law. Acting on this theory, Simon explored new areas of preventive medicine, expanding the basic concepts of public health. Under his direction, the able and industrious Privy Council medical staff made inquiries into pulmonary deaths among factory workers, into infant mortality, and into the housing of the poor. Simon also undertook a vigorous campaign against smallpox through a wide-scale government vaccination program.

Meanwhile, a large number of special acts for sanitary reform were successfully shepherded through Parliament—legislation such as the Burials Act, Factory Acts, Nuisances Removal Acts, Common Lodging House Acts, the Adulteration of Food Act, the Pharmacy Act, and the Alkali Works Act. The first local medical officer of health was appointed in 1847 in the teeming immigrant city of Liverpool, and over the next ten years, medical officers of health were appointed in increasing numbers in urban areas.

In the mid-sixties, however, no one national health authority administered the government's multiplying activities in preventive and curative medicine. The Medical Office of the Privy Council had extended its sanitary surveillance and control of infectious disease. But John Simon had no responsibility for medical relief to the poor which, since the passage of the Poor Law Amendment Act of 1834, had been administered by the Poor Law Board. Poor law medical officers existed in every parish, some serving full-time, others part-time, receiving fixed salaries and additional payments per case from the parish "Boards of Guardians." The Poor Law Board exercised very little supervision over the work of these "parish doctors"; and the medical reformers in the first half of the nineteenth century showed little interest in improving the state's role in curative medicine. From time to time medical journals carried complaints on the quality of treatment permitted by Boards of Guardians. More frequently the journals denounced the Guardians for underpaying parish doctors. The "sanitary idea," or Chadwick's principle that improvement in the material environment would advance the physical well-being of the English people, seemed far more important to midcentury sanitary reformers than did the extension or improvement of public medical care.

The most important piece of general health legislation during the period immediately preceding the Royal Sanitary Commission was the great Sanitary Act of 1866. Passed during another cholera outbreak, the Act of 1866 embodied the important principle of compulsion by the central authority (the Secretary of State) if local sanitary authority failed in its duty. Other detailed provisions of the act extended and improved legislation relating to public lodgings, sewers, nuisance removal, and infectious disease.

The considerable sanitary progress, thus achieved in England by the mid-sixties, contrasted markedly with conditions in American cities. New York in 1865, wrote Dr. Stephen Smith (1823–1922), founder of the American Public Health Association, was a city with practically no sanitary government. In some sections of this city of 1,000,000 persons garbage accumulated in the streets to a depth of two or three feet. Dwellings were interspersed with some 200 slaughter houses for hogs, cattle, and sheep.[2] Even by the early seventies no good sewerage system had been installed in any American city.[3] Less than twenty per cent of the states had compulsory registration of marriages, births, and deaths.

Chadwick's Report of 1842 and the work of English sanitary leaders like Thomas Southwood Smith, Farr, and Simon profoundly influenced American public health legislation—far more than did the work of such Continental sanitary pioneers as Johann Peter Frank (1745–1821) or Max von Pettenkofer (1818–1901). The U.S. public health movement is usually considered to date from 1850, with the publication of the brilliant *Report of the Massachusetts Sanitary Commission,* drawn up by Lemuel Shattuck. This document drew heavily upon the work of Chadwick and Simon.[4]

In England the Sanitary Act of 1866 had provided central sanitary legislation which represented more than clauses on paper. It was now the duty of local authorities to inspect and remove sanitary nuisances, to supply water, and to construct sewers. But the Act of 1866 by no means met all of the nation's sanitary problems. There was still no central administration for health, and there was still an astonishing confusion of sanitary statutes and overlapping authorities. By 1868 the deficiencies of both legislation and authorities led sanitary reformers to call for a complete investigation of the system and an overhaul of legislation. A clearer definition of the central government's role in public health was required—and the time was favorable for its formulation.

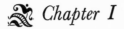 *Chapter I*

The Profession, Parliament, and Public Health in the Seventies: Three Legislative Landmarks

A LIVELY SPIRIT of progress charged the British political scene of the late eighteen-sixties. Following the Franchise Act of 1867, which gave the vote to almost 1,000,000 male householders in towns and cities, a new electorate, double the size of the old, carried in a government pledged to administrative reform. Within the next few years, the civil service, the army, the judicature, and the schools felt the impact of the Liberal Party's promise. Gladstone at the height of his powers moved briskly against old bureaucratic entrenchments. And for a few years at least, the central administration was infused with a new vigor.

Sanitary reform was only one of the manifestations of the changing concepts of the individual and the state, but it was an important and fast-growing indication. Many of the public health problems faced nationally in the late sixties had been explored earlier in local communities. Manchester and Liverpool had pioneered in early sanitary measures. Now, in Liverpool, the City Health Committee set up a municipal scavenging service and refused after 1865 to approve plans for new houses without water closets.[1] Voluntary organizations like the Manchester and Salford Sanitary Association took up the banner of the older Health of Towns Association, delivering lectures and issuing tracts to the working classes.

Despite such signs there was as yet no clearly perceptible public mandate for broad-scale coercion from London to rid the country of dirt or disease. Those opposed to spending public money on sanitary reform complained with some justification that exact methods of preventing disease were still being disputed. The sanitation of the sixties and seventies as yet had no sound scientific basis. John Snow and Wil-

liam Budd had put forth theories on the transmission of cholera, but
Robert Koch was still many years from identifying the comma bacillus.
When Dr. Snow called for sanitary reform with the words: "Our present machinery must be greatly enlarged, radically altered, and endowed with new powers," in particular with that power of "doing
away with that form of liberty to which some communities cling, the
sacred liberty to poison unto death not only themselves but their
neighbours," [2] *The Times* editor responded cautiously:

> What this means is tolerably clear, but, considering that we have
> hardly yet succeeded in making vaccination compulsory, the pros-
> pect is by no means clear also. When Dr. Budd calls for a "standing
> army, well-trained, and able to garrison the land," he will too
> certainly alarm all but those soldiers, in other words, our doctors
> themselves. . . . What is needed is first information and then faith
> on the part of the public, and doctors must agree among them-
> selves, if that be possible, before the outside world can be expected
> to agree with them. It may be that after a series of errors we have
> at length arrived at the truth, nor is that truth of a discouraging
> character, for though the terrible theory of contagion is revived
> once more, the antidote is presented by its side. But every age has
> its own persuasions on this subject, and the stage of universal
> consent has never been reached.[3]

Clearly, as *The Times* recognized, leadership for sanitary reform
had to come from the medical profession, from the group whose training best equipped them to know what sanitary reforms were needed.
The medical response to this public want had already found expression, in and out of the government, by 1868.

The Royal Sanitary Commission, 1868–1871

The appointment of the Royal Sanitary Commission, whose recommendations had a profound affect on sanitary legislation of the next
decade, was directly attributable to medical men, both within and
without the government, who were still dissatisfied with sanitary conditions in England.

GOVERNMENT MEDICAL REFORM PLANS

Within government circles the most influential spokesman of the
period was John Simon, Medical Officer of the Privy Council. Like

Chadwick, Simon is a giant figure in public health history. The son of a shipbroker, Simon grew up in comfortable circumstances. His father, of French ancestry, maintained ties with the Continent, and at sixteen Simon was sent to Germany for a year to study foreign languages. On returning to London, he undertook medical studies at King's College and St. Thomas' Hospital. Simon's abilities were quickly recognized, and he soon became a practicing surgeon at St. Thomas'. At 29, he was elected a Fellow of the Royal Society; at 30, in 1848, Simon became the first Medical Officer of Health for the City of London. Ten years later, he was appointed Medical Officer of the Privy Council.

A man of considerable culture, John Simon was at home in a brilliant circle of Pre-Raphaelite artists and writers, while his professional stature commanded the deep respect of his medical colleagues.[4] Gifted with a remarkable power of verbal expression and the integrity and determination of the dispassionate scientist, Simon wielded considerable influence on the Privy Council's health policies.

Simon's position gave him an unequaled opportunity to survey the health needs of the nation. Throughout the sixties, he employed the trained medical staff of the Privy Council's Medical Office to examine sanitary conditions in various parts of the country and to make inquiries into the housing of the poor and into epidemic outbreaks of disease. Repeatedly, in the detailed annual reports issued by the Medical Office of the Privy Council, Simon exposed national sanitary defects. Unwilling to rest on the partial gains of the Act of 1866, in the late sixties he renewed his efforts to widen the standards of sanitary well-being.

The formal program of reform, which originated in government medical circles, was published in the *Eleventh Annual Report of the Medical Officer of the Privy Council.*[5] Sanitary law, Simon warned, was still chaotic. Lack of communication between central and local health authorities, failure to enforce both permissive and mandatory nuisance statutes, and the lack of uniformity in the existing sanitary law—all shared responsibility for the confusion. Simon then suggested a six-point reform program. The first essential was a clarification of the areas of jurisdiction in the operation of the nuisance law. Next, he proposed that medical relief during epidemics become the responsibility of the poor law authorities. Going on to consider public protection against commercial malpractices, Simon stressed the need for larger areas of jurisdiction and for authorities of the magisterial type, rather than the popularly elected (and more easily influenced) boards. Shrewdly he advocated "an elastic margin of . . . law in reserve" to permit greater ease in applying the law.[6] As his fifth suggestion, Simon recommended a number of additions to the laws dealing with the circulation of birth and death statistics. His final recommendation was a systematic co-ordination of all sanitary administration.

The Simon proposals demonstrated that by 1868 medical men within the central government recognized that further reform of England's sanitary system was necessary. Indeed, as early as January 1867, the Privy Council circulated a confidential memorandum describing the diffuse administration of the sanitary acts and stressing the need for centralization and consolidation.[7]

THE MEDICAL PROFESSION'S CALL FOR REFORM

Although government medical authorities were well aware of the need for improvement, the immediate push for reform came from members of the medical profession outside Whitehall. Foremost in the drive for a national investigation of the sanitary law was Henry Wyldbore Rumsey, F.R.C.S. (1809–1876). Rumsey was a man of broad education and experience, esteemed by the medical profession at large. He had published several essays dealing with state medicine, and it was at his instigation that a Joint Committee of the British Medical Association and the Social Science Association was appointed in 1868 to promote the improvement of public health.

The Joint Committee's deliberations produced a memorial which was presented to the Disraeli Government in the spring of 1868, calling for an impartial and comprehensive inquiry by a Royal Commission into the existing sanitary organization, and the revision and consolidation of the sanitary laws.[8]

The memorial was favorably received. In November the government, under royal warrant, appointed a commission to be headed by Lord Northbrook. The fall of the Conservatives in the general election shortly afterwards left the warrant inoperative. However, by spring of the following year (1869), the Gladstone Government appointed a new Royal Sanitary Commission, chaired by Sir Charles Adderley (1814–1905), subsequently Baron Norton. Its purpose was to inquire into and report on the operation and administration of the sanitary laws of the nation, together with suggestions for improvements. Barred from the Royal Commission's jurisdiction was the operation of sanitary law in the city of London. Four medical men were named as members of the Royal Sanitary Commission, all physicians of distinction: James Paget, Henry Wentworth Acland, Robert Christison and William Stokes.

The *British Medical Journal* cheered the establishment of the Royal Sanitary Commission and paid tribute to Acland, Rumsey, and the Joint Committee.[9]

Throughout the spring of 1869 medical leaders continued to look upon the Royal Sanitary Commission as a creation of the medical profession. By July this attitude had become prevalent to the extent of a lament (published in the *British Medical Journal*) on the "secrecy" with which the Royal Commission's investigations were being carried out:

> As it was avowedly in consequence of the earnest and persevering solicitations of the Joint-Committee that the Commission was appointed, it was naturally supposed that those who had paid special attention to Public Medicine, and had not grudged years of profitless toil and considerable pecuniary outlay in the service of the public, would at all events be welcomed as spectators, if not occasionally consulted as confidential advisers. Yet we have been informed, on credible authority, that the entrance to this Star Chamber is jealously guarded against all comers except those who are summoned to give evidence, and such as may be admitted by special favour of the chairman.[10]

MEDICAL TESTIMONY BEFORE THE ROYAL COMMISSION

Despite such momentary pique, expert medical testimony was being collected by the Royal Commission—evidence which supported the need for broad-scale reform by the central government. While the tales of filth and overcrowding were not as shocking as those in the 1842 Chadwick Report, it was evident that the sanitary laws passed by the early reformers were not producing results.

Henry Day, M.D., Physician to the Stafford Infirmary, testified that there was no medical officer of health in Stafford. Stafford drainage, said Dr. Day, "was as bad as it is possible to be . . . excrement may be seen floating down the gutter in the daytime," and the water supply was "as bad as the drainage." [11] Day called for compulsory sanitary legislation throughout England. The medical officer of health for Liverpool, Dr. William Stewart Trench, described the difficulties of operating the sanitary system of the city under the Sanitary Act of 1866. Poor sanitary conditions were the rule rather than the exception in Liverpool.[12]

The chief criticisms levied by medical witnesses were the inactivity of local authorities and the need for broader compulsory regulation to cover such conditions as overcrowding of workshops and factories, lodging houses and nuisances on public and private property, smoke pollution, and poor privy facilities.[13] One medical officer of health who favored centrally administered, compulsory legislation pointed out that members of local boards of health and Boards of Guardians were usually "large rate-payers, and they like to save their own pockets, and simply decline to tax themselves for any improvement." [14] Others blamed the sanitary sluggishness of some local boards on ignorance and innumerable petty jealousies.[15] Some witnesses recommended that medical officers of health should be freed from private practice, given adequate full-time salaries of £500 to £1,000, and a staff of sanitary police to help carry out their duties.[16]

A number of medical witnesses advocated a strong central health authority, capable of moving the local boards to real sanitary effort. The testimony of John Simon was, of course, persuasive on this point. But Simon made it clear that such a central authority would not be merely a revival of the unpopular General Board of Health. Instead he suggested a medical department, headed by a medical officer as the country's "superintendent-general for health" who would act immediately under the minister to whom he was responsible. In stressing the need for a clarification of overlapping sanitary authorities, Simon pointed out that in all country districts there was "one authority for every privy, and another authority for every pigsty; . . . one authority is expected to prevent the privy's being a nuisance, and the other to require it to be put to rights if it is a nuisance." Simon was supported in the desire for a strong central health authority by the articulate Dr. Henry Rumsey and by Dr. William Budd.[17]

Medical practitioners testifying before the Commission also urged the adoption of a national plan of registration of disease and improvements in registration of deaths.[18] Dr. Robert Druitt, President of the Association of Medical Officers of Health, testified at length on death registration. Citing the fact that many bodies of dead children were found in streets, parks, and dust heaps, "a constant factor in the number of deaths," he attributed this not to murder, but to the fact that it cost five shillings to bury an unbaptised child and seven shillings sixpence to bury a baptised child. These corpses, he felt, had been merely thrown away to save the expense of burial.

RECOMMENDATIONS OF THE ROYAL COMMISSION

The final report of the Commission was not issued until 1871, and, as John Simon pointed out, some of the most important of its recommendations "may have seemed to come at last as mere matters of course." [19]

The Royal Sanitary Commission recommended a consolidation of the fragmentary sanitary legislation, the centralizing of sanitary powers in towns and counties in one fully responsible local authority, and the setting up of a central authority of ministerial rank to direct the nation's sanitary program. The central authority was also to be responsible for the relief of the poor.[20] Each local authority was to have a minimum of one medical officer of health. The Commission felt that in rural districts the offices of medical officer of health and poor law medical officer might be combined.[21] A number of sanitary necessities for minimum national health were listed by the Commission, covering specific sanitary abuses scored by the medical witnesses, such as inadequate drainage, poor and unwholesome supplies of water, and overcrowding.

The Commission emphasized, however, that "we would leave *direction* only in the Central power. It must steer clear of the rock on which the General Board of Health was wrecked; for so completely is self government the habit and quality of Englishmen, that the country would resent any Central Authority undertaking the duties of the local executive." [22]

The Royal Sanitary Commission's recommendations, for the most part, were favorably received by the medical journals.[23] While it was recognized that they were not the final answer to sanitary reform, they were acceptable to most members of the government,[24] and Whitehall moved to draft legislation to implement the Commission's suggestions. With the completion of the report the inspiration for sanitary reform passed for the moment into the hands of the professional lawmakers. Three great legislative acts in the period 1871 to 1875 implemented the Royal Commission's recommendations and provided the framework for central sanitary administration for more than forty years.

The Local Government [Board] Act of 1871

With the Report of the Royal Sanitary Commission, England had, for the first time, a comprehensive national sanitary plan.[25] The patchwork quilt, which had been pieced together over so many years and by so many hands, was finally to be taken apart; strong materials were to be added to a substantial frame-sheet, and a new and ambitious design worked out—or so the sanitary reformers hoped.

But again the old problem of how much legislation could be pushed through Parliament at one time arose, and the government decided first to set up the frame-sheet. The plan was simply to establish a central organization which would concentrate the central health responsibility and leave the working out of the rest of the sanitary reform to Parliament and the head of the new central organization. The problem of drafting the legal frame for the new central board was allocated to the President of the Poor Law Board, which under the recommendation of the Commission was to be merged with the new central board.

To authorize the new plans for centralization, a short bill was introduced into Parliament on July 6, 1871, providing for a merger of the staff of the Poor Law Board, the staff of the Local Government Act Office, the staff of the Registrar-General's Office, and the staff of the Medical Office of the Privy Council, into one, new Local Government Board, which was to exercise the functions of its old components.[26]

Sir Charles Adderley, who presented the bill at its first reading, emphasized that it was merely the first step in carrying out the recommendations of the Royal Sanitary Commission. The unofficial parliamentary spokesman of the medical profession, Sir Lyon Playfair,* supported the measure heartily, stating that "the Bill would extend the same protection to human beings that Parliament had already given to cattle. . . . It was a Bill to get order out of disorder, and though it gave no new powers which have not already been enacted, it made a new health department of the State which would be more powerful in administration." [27]

---

* Sir Lyon Playfair (1818–1898) studied medicine at Glasgow and Edinburgh but never took a medical degree. He was, however, a distinguished chemist, a professor of chemistry at the University of Edinburgh, the organizer (with Prince Albert) of the Royal College of Science; in addition, he served as the Liberal Member of Parliament for the university seat of Edinburgh and St. Andrews. See Wemyss Reid, *Memoirs and Correspondence of Lyon Playfair* (London: Cassell & Co., 1899), *passim*.

The bill became law on August 14, 1871, and four days later Queen Victoria appointed Mr. James Stansfeld President of the new Local Government Board.

Most of the medical journals approved the passage of the Act of 1871, although they took some exception to the consolidation of the Poor Law authority. It is a characteristic of these journals throughout the second half of the nineteenth century first to accept a proposed sanitary reform enthusiastically, and later, in more considered editorials to point out defects in the proposal. In the case of the more articulate publications like *The Lancet* and the *Medical Press and Circular,* this gives a curious impression, as of the fond parent who has been urging its child to a new and difficult accomplishment, first praising the offspring in a burst of reflected glory, and then scolding irritably because the performance is not perfect.

The Local Government Act of 1871 was the first legislative step to implement the recommendations of the Royal Sanitary Commission. It passed without great difficulty but was only the start of what was necessary to bring about a fundamental change in the sanitary state of England and Wales.

The Public Health Act of 1872

A severe epidemic of smallpox raged throughout England from 1870 to the end of 1873, reaching its crisis during 1872. Historically, contagious disease was the spur to public health reform. Public anxiety aroused by the serious attack of typhoid fever suffered by the popular Prince of Wales also created a demand for a systematic attack on preventable disease. But these were only precipitating factors. The public health movement had gathered too much momentum by this time to rest on the gains of the Act of 1871. And merely to implement its own administrative machinery, the Local Government Board had now to present to Parliament some organized plan for further sanitary legislation.

On the sixteenth of February, 1872, the new President of the Local Government Board, James Stansfeld,* brought in a bill, ostensibly

---

* James Stansfeld (1820–1898), a graduate of University College, London, was an enthusiastic admirer of Jeremy Bentham, and through his wife, became a close friend and supporter of Mazzini and the cause of Italian unity. He served as the Liberal Member of Parliament from Halifax, 1859–1895.

based on the Report of the Royal Sanitary Commission. The Bill proposed to divide England into urban and rural sanitary districts, with an additional provision of port sanitary authorities. To these new administrative units were to be given the powers and obligations of sanitary law authorized in such earlier sanitary acts as the Sewage Utilization Acts, Nuisances Removal Acts, Common Lodging House Acts, Artizan's and Labourer's Dwellings Acts, and Bakehouse Regulation Acts. John Simon observed that the Bill was drafted to favor the appointment of poor law medical officers as the health officers of the newly created districts, and it was precisely about this point that a medical storm arose. But further, the bill proposed to employ the same sanitary law which had already been proven ineffective by the investigations of the Royal Commission. Again the complaint went up that the legislators would not go far enough to meet the country's sanitary needs.

The medical journals rushed to the attack. The *British Medical Journal* deplored placing the poor law medical officers "precisely in that position which they have beforehand deprecated," and caviled at a proposal which would employ the same old fragmentary machinery in a new scheme.[28] *The Lancet* feared that a new, unwelcome class of state physicians might develop as a result of the Act.[29]

More concretely, the Joint Committee of the British Medical Association and the Social Science Association, watchdog of health legislation, sent a deputation to James Stansfeld. They pointed out the need for a broader bill than that which Stansfeld had introduced in Parliament. They were opposed to poor law medical officers being appointed as the only health officers, especially in rural districts. They advocated the creation of supervisory county boards to control the local authorities, and reiterated the need for trained medical officers of health, serving full-time and paid substantial salaries.[30] The President of the Local Government Board received the deputation courteously but explained that he believed there were greater advantages in using existing machinery.

The protests grew. The Parliamentary Bills Committee of the British

---

Stansfeld resigned from his Local Government Board post in 1874 to devote his life, with Josephine Butler, to the repeal of the controversial Contagious Diseases Acts, which required compulsory medical inspections of prostitutes in areas around naval and military stations. See J. L. and Barbara Hammond, *James Stansfeld, A Victorian Champion of Sex Equality* (London: Longmans, Green & Co., 1932), *passim*.

Medical Association, together with the Joint Committee, appraised the bill carefully in March and concluded it needed serious amendment. It did not, they felt, provide for sufficient medical counsel in the central department; it lacked a sufficiently uniform sanitary authority; moreover, they feared that urban and rural sanitary authorities would not use sufficient discrimination in appointing medical officers of health.[31]

The poor law medical officers also entered the ring. Meeting in the second week of March, 1872, the Poor Law Medical Officers' Association listened as Dr. Henry W. Rumsey commented irritably on the defects of the bill:

> The provision for dispensaries was only permissive, and only applicable to places, which in the opinion of the Local Government Board might require them, and it would, therefore, be only a mere sop in the pan to the medical officers who were weak enough to trust Mr. Stansfeld. The provision for officers of health was simply execrable. The clauses about hospitals were most absurd. Urban authorities were to provide these hospitals; and in the very same place the rival authorities—viz., The Board of Guardians would have their workhouse-infirmaries and their regular medical relief. There would thus be two rival authorities managing medical poor relief in the same union.[32]

In June, the Poor Law Medical Officers' Association sent out a query to its members, and found that 195 of the 200 replies were opposed to the bill.[33] *The Lancet* summarized the main issues succinctly:

> Does even Mr. Stansfeld believe for one moment that the average parish medical officer (who is no better than the average man of his rank in any other profession or business) would have moral courage to tell his vestrymen and other patients that the filthy house property of which they were the landlords was unfit for human habitation, and must be pulled down or greatly remodelled?[34]

The Lancet urged again that some provision be made for the appointment of superior health officers in supervising certain districts.

Not only did these complaints go unheeded, but the government replaced its February bill with a second bill on June 27. It was this second bill which was to be enacted into law, and it dropped a number of the stronger clauses of its predecessor. Simon attributed the change to Stansfeld's desire to lighten his task.[35]

The Public Health Act of 1872 passed, despite the protests of the medical profession, but as the months went by signs began to appear that the measure was viewed more tolerantly. At least, *The Lancet* said, sanitary authorities were now established everywhere except in London.[36] By September, Dr. H. W. Acland, F.R.S., President of the Health Department of the Social Science Association, echoed *The Lancet's* acceptance of the Act of 1872: "it appears to me that the Government of Mr. Gladstone proceed upon the wise principle, that instead of waiting until they could construct a perfect theoretical system they should avail themselves of the existing institutions and habits of the country." [37]

The Public Health Act of 1872 set up a new sanitary organization for the country, supplementing the central organization established by the Local Government Act of 1871. Many overlapping functions were still a source of confusion, and no provision had been made for strengthening particular sanitary laws. But the legislators were still in midstream.

The Public Health Act of 1875

In January, 1875, leaders in the sanitary movement gathered in Birmingham at a conference called by Joseph Chamberlain, the city's reforming mayor. The conference aimed at arousing a national awareness of the sanitary evils which still plagued the country, and the *British Medical Journal* felt it was well-timed. "The Government needed a strong reminder that the Premier's motto of *sanitas sanitatum* must be strictly adhered to if the Augean evils which now exist are to be remedied." [38] (*Sanitas Sanitatum omnia sanitas,* uttered as a party war cry in 1872, was, of course, one of Disraeli's touches of genius.) The *Medical Press and Circular* hailed the Birmingham conference, urging that other cities follow the example: "It is most immoral to allow so many miserable quarters to exist in all places, of our large cities, where human life is a sordid, unhappy lot, compared with which the existence of a sheep in a good pasture seems to us a paradise." [39] The *Medical Press and Circular* did not dramatize the sanitary situation. At the Birmingham conference the Medical Officer of Health for Manchester stated that the average age of death of the laboring classes was seventeen, and that of the middle classes thirty-eight, while in Liverpool the average working class age at death was fifteen, and that of the middle classes thirty-five.[40]

But the last of the great sanitary landmarks of the seventies was at hand. On February 11, 1875, a government bill was introduced into Parliament "to consolidate and amend the acts relating to the public health." This bill represented much of the legislation postponed in 1871 and again in 1872. The sweep of past legislation which the new bill proposed to consolidate was impressive: the Public Health Acts of 1848, 1859, and 1872; the Sanitary Acts of 1866, 1868, and 1870; the Nuisances Removal Acts; the Local Government Acts from 1858 on; the Sewage Utilization Acts; the Towns Improvement Acts and many others.

The Liberal Government had fallen in 1874, putting an end to Stansfeld's administration and bringing in, under the Disraeli Government, George Sclater-Booth (later Lord Basing) as President of the Local Government Board. The 1875 Public Health Act, however, was, rather than a Conservative political coup, the final major step in implementing the recommendations of the Royal Sanitary Commission. The bill was framed as a departmental measure at the Local Government Board, with the advice and assistance of John Simon.[41]

By mid-March 1875 the two leading medical journals found time for detailed studies of the proposal. *The Lancet* cheered the principle of consolidation.[42] The *British Medical Journal* acknowledged the importance of consolidating sanitary law, but pointed out that the bill failed to eliminate many defects in the old acts now to be consolidated.[43] The Society of Medical Officers of Health submitted a series of suggested modifications to the President of the Local Government Board, together with plans for subsequent amendments to sanitary law. But the Society, too, conceded that consolidation of the sanitary law, even if that law were still imperfect, would be a big step forward.[44]

Medical men in Parliament were not entirely happy about the bill, and Lyon Playfair criticized the Conservative Government for unwarranted trumpeting of the proposal. He noted inefficiencies in the provisions relating to sewage and nuisances, and condemned the section on contagious diseases as giving the government illusory powers.[45]

Sclater-Booth, replying to Playfair for the government, said flatly that the government had no intention of proposing "violent changes" in the sanitary legislation, because they saw no prospect of implementing them. Mr. Sclater-Booth thought his right honorable friend Playfair "a little forestalled the opinion of the country in the matter, and was in too great a hurry to believe that private individuals were anxious to be controlled and directed to the extent he suggested." [46]

The objections of medical men in Parliament did not prevail. Indeed, it was apparent from Playfair's speeches, that the objections were advanced without any real hope of altering the law. And on the final passage of the bill, *The Lancet* in August, 1875, summed it up by commenting, "it is cheering to know that our sanitary laws are now at all events packed up in but one parcel." [47]

The Public Health Act of 1875 was the last of the major acts to develop from the recommendations of the Royal Sanitary Commission. It had not met any determined opposition. By 1875 it was generally acknowledged that consolidation of the sanitary laws was necessary.[48] For the first time there was now a comprehensive act embodying the great number of sanitary statutes which had, in their time, been so laboriously passed. A number of amendments to these acts had also been included in the new over-all statute, some clarifying provisions in the old statutes, some enlarging the powers and obligations of the sanitary authorities. The Act did nothing about the notification of disease, although both John Simon and the Royal Sanitary Commission had advocated such legislation. But despite the many weaknesses remaining in the sanitary law, there was still nothing comparable to the Public Health Act of 1875 anywhere in Europe.[49]

The medical men who were so largely responsible for the passage of the three great pieces of sanitary legislation of the seventies knew how much still remained to be done. In May, 1876, the Joint Committee of the British Medical Association and the Social Science Association sent out a call for a new sanitary conference to consider revision of the Act of 1875. Held at the end of May, the conference was attended by many medical officers of health, as well as some members of Parliament. It passed resolutions calling for improved organization of sanitary machinery, a greater uniformity of sanitary powers, the provision of water supply, the extension of legislation on infectious diseases, and making the administration of such legislation compulsory. Again, consolidation of local sanitary authorities into county boards was recommended. But such reforms had to wait for later years, and for a further development of compulsory central health legislation.

In November, 1875, the *Medical Press and Circular* summed up the situation:

> we cannot fail to draw the conclusion that medicine, nothwithstanding its many deficiencies, is, at present, and is likely to remain for some time to come, far in advance of public opinion and support. Aspersions are frequently cast both upon medical men and the art which they practice, and by no class more so than by those

who refuse or neglect to avail themselves of those very means of cure or of prevention which science has placed in their hands. We may have discovered the best means of curing or preventing a disease, but we cannot force either the individual or the community to employ them. The State can, and undoubtedly does a great deal to rectify this anomoly in our social economy, but it is evident that there are many things materially influencing the health of the public with which no Government will ever be able to interfere.[50]

Chapter II

The Medical Department of the Local Government Board: Formulation of Policy, 1871-1900

WHILE THE legal framework of sanitary reform in the seventies evolved in Parliament, medical practitioners within the administration were slowly developing a national health program. The extent of the government's service depended partly upon the quality of medical men employed, partly upon the administrative framework in which they were placed, and partly upon public opinion.

Theoretically, the government doctor could do much to forward government action for the public health. It was within his ability to throw the light of science on such recognized public problems as the control of contagious and industrial disease, the treatment of the sick poor, and the improvement of insanitary housing. But the degree to which science could improve the public health was dependent on the influence government medical men could exert upon policy making. An unfortunate series of interpersonal struggles within the new Local Government Board strangled John Simon's hopes for the development of any real "superintendent-general for health" in England in these years.

The Privy Council Background

When the Local Government Board was set up in 1871, with John Simon as Medical Officer, the small medical band who had served under Simon in the Privy Council was transferred to the new Board's

Medical Department. The Privy Council group had been a capable one, headed by a man who would have been exceptional in any community. Many of the principles Simon established in the Privy Council carried over into the work of the Local Government Board even after his resignation in the summer of 1876.

As Simon reviewed the work of the Medical Office of the Privy Council he felt it had resulted in a threefold contribution, by providing a wider and more exact knowledge of sanitary law, by stimulating new sanitary legislation, and by conquering much hostility hitherto aroused by the mention of sanitary progress.[1] But the chief contribution was Simon's development of government research and inquiry into the health conditions of the population of England and Wales. In this he had been greatly aided by the steady flow of statistical reports issued by William Farr and the office of the Registrar-General.[2] From 1858 to 1871, Simon and his medical staff had gathered masses of evidence, had piled up example upon example of inadequate nuisance abatement measures, of the deplorable housing of the poorer members of the community, of the government's failure to take preventive action to reduce the incidence of disease.

As Privy Council Medical Officer, Simon had been working toward a co-ordinating national medical authority both to inspire and supervise local sanitary authorities. The Royal Sanitary Commission had agreed on the necessity for such a command, and in 1871 it must have seemed to Simon as if his hopes were to be fulfilled. Behind him was the scientific weight of his eminent colleagues in the Privy Council. And the organization which could eventually bring about a long-range program of national health based upon improved social conditions had finally been created.

But the merger of the Privy Council Medical Office into the Local Government Board did not even begin to approximate Simon's dream. Instead, it marked the eclipse of his personal role in sanitary administration.

The New Administrative Picture

By the union of the old Poor Law Board and the Privy Council Medical Office, a variety of health activities were brought under the jurisdiction of the Local Government Board: medical administration under the poor laws, the responsibility for public vaccination, the supervision of health in relation to excess of disease, and responsibilities in relation to local sanitary officers.

It was a confused atmosphere in which the new Board commenced its operation. Endless difficulties were encountered in setting up the new organization, and the administrative confusion was not lessened by the appointment of a single secretariat composed primarily of the former Poor Law Board officials. Simon had hoped for a separate department for medical activities within the Local Government Board. The Royal Sanitary Commission had commented that separate secretariats would probably be found necessary, one for public health and one for the relief of the poor. But this arrangement was not followed. As a result, the Privy Council medical staff found themselves in a situation where their experience was not taken into account, and Simon was unable to exert any influence upon the main health policies of the Local Government Board. Joseph Rogers, the distinguished leader of the poor law medical officers, was made aware of Simon's situation when a deputation of medical men called upon the new President of the Local Government Board. Wrote Rogers: "I saw Mr. H. Fleming and Mr. Lambert sitting together with the President, whilst . . . Mr. John Simon and his staff, who were the only intellectual element of the new Board, were relegated to distant seats in the corner of the room." [3]

Not only was this a great waste of technical skill, but some of the poor law officials who now directed national health policy were less than efficient.[4] James Stansfeld, while well-intentioned, was wholly unfamiliar with the medical needs of the nation. His previous experience in the Admiralty and Treasury gave him little acquaintance with local government, and he relied almost completely upon the old poor law advisers, primarily John Lambert.*

Lambert, the son of a Hendon surgeon, had far more direct knowledge of local conditions. He had served as a poor law inspector since 1847, and was also a member of the Royal Sanitary Commission. But his strong influence with Stansfeld resulted in the Local Government Board's being organized on the stultifying outlines of the defunct

* Afterward Sir John Lambert (1815–1892). Lambert had been closely associated with Charles Villiers, President of the Poor Law Board. In 1865 and 1867, he had prepared statistics in connection with the reform bills, and was a recognized authority on the franchise and distribution of seats. He was also a gifted musician and the author of many works on church music. See Algernon West, *Contemporary Portraits* (London: Thomas Nelson & Sons, 1920), p. 159ff.

Poor Law Board. John Simon and his medical staff from the Privy Council, which had been incorporated into the new structure, were pushed to the background. As a consequence, Simon's broader sanitary program was buried in the files of the Local Government Board. The sharp conflict between the two men underlay much of the Board's ineffectiveness in its early years.

Stansfeld acknowledged openly that his policy was first of all one of local health self-government.[5] The perceptive Local Government Board inspector, Mr. Herbert Preston-Thomas, described the resulting impasse:

> If it was unfair to say of him that he [Stansfeld] knew about as much of science as a cow does of conic sections, it is yet undeniable that at the time he failed to appreciate the possibilities of preventive medicine, and the importance of dealing in a comprehensive fashion with the public health of the country. Simon and his department were relegated to a subordinate position, and he complained bitterly that if a town wished to avail itself of his advice as to some sanitary question, he was not even allowed to write a direct reply, since officialism required that all letters should proceed from the secretariat.[6]

Unquestionably, this must have been a very difficult period for the brilliant former Medical Officer of the Privy Council. The internal memoranda and correspondence of the Board record the struggle between Lambert and Simon clearly. In many ways, John Lambert was an admirable civil servant, precise, controlled, careful to avoid risk. He was also a powerful and determined man. As Permanent Secretary of the Local Government Board, he was able to set up its administrative procedures, one of the most important being the routing of mail. It is obvious, from Lambert's notes and instructions on the thousands of documents preserved in the files of the Local Government Board, that he organized the flow of memoranda and correspondence so as to enable him to exercise primary control over the Board's activities. No detail was small enough to escape Lambert's meticulous attention; he even answered, personally, requests to the Medical Department from public health groups for copies of official reports.[7] Occasionally, Lambert referred sanitary problems to Simon and his staff without comment. An inquiry as to the minimum number of cubic feet of air space per adult considered necessary by the Board for maintaining the health of a building's occupants might be routed to Simon.[8] But any matters directed by Simon to the attention of the Board's President went first through Lambert's hands. And a notation in the Permanent Secretary's neat handwriting would then be appended to advise Stansfeld of the action to be taken.[9]

It is impossible to read through the correspondence of the Board and not acknowledge Lambert's abilities. But it is also easy to understand what a formidable opponent Simon faced—an opponent who was virtually the sole official channel of communication to Stansfeld. Lambert also enjoyed the high esteem of Gladstone, who had appointed him to the post of the Board's Permanent Secretary.[10]

Outside the Board, two other powerful enemies—Edwin Chadwick and Florence Nightingale—jealous of Simon's position in state medicine and opposed to his approach to sanitary reform, attacked him sporadically in letters, during visits to Stansfeld, and in the medical press.[11] Simon had never seen fit to consult Florence Nightingale in his plans for sanitary reform, and she became an implacable enemy.

In November 1873, Simon drafted a lengthy letter to the President of the Local Government Board on the status of the medical staff—a letter that was at once a lament and a justification. He described the "unclear, provisional hand-to-mouth, unsystematic state of things" under which the medical staff worked. He deplored the fact that he was unable to see Stansfeld in day-to-day contact. "I have really no chance of giving you that kind of information which the head of an office absorbs almost insensibly from the officer whom he sees day by day." Simon requested a fixed time each week in which he might brief Stansfeld on medical activities. He continued: "I think I ought not to withhold from you . . . that the unsettled and controversial state in which we have been going on for the last two and a half years has been a most depressing and bewildering influence." [12]

As Simon described the Board's medical staff, seven district medical inspectors were employed. "Four and a half" of these were assigned to the inspection of vaccination, and the remaining strength given to general sanitary purposes. In addition to the inspectors, Dr. Edward Seaton devoted much of his time to vaccination problems, except when he substituted for Simon in the latter's absence. Dr. George Buchanan, with the title of Assistant Medical Officer for General Sanitary Purposes, advised on matters relating to the Registrar-General's quarterly death returns and handled port sanitary arrangements. Dr. Edward Smith "so far as not engaged in the Poor Law Purposes for which he is Assistant Medical Officer, is assigned by the President for general sanitary employment." [13] Mr. John Netten Radcliffe served as Chief Inspector for General Sanitary Purposes, assisting Simon in the office, digesting information on quarantine and foreign epidemics, and carrying out major sanitary inspections.[14]

The following month, December of 1873, Simon submitted additional information on his staff's activities to the Board's President. But there is no evidence that this, or the earlier effort to call Stansfeld's attention to the plight of the Medical Department, met any success. Stansfeld relied heavily upon his Permanent Secretary and could not afford to cross him on the basic question of who was to make health policy.

However, as in most difficult situations, there were two sides to the picture. While Lambert was an unyielding man, Simon, accustomed to a large degree of autonomy in the Privy Council, was not wholly co-operative in the new organization. Dr. Edward Smith (1818–1874), formerly the Medical Officer of the Poor Law Board, had been assigned to Simon's department under the merger. Smith, who had served with Simon in Privy Council days, had earlier carried out excellent surveys of the tailoring industry and of dietary conditions. His readable yet authoritative publications on the poor law and on prison diets had led to his subsequent appointment as Medical Officer of the Poor Law Board. According to the table of duties outlined by Simon after the amalgamation, Dr. Smith appears to have been largely independent of his nominal new chief. Smith, in his new position, proceeded to publish in quick succession several manuals and handbooks for medical officers of health and inspectors of nuisances. There is some indication that Simon resented this state of affairs, and at one time went as far as to remove Smith's furniture and take away his private office. The irascible but sorely tried Dr. Smith wrote an outraged letter to the Board upon this occasion. No record of the immediate solution has been preserved, and Smith died of pneumonia a year later in November, 1874, at the age of 56.[15]

Despite his intellectual brilliance and solid professional attainment, Simon was not able to muster adaptive mechanisms of aplomb, detachment, and compromise which would have helped ease his situation at the Local Government Board. At a crucial time in his life, his early skills in persuading and in making perceptive judgments of his colleagues [16] failed him. Difficulties in his personal life from 1872 to 1876— his illness and that of his devoted wife, and the divorce of a wayward stepdaughter—added to his unhappiness.[17] Simon, seemingly frustrated on all sides, gave way "to that extraordinary but dangerous power of sar-

casm which he had cultivated at the zenith of his fame." [18] No longer
could he embrace a philosophy of gradualism and patiently overlook
"the constantly recurring pinpricks of official interference." [19]

With such an over-all state of affairs within the Board, it is not surprising that no spectacular program of health reform was initiated.
No record, however, has survived in the Board's files of any further
health reform measures proposed within the secretariat by Simon or
his staff. Increasingly aware of the strictures under which he labored,
Simon may have felt that any further suggestions would have no chance
of fulfillment.[20]

Limitations in Contemporary Views of State Medicine

The medical officers of the Local Government Board found themselves confined in an administrative strait jacket. In addition, they had
to conduct their affairs within the framework of contemporary thought
on the state's function in public health.

By the 1870's, the concept of government action in preventive public
health measures was fairly well accepted by the medical profession and
informed laymen. The earlier reformers had demonstrated that prevention of disease was economically desirable and that a central health
authority was a needed spur when it came to local application of sanitary law. Disease prevention was thus the key to government intervention in public health. "All the aim of state medicine is the prevention
of disease," stated Dr. François de Chaumont in his lectures on state
medicine in 1875.[21] By the 1880's, when Arthur Newsholme * started
practice as a medical officer of health, the situation was much the
same. Dr. Newsholme later wrote: "in the earlier years of my practice
of preventive medicine, it was tacitly assumed that public health was
concerned chiefly, if not solely, with the prevention of infection." [22]

---

* Sir Arthur Newsholme (1857–1943) was one of the most distinguished
public health reformers of the period. Graduated from St. Thomas' Hospital
in 1879, he qualified for an M.D. in 1881, was appointed as a part-time medical officer of health for Clapham in 1883, and in 1888 became the first full-
time medical officer of health in Brighton, where he investigated the
epidemiology of tuberculosis, scarlet fever, and diphtheria and introduced
voluntary notification. Newsholme served as President of the Society of Medical Officers of Health from 1899–1900. He became Medical Officer to the
Local Government Board in January, 1908, and was awarded the K.C.B.
in 1917.

It could not be expected that government medical officers would be too far in advance of public opinion. But even with its constricted view of state health, the Local Government Board did not rise to any great heights of medical endeavor, and contemporary medical opinion was sharply critical. Numerous complaints about the inactivity of the Local Government Board turn up in the medical periodicals of the seventies and eighties. At the annual meeting of the British Medical Association in 1875, the experienced parliamentary spokesman, Sir Lyon Playfair, commented on the limitations of the four-year-old Local Government Board:

> That Board has two main purposes to discharge—viz., to super-intend public health and pauperism. It is reasonable to join them under one administration for they are closely connected as cause and effect. But though both should be made subjects of preven-tion, pauperism is an existent evil of such persistence that it is treated as one of economical administration, and thus it happens that sanitation is viewed in the same light, although its chief re-lation to public interests is in the prevention of disease. The Local Government Board has never yet recognized its preventive func-tions.[23]

The old poor law administrators who now controlled the Local Government Board embodied the spirit of retrenchment. The poor were an ever-present problem; society still frowned upon too much state assistance. But the combination of the do-little spirit of poor law administration on the part of the public health authority and the failure to apply existing knowledge had unfortunate results. Even in-telligent laymen were dissatisfied with the inadequate work of the Board.

Simon's Resignation

Although contemporary views of state medicine may have partially explained the inactivity of the Local Government Board in some pub-lic health fields, the primary fault lay within the Board's administra-tive structure. For the rest of the short time he remained with the Local Government Board, Simon continued in his yearly reports to urge the adoption of broader preventive health measures. He estimated in 1874 that, of the 500,000 annual registered deaths, fully 125,000 were caused by lack of reasonable application of existing knowledge of disease prevention.[24] And cases resulting in death represented only a portion of the yearly suffering and loss from preventable disease.

Simon resigned as Medical Officer of the Local Government Board in July, 1876. Technically, he asked and obtained leave to retire. As he noted in his *Personal Recollections,* "It was with extreme pain that, in 1876, I found I could no longer hope to be of official use in public service." [25]

With Simon's resignation the old Medical Office of the Privy Council ceased to struggle for policy control and obediently allowed itself to come under the Board's administration. Simon's letter requesting retirement has not been preserved in the files of the Local Government Board, but it is clear that it was the inevitable outcome of the painful clash with Lambert and Stansfeld. Simon was only sixty years of age at the time and had many more capable years before him. Not only had he been prevented from using his abilities and experience in the Board, he had been forced to observe daily the apathy and inadequacy of the local sanitary inspection services. In his own words:

> The opportunity which circumstances at that critical time had offered to the new department to become a widely authoritative influence for the bettering of local sanitary government, and the moral claim which the existence of such an opportunity constituted, had, so far as I can see, been met with but poor appreciation; and especially it seems to me that, in relation to local neglects and defaults in matters of sanitary duty, there had been created, instead of the effective supervising authority which the Report of the Royal Commission had prefigured to the hopes of the sanitary reformers, an authority of but doubtful courage for unpleasing responsibilities, an authority "bestilled almost to jelly" at points where the chief need for initiative usefulness existed, an authority not even so far organized as to command full cognizance of the evils against which its organization was to have been our strength.[26]

Simon was replaced in this "authority of but doubtful courage" by Dr. Edward Cator Seaton,* one of his valued Privy Council assistants. Seaton had been greatly interested in the establishment of public vaccination, one of the more successful ventures of the Privy Council

---

* Edward Cator Seaton (1815–1880) took an Edinburgh M.D. in 1837 and began practice in London in 1841 as surgeon at the Chelsea Dispensary. He was an active supporter of the compulsory Vaccination Act of 1853, and in 1858 was appointed the first vaccination inspector under the General Board of Health. Between 1865 and 1871, he served as superintendent inspector and then as Director of the National Vaccine Establishment. In 1871, Simon appointed him Senior Assistant Medical Officer to the Local Government Board.

and Local Government Board. But, as Simon wrote later, "Even Dr. Seaton's experience and unsparing industry could not bring into much effectiveness the very circumscribed office to which he had been called." [27]

The Local Government Board's files contain almost no material on the initiation of health policies during Dr. Seaton's short term as Medical Officer. This supports Simon's belief that the Medical Department was completely subordinated in matters of policy during the Seaton administration. Even in the preparation of his annual report, Seaton was forced to limit his discussion to "special matters," and at Sclater-Booth's direction to leave for the Board's general annual report all other business of the Medical Department.[28] Failing health caused Dr. Seaton to resign three years after his appointment, and his position was taken over by his son-in-law, Dr. George Buchanan (1831–1895).

The Buchanan Administration, 1879–1892

Simon felt that Dr. Buchanan was a man of extraordinarily active and discriminating mind. A distinguished medical student at the University of London, Buchanan became Resident Medical Officer at the London Fever Hospital at the age of twenty-three. Three years later, he accepted an appointment as Medical Officer for St. Giles, one of the poorest and most unsalubrious of London districts. Buchanan's careful researches and clear reports on the origin of disease in St. Giles attracted the attention of government medical men, and he was asked by the Privy Council to undertake sanitary investigations in many parts of England.[29] In 1869 Buchanan had been appointed a permanent medical inspector to the Privy Council. Simon and Seaton subsequently persuaded him to join the Medical Department of the Local Government Board in 1871.

After the fall of the Liberal Government in 1874, Stansfeld had been replaced as President of the Board by Mr. George Sclater-Booth. The indomitable Lambert, however, was to remain on the Board until 1882, when he resigned on grounds of impaired health and advancing years. Thus, when Buchanan was appointed Medical Officer of the Board, Lambert's rigid bureaucracy was still in force. Buchanan, however, was able to prevent a total loss of the Simon ideal. Considerable progress was also made in curtailing the spread of infectious disease under his administration.

There is some evidence in the files of the Local Government Board to indicate that Buchanan envisaged a wider state role in public health than developed under the Board's rule. And upon one occasion he wrote to Arthur Newsholme, "We shall never get a proper recognition of Medicine by the State if we continue to limit 'State Medicine' to the area of a statutory health officer's business, and we shall continue to confuse . . . 'sanitation' with privy arrangements." [30] But, whatever Buchanan's personal feelings on the place of the state in medicine, few radical changes or improvements in the central health policies of the Local Government Board took place.

What influence on policy did the medical staff exercise then in the Board during this period? In a few matters Buchanan seems to have been permitted a large degree of autonomy—such as the appointment of medical personnel to the Board and the publication of scientific reports.[31] More important, however, Buchanan started a Local Government Board inquiry into the evils of back-to-back housing. He was also much concerned with the establishment of vaccination stations for educating medical students and made careful inquiry into the qualifications of those appointed as public vaccinators.

However, for the few examples of direct initiatory action taken by Buchanan and the medical staff, there are many others to indicate that the major role was taken by the lay secretariat. Lambert personally handled many of the requests to the Board for advice on sanitary matters and for copies of medical reports and regulations. From time to time the Permanent Secretary consulted the Medical Department on requests for sanitary information. But he retained the right of revising their replies. In 1881 the Colonial Office transmitted a request for advice on how to handle a smallpox epidemic in New South Wales. Buchanan was allowed to draft the answer, but the draft was freely revised by the omnipresent Lambert before the final copy was sent to the Colonial Office.[32] In 1883, the Home Office, responding to pressure from the Manchester and Salford Sanitary Association, queried the Local Government Board as to whether local sanitary authorities could prevent abuses of sanitation in bakehouses. The Local Government Board's affirmative reply to this was drafted wholly without reference to the Medical Department.[33]

There were occasions during the Buchanan administration when the Board's Medical Officer was given the opportunity to express his views on sanitary matters. In November 1887, a Mr. H. March Webb wrote a long letter to the President of the Board, demanding the reform of sanitary conditions in private hospitals and nursing homes of

London's West End. Asked for his opinion, Buchanan noted: "It does not seem to me that the time has come for any Governmental dealing with such private establishments as these. I do not see why, however, local sanitary authorities should not have power for regulating these establishments, supposing that the health institutions in their districts call, in their opinion, for the regulation of them." [34] But the Permanent Secretary advised the President, "I presume you would not be prepared to propose legislation on this subject," and the letter was filed without further action.

Buchanan was fortunate in having as the Board's President from 1882 to 1884 Sir Charles Dilke (1843–1911), a friend and disciple of John Stuart Mill. Dilke infused a more energetic spirit into the Board. He refused to make political appointments to the secretariat and adopted a policy of promoting able men from within the staff.[35] A Liberal, Dilke had supported parliamentary efforts to provide a minimum of protection for the working classes, and his personal interest in housing reform led to the appointment of the Royal Commission on Housing. He was also concerned about deaths and disabilities in the pottery industry.

Such a figure was at least more approachable by the permanent medical staff of the Board, and Dilke also had the advantage of greater political backing than did his predecessors. This proved to be especially useful during the cholera outbreak of 1884, when Dilke defeated an attempt by the Chancellor of the Exchequer to cut down the Board's budget estimate for cholera control measures.

The Board's medical staff was enlarged under Dilke's administration and a valuable survey of ninety-two port health authorities carried out. Much of the success of controlling the cholera outbreaks of the mid-eighties was due to this survey. But even Dilke's regime had its limitations. His main policy in local government was decentralization. Although Dilke recognized the fallibility of local authorities, it was his belief that "public interest is often best served by allowing such errors to correct themselves." [36]

By Simon's account, the flurry of efficiency which passed through the Board under the Dilke administration lasted only until the close of 1886, when the cholera alarm had passed. Once again, the system of "how *not* to do it was tranquilly resumed." [37] Nevertheless, there was evidence that the medical staff in the late eighties was able to expand its role slightly. The Medical Officer's supplements to the annual reports of the Board list a growth in the number of inquiries on sanitary affairs. The annual reports, however, do not elaborate on the composition of these requests or inquiries. And Simon's comment on the value of these listings was somewhat critical.

From about 1884, the medical staff began to take a more active part in conferences with local sanitary authorities. The early conferences dealt largely with the provision of hospital accommodation for infectious cases and the applicability of bylaws to the needs of particular communities. By 1888, the Medical Officer recorded fifty-two instances of this type of consultation, noting with satisfaction the increasing degree to which the Medical Department counsel was being sought.[38] Five years later, the new Medical Officer of the Board, Dr. Richard Thorne Thorne,* stated that conferences were still on the increase.[39]

Any policy which might have developed as a result of these conferences with the Medical Department, however, suffered from the lack of such basic information as would have resulted from a national system of health inspection. It is also difficult to estimate the significance of such consultations in policy making, as almost no detailed records of the meetings were kept. Simon went so far as to say that "suspicion will perhaps arise that they who make these references to the Medical Department may at times go through their official ceremony with the smile of augurs." [40] It is probable that many of these transactions, whose total reached such impressive numbers, were largely routine.

Health Policy in the Nineties

Richard Thorne Thorne, who, as a young man in his twenties, had joined Simon's brilliant medical band at the Privy Council, was to achieve international recognition as a public hygienist. The son of a banker, he received his early education in Prussia and France. As the years passed, he developed into a man of considerable personal charm and urbanity. Dr. Thorne Thorne served as President of the Epidemio-

---

* Dr. Richard Thorne Thorne (1841–1899), who became Medical Officer of the Board in 1892, trained at St. Bartholomew's Hospital, London. He was appointed Physician to the London Hospital for Diseases of the Chest in 1868. He entered the Privy Council as an inspector in the Medical Office in 1871. He was well known for his research on typhoid as a water-borne disease. Dr. Thorne Thorne became a F.R.C.P. in 1875, a F.R.S. in 1890, and a K.C.B. in 1897.

logical Society from 1887 to 1889, and was respected both by his scientific colleagues and his political superiors at the Local Government Board.[41]

Despite his personal stature, Thorne Thorne's appointment as Medical Officer did not seriously change the role of the Board's Medical Department. The internal papers of the Local Government Board during the final decade of the nineteenth century continue to show little evidence of Medical Department participation in the formulation of major health policies. Indeed few questions of policy seem to have been raised. This was largely a period of continuing consolidation and the slow building up of evidence, supplied mainly by outside pressure groups, in favor of future change.

Reading through the memoranda and correspondence of a government office in the late nineteenth and twentieth centuries, one is impressed forcibly by the ponderous weight of the machinery to be set in motion before a reform could be transmuted into legislation. Like drops of water on stone, each petition and letter, each experience recorded by the officers concerned, had to wear away a tunnel through which the accumulated pressure could be brought to bear on the needed reform. Even when the necessity for change was at last recognized, qualifications must be applied by the legal department; the measure must be snipped here and there to make it more acceptable to special interest groups. Finally came the presentation to a Board or to Parliament, whose collective mind might well be concentrated upon matters more politically expedient.

When the Board's files are surveyed, it is at once apparent that the Medical Department exerted very little influence on sanitary legislation of the nineties. In July of 1890, the Board considered a "Bill to Consolidate and Amend the Acts Relating to Artizans and Labourers Dwellings and the Housing of the Working Classes Act." Although this contained a number of clauses which were sanitary in nature, and others concerning the responsibilities of medical officers of health, there is no evidence of the file's being circulated to the Medical Department.[42] The following year, the Public Health of London Law Amendment Bill was considered by the Board's secretariat. This bill was finally sent in draft to the Medical Department, but its existence was merely noted there by Dr. Buchanan.[43] In 1895, the Board scrutinized a Sanitary Registration Bill whose object was to require improved water drainage and water supply in new buildings. Like its predecessors of

1890 and 1893, this Bill was never sent to the Medical Department for comment. And the Board turned the bill down on the grounds that it was in advance of public opinion.[44]

Although none of these bills was technically medical, their sanitary character certainly brought them within the sphere of Medical Department interests. The Medical Officer does note in the Board's annual reports for 1898 and 1899, that the Medical Department examined bills for new schemes of water supply. But this was only a small part of public health legislation at the end of the century.

Unquestionably, the Local Government Board's medical staff in this period was subordinated to the lay secretariat, and was unable to exert more than a sporadic influence upon the Board's policy making. Other features of national health, still to be considered, took up much of the time of the Medical Department: disease control, the sanitary inspection service, and scientific research. But it is apparent from the internal correspondence of the Board that in policy matters the Medical Department acted, for the most part, only on the sufferance of the lay secretariat. Despite the high professional caliber of the four successive Medical Officers—Simon, Seaton, Buchanan, and Thorne Thorne—the medical staff was unable to lead the country in sanitary reform. After Simon's departure, there is no evidence that his successors waged any real struggle for a greater share in policy formulation.

The Medical Department of the Board must be viewed from another perspective before a more complete estimate of its work can be arrived at—a perspective that should include the primary duties of the nineteenth century government medical officer: disease control and sanitary inspection.

Chapter III

The Medical Department of the Local Government Board: Disease Control, 1871-1900

EPIDEMIC DISEASE was a constant and severe problem in nineteenth century England. In one of its most sensational forms, cholera, it had forced the premature establishment of the first General Board of Health. By 1871 disease control was accepted, almost without question, as a primary function of the new Local Government Board.

The Board's medical staff was well aware of the need for a centrally co-ordinated program against infectious disease and devoted much time to this area of public health. Cholera, smallpox, diphtheria, scarlet fever, and the enteric fevers repeatedly broke out in epidemic waves in the nineteenth century. Their control, while linked to general sanitary improvement, came finally from the great bacteriological discoveries made toward the close of the century—the isolation and identification of specific living organisms as the cause of disease.

The Coming of Bacteriology

Public health administration in England and elsewhere was greatly reinforced by the rapid advances in medical bacteriology in the eighties and nineties. It was not until the last twenty years of the nineteenth century that the germ theory of disease took hold. As a contemporary physician, Dr. Charles Cameron, pointed out in 1881, "It is only recently that the organisms have been identified, and it is only within a period to be reckoned in months rather than by years that their habits have been so exposed to us that it is already in our power to isolate them from the living body . . . to multiply, to destroy, modify, weaken or intensify them at our pleasure." [1] Cameron was oversanguine about contemporary powers to control bacteria. But it could not be doubted that the new knowledge of bacteria gave another dimension to the value of isolation and sanitation in infectious disease—the public recognition that every person suffering from contagious disease was a "hotbed, swarming with living organisms which caused and spread the disease."

Throughout the nineteenth century there could still be found persons who believed plague and disease to be a punishment, dispatched directly from an irate heaven.[2] But by midcentury three distinct scientific theories were supported by those seeking to explain infection and disease. A majority of the English sanitary reformers accepted the vague but popular pythogenic theory, whereby miasmas and gases—air compounded of unhealthy exhalations from decomposing filth, garbage, and sewer gas—created infectious disease. Chadwick and Simon both based their sanitary convictions on this miasmic theory of an "epidemic atmosphere," and it was officially accepted by the Privy Council. On the Continent the chemical theory of spontaneous generation of disease in the blood attracted more supporters than in England. Even though the experiments of Francesco Redi (1626–1697) and Louis Joblot (1645–1723) almost two centuries earlier proved spontaneous generation to be improbable, the concept survived well into the nineteenth century, supported by the internationally renowned chemist, Justus von Liebig (1803–1873).

The third major contemporary explanation for disease was the germ theory—or infection by a living organism, a *contagium vivum*. Some two hundred years before the findings of Pasteur and Koch, Antony van Leeuwenhoek (1632–1723) turned up a wonderful new world of "incredibly many very little animalcules of divers sorts" in his microscope—a world anticipated by ancient explorers. Other microscopists in the eighteenth and early nineteenth centuries extended the classification of bacteria. And in eighteenth century France advances in pathological anatomy and the classification of diseases set the stage for the subsequent nineteenth-century linkage of specific causative agents to specific diseases.

By the 1840's scientific observers like Jakob Henle (1809–1885) the Heidelberg anatomist, and Agostino Bassi (1773–1856) had set forth reasoned statements on the role of animalcular factors in the etiology of contagious disease. Not long afterwards, Theodor Schwann (1810–1882) established the basis for the germ theory of fermentation. By the eighteen sixties the careful researches on fermentation of Louis Pasteur (1822–1895) had finally demonstrated that the theory of spontaneous generation of microorganisms in the blood was false and had confirmed the theory that fermentation was due to live organisms.[3]

In a wave of scientific activity, Continental scientists started the search to link bacteria with specific diseases. Following Pasteur came the work of Obermeier with spirochetes and relapsing fever, Neisser's discovery of the relation of the gonococcus to gonorrhea, and Koch's identification of the tubercle bacillus in 1882, and of the dread cholera vibrio, or comma bacillus, in 1883. The next year, Loëffler identified the diphtheria bacillus, Nicolaier the tetanus bacillus, and Fraenkel the pneumonia bacillus. The origin of epidemic cerebrospinal meningitis was discovered in 1887 by Weichselbaum, and in 1894 the bacillus of bubonic plague was brought to light. Robert Koch's improvements in staining techniques, followed by his development of a method to achieve pure cultivations of bacteria, led the way in the eighties to many other methodological advances in bacteriology.

The scientific developments in the early eighties were primarily the work of Europeans. Midcentury Americans were indifferent to basic research,[4] and the new bacteriological discoveries were not widely recognized in the United States until 1885. But by that year medical schools began to offer courses in bacteriology.[5] By the eighteen-nineties American scientists, many of whom trained in German laboratories, were actively contributing to the development and practical application of bacteriological knowledge.

Meanwhile, in England, the medical staff of the Local Government Board in the eighties and nineties brought the bacteriological discoveries to the attention of local authorities through information-memoranda directives, through medical inspections, and through direct staff consultations, particularly during epidemic outbreaks. The auxiliary scientific investigations, carried out by the Board's Medical Office, added further valuable information on the control of disease.[6]

Steady gains from 1870 to 1900 in the nationwide sanitary movement also helped to reduce disease-breeding conditions. Large-scale improvements in drainage, ventilation, and in the supply of drinking water took place in London and many of England's large cities during these years. The broad program undertaken by the Metropolitan Board of Works, which, between 1856 and 1887 spent £14,000,000 on the destruction of condemned dwellings, contributed substantially to sanitary improvement. And work in the building of model dwellings by such private bodies as the Peabody Trustees, the Artizans and Labourer's General Dwelling Company, and Sir Sidney Waterlow's Company had considerable sanitary by-effects.

Capital loans for sanitary improvement were also made available by the Local Government Board. During the years 1874 through 1888, the annual amounts spent by the rural and urban sanitary authorities grew from £11,955,032 to £17,854,696. The greater part of this money was borrowed from the Local Government Board.[7]

It was in this framework of developing awareness of the role of microorganisms in sickness, and of steadily increasing public support for sanitary improvement, that the Local Government Board directed England's program for disease control.

Cholera

Epidemic cholera had been one of the most effective stimuli in the early sanitary movement when it first reached England in 1831. The sudden onset and alarming symptoms—livid face, clammy skin, vomiting, cramps, severe diarrhea, shrunken features, and convulsions—were a source of terror to those near the victim. Despite acute public fear of cholera, any early central government campaign against the disease was hampered by uncertainty as to its cause, reluctance to spend public funds on sanitary improvements, and strongly localistic feelings.

The year 1849, the year of the most severe and widespread cholera epidemic England ever experienced, was also the year in which a new theory of the transmission of the disease was published—Dr. John Snow's demonstration that cholera was water-borne, the carrier agents being the excretions of cholera victims.[8] Snow (1813–1858) made his professional living principally as an anesthetist. Although his views found little favor with his medical colleagues, Snow continued his investigations and submitted his conclusions in a more detailed form following the cholera outbreak of 1853.

At the time Snow first announced his theory, there was a generally recognized analogy between infection and fermentation, and it had been demonstrated that a number of communicable diseases could be transmitted through the inoculation of a small quantity of morbid matter. This had not been demonstrated in the enteric infections, however, and the variable patterns of cholera outbreaks made difficult any simple solution. Four weeks after Snow's pamphlet was published, William Budd (1811–1880), who had been working independently, published the same conclusions.[9] It was not until 1883 that Robert Koch (1843–1910) in Germany was to identify the cholera vibrio, and put his scientific weight behind the theory of a water-borne pollution.

Meanwhile studies of cholera became more frequent—in reports by William Farr on the 1848–1849 and 1853–1854 epidemics, in reports by the Royal College of Physicians, in Dr. Henry Acland's distinguished *Memoir on the Cholera at Oxford in the Year 1854,* and in the *Report of the General Board of Health.* This last report bore out the Snow theory of infection by water supplies. In 1853, acting as a Special Cholera Committee of the General Board of Health, Doctors Arnott, Baly, Owen, Simon, and William Farr admitted the organic pollution of drinking water to be dangerous, although their findings were hedged with reserve in the absence of conclusive proof. Simon, while he served on this committee, was reluctant to accept the Snow theory, and placed more reliance upon Southwood Smith's sanitary teachings, which attributed cholera to general insanitation. In 1866, Simon still upheld the theory that filth and excremental uncleanliness were the epidemic sources of cholera. William Farr, however, in 1866, blamed London's cholera on the distribution of unfiltered water by the East London Company. According to the *Medical Press and Circular,* which commented two years later on the Farr Report, this view was not then generally accepted in England.[10]

CHOLERA UNDER THE LOCAL GOVERNMENT BOARD

At the time of the Board's establishment in 1871, cholera control was thus a recognized function of the central health authority. While the actual cause of the outbreaks was still uncertain, measures based both on the theory of contagion and upon the miasma concept were being applied. The newly industrialized, and heavily congested, cities were vulnerable targets to an outbreak of cholera. It was publicly recognized that the enormous growth of population, which had transformed England between 1800 and 1875 into a country with 13 cities (apart from London), each with over 100,000 inhabitants, and 103 towns with over 20,000 inhabitants, constituted a threat to the health of the new England.[11]

Under the Board of Health, regulations for dealing with a cholera epidemic had been issued to local authorities, many of whom were wholly unprepared for the exercise of such duties.[12] The program dealt then with daily house-to-house inspections, quarantine, orders on burial, and prescriptions for disinfecting cholera-contaminated dwelling places.

A new threat of cholera from the Continent in 1871 led the Local Government Board to ask the Royal College of Physicians to prepare a list of instructions which might be circulated in slum areas by nurses and district visitors. The solemn response from the College recommended to the poor of England that their houses must be "clean, light, thoroughly dry and well ventilated"; that three or four "nourishing and ample meals" must be eaten "with undeviating regularity," that soup, cheese, and indigestible things should be avoided, and alcoholic beverages consumed in moderation. Fatigue, undue mental strain, and emotional excitement must be rigidly shunned, and the aim should be a "tranquil life." [13] As a disinfectant, the College recommended corrosive sublimate which, by Act of Parliament, was prohibited in general sale. These instructions were never issued, however, by the Board, which contented itself with sending a general warning of the outbreak to local authorities, more especially the port authorities.[14] Customs officials were authorized to stop ships suspected of carrying cholera, and arrangements were made for the detention of suspected persons and the disinfection of ships.[15]

Year by year, the Board's Medical Department kept close watch upon any outbreaks of cholera in Europe which seemed to offer a threat to England, and the annual reports summarized cholera conditions abroad with regularity. Without question, the medical officers of the Board were aware of the major role to be played by the central government health authority in preventing cholera. In April of 1874, upon his own initiative, Dr. George Buchanan addressed a lengthy memorandum to John Simon, dealing with the dangers of transmission of cholera by foreigners visiting England, and stressed the necessity of proper lodging under medical supervision for suspected cases to be kept apart from the general population of port towns. Simon gave the matter his full endorsement and communicated the proposal to the Emigration Commissioners.[16]

Dr. Buchanan took a lively personal interest in central control of epidemic disease, and on one occasion rushed to Birkenhead without notifying his family in order to advise local authorities on steps to meet a cholera outbreak among emigrants on ships in the Mersey.[17]

Quarantine, however, was of limited value and was a serious disruption to foreign trade when vessels were interned for long periods. From 1875 on, with the creation of Port Sanitary Authorities, medical inspection of ships' crews and passengers, and disinfection of the ship where necessary, were emphasized, rather than full-scale quarantine, which was finally abolished by the Public Health Act of 1896.[18]

Up to 1893, the Local Government Board Medical Office periodically prohibited the importation of rags, in bales, from countries in which cholera had broken out. However, as a result of a decision of the International Sanitary Conference at Dresden in March and April of 1893, the wholesale prohibition was moderated to prohibitions against body linen, worn clothes, and bedding. Dr. Koch at this conference had declared that "in no single instance had there been to his knowledge, an authenticated case of the transmission of cholera by means of rags of commerce," and this view was supported by the leading European medical delegates.[19]

The Board's cholera control measures were particularly effective in 1884, when a severe cholera epidemic on the Continent alarmed all England. In the summer of that year, 11,000 died in Italy from the terrible disease, 4,600 in Paris, and numbers more in Spain.[20] The Board took immediate action. A circular letter was sent out warning all sanitary authorities in England. Special inspectors were detailed to the ports, and the importation of rags prohibited. On July 11, the Medical Officer of the Board applied to the Royal College of Physicians for a revision of cholera instructions, and this time the College responded with more practical measures which were incorporated into an instruction sent out by the Board. They urged attention to pure water supplies, prevention of water contamination with sewage, free ventilation, great cleanliness, avoidance of overcrowding, and thorough drainage in towns, villages, and dwellings.[21] At the request of the Chief Inspector of Factories, Alexander Redgrave, the Board also prepared a special memorandum for cholera prevention in factories.[22]

But the memoranda, exhorting local authorities to look to drainage, water supplies, disposal of filth, and overcrowding, might have been merely so much paper, had not the Medical Department been able to find strong political support in the President of the Board, Charles Dilke. Against the opposition of the Chancellor of the Exchequer, Dilke was able to push through financial allotments for the Board, which authorized the increase of the medical staff to meet the threat of cholera and also resulted in a sanitary survey of the entire coast.

The survey permitted a careful examination by the Medical Department of the condition of 92 port towns, and the precautions observed for preventing the spread of infectious disease cases arriving by ship.[23] The results were highly beneficial. As Inspector Preston-Thomas saw it:

> The authorities of the ports were to some extent brought into line; they were impressed with a sense of their responsibilities; not only did they organize special arrangements for the inspection of ships from infected countries, but they also recognized the necessity of setting their own houses in order in a literal sense, and many of them for the first time displayed activity in providing pure water, efficient sewerage, and a system of prompt removal of nuisances.[24]

The doctrine of "sanitation by anticipation," urged by Dr. William Budd, and set up as a motto by the President of the British Medical Association at the Belfast meeting in 1884, was strengthened in the campaign against cholera.[25] As a result of the immediate steps taken by the central government medical staff, England escaped the 1884 cholera completely, with the exception of one isolated case in Cardiff.

Watchful precautions were continued throughout the eighties, and the medical office maintained a routine check on European outbreaks. An epidemic on the Continent in 1892 brought 35 cholera victims to English shores within two months, but so successful were the precautions taken that no further infection took place in England except among those arriving from abroad. However, the following year, fears of a new European epidemic led Dr. Thorne Thorne to persuade the Board to institute a cholera survey, and to this end four additional inspectors (two permanent and two temporary) were added to the medical staff. The Board also announced to local sanitary authorities its willingness to provide bacteriological analysis in attempting to distinguish between Asiatic cholera and diarrheal disease.[26]

The cholera survey at first embraced only 60 port and 75 riparian districts, but later was extended to inland areas. In all, a total of 396 districts came under the inspection, including the more important mining and manufacturing districts of the North and Midland counties.[27]

The report served its primary purpose of rousing local authorities against cholera infection and was a valuable index to the sanitary state of the country as well. By 1893, it was generally conceded by bacteriologists that the comma bacillus was the cause of the disease, although a few still looked upon the organism as a consequence of the illness.[28]

In forwarding the survey to the President of the Local Government Board, Dr. Richard Thorne Thorne commented that the study emphasized the need, not for futile quarantines, but for urging upon all who were responsible for the health of rural and urban communities the need for higher standards of cleanliness in regard to the air, soil, and water in their districts.[29]

In all, the Local Government Board was highly successful in controlling cholera in England. During 1894 and 1895, when 42,000 died of the disease in Russia alone, no English inhabitant succumbed.[30] Thorne Thorne credited their success to the steadily improving sanitary conditions throughout the country.

The abandonment of quarantine and emphasis on port security measures were, he felt, major steps. "So long as Government tell their peoples that a line shall be drawn around them across which disease shall not pass, so long will those peoples be reluctant to spend their money on the promotion of true measures of prevention." [31]

But more than the elimination of cholera from England had been achieved in times of its threatened invasion from the Continent. The dreaded name acted as a powerful weapon for the sanitary reformers and loosened civic purse strings where all other appeals had failed. Cholera scares had been of great service to the advancement of English sanitation. Reporting in 1895 to the Parliamentary Bills Committee of the British Medical Association, on water-borne typhoid, Dr. Ernest Hart noted:

> An apparent paradox has now been for some time promulgated to the effect that cholera in this country saves more lives than it costs, but the assertion is true. All sanitary measures that go to lessen the likelihood of cholera-spread go also to lessen the chance of the spread of diseases which are disseminated in like manner . . . Yet when cholera threatens our coasts, there is but little difficulty in securing the co-operation of sanitary bodies and the public in carrying out these measures which are thought to be necessary.[32]

In 1883, Dilke observed the same useful purpose of cholera:

> I circulated a draft of a Bill to meet the cholera scare, which I carried into law as the Disease Prevention Act. I did not much believe in cholera, but I took advantage of the scare to carry some useful clauses to deal with smallpox epidemics.[33]

The "filth theory" of disease origin was gradually replaced by germ discoveries of the eighties and nineties. Cholera outbreaks, however, had been held in check by preventing the contamination of water supplies some years before the bacillus was isolated.

No discrepancy existed between the public and the official medical views on the necessity of central government intervention for cholera control. The Local Government Board inherited a body of precedent for action in this field and extended it through use of such tools as scientific investigation, medical inspection, coercion of local authorities, and international co-operation.

Smallpox

Pitted and disfigured faces were a common sight in nineteenth-century England, and for those persons who escaped with only scarring, hundreds more died every year from smallpox. During its first years, 1871–1873, the Local Government Board faced a smallpox epidemic more severe than any in the century.[34] Moving swiftly and virulently throughout Europe, the epidemic killed thousands. In England and Wales alone, 23,126 persons died of smallpox during 1871. Before the wave spent itself in the first quarter of 1873, a total of 44,079 succumbed; over a quarter of the deaths were in the city of London.[35] Although handicapped until the end of the century by the absence of a national system for compulsory notification of infectious diseases, the Board, by sponsoring compulsory vaccination and the fostering isolation hospitals, played a major role in the reduction of smallpox.

BACKGROUND OF NINETEENTH-CENTURY SMALLPOX CONTROL

Some attempt to control this disease had developed in the eighteenth century through the introduction of inoculation into the English Court by the redoubtable Lady Mary Wortley Montagu on her return from Turkey. By the early nineteenth century, vaccination had replaced the clumsier, and less reliable, process of inoculation.[36] Jenner's application of the new method was first rewarded in 1802 with a £10,000 grant from a grateful Parliament, and six years later, England set up a National Vaccine Establishment to maintain and distribute lymph supplies.

By 1840 Parliament had passed an act establishing free vaccination in each poor law parish. It would be misleading to interpret this as the setting up of a real national vaccination program, however, as local authorities varied considerably in applying this law. Subsequent legislation made infant vaccination compulsory under penalty (1853), regulated the performance of vaccination (1858), set up a vaccination inspection system (1860), and, in 1867, consolidated and amended the Vaccination Acts.[37]

VACCINATION

The Local Government Board thus inherited a well-established system of preventive measures for dealing with smallpox. The vaccination program which the Board supervised from 1871 to 1900 was carried out against not inconsiderable harassment from the anti-vaccination movement, but with warm support from Parliament. Shortly before the Board's establishment, the House of Commons had appointed a Select Committee to consider the state of vaccination administration throughout the country. The appointment was inspired by public attacks during 1870 of the anti-vaccinationists on the practice of compulsory vaccination of infants. Anti-vaccinationists clamored that vaccination was dangerous and offered no real protection against smallpox. These charges echoed nineteenth-century concepts of private property rights. One cartoon of this period pictures the devil chuckling and waving his tail gently at the spectacle of a father imprisoned for refusing to "poison his child's blood" by vaccination.

The public hearing afforded to the anti-vaccinationists by the Select Committee came, as Simon pointed out, at a fortunate time.[38] For the smallpox epidemic raging throughout England in the early seventies furnished an excellent background against which to test the effectiveness of the vaccination system that had been in effect for the past thirty years. Although the Select Committee devoted eight of its twenty sittings to the anti-vaccinationists, it also heard local administrators and medical witnesses. The final report swept out the claims of the antivaccinationists, stating unequivocally that "it is the duty of the State to endeavour to secure the careful vaccination of the whole population." [39] The Select Committee's report also recognized the need to vaccinate children, both for their own and the community's protection. Their over-all recommendations were incorporated in the Vaccination Act of 1871, which made compulsory the appointment of paid vaccination officers in every Poor Law Union.

Although the anti-vaccinationists renewed their charges from year to year, the Local Government Board started its administration with full parliamentary backing for a strong national program of vaccination. Supervision of the program was regularly, and carefully, carried out by the central health authority.

Successive annual reports from the Board's Medical Department dealt at length with the vaccination system. In 1874, the Medical Officer noted that the 647 Boards of Guardians of England and Wales, who constituted the local vaccination authorities, employed more than 3,000 medical practitioners for public vaccinations, and another 1,400 nonmedical "vaccination officers." A representative of the Board individually inspected these authorities at least once every two years, more frequently in London.[40] By 1890, nine medical inspectors were employed on a part-time basis in this work—examining the work of each vaccinator, his methods, and his register of public vaccinations. Where faults existed, the central inspectors notified the Board of Guardians concerned. The Board's inspectors also carried out special inquiries upon receipt of complaints.[41]

The Local Government Board, in addition, administered the National Vaccine Establishment, charged with the distribution of lymph supplies to public vaccinators and private practitioners. Calf lymph was first distributed by the Establishment in 1881. By 1896, it was issued in the more satisfactory form of glycerinated lymph. The National Vaccine Establishment also opened a variety of educational vaccination stations throughout the country, to instruct and certify medical practitioners in performing the approved methods of vaccination.

The test of the effectiveness of the vaccination program lay in the steady reduction of smallpox throughout the country in the period following the 1870–1873 epidemic. This severe outbreak had demonstrated the need for revaccination in adults, and the Board repeatedly urged public vaccinators to make this a regular part of their program. During epidemic periods, the vaccination officers and their assistants, carried out house-to-house visitations to vaccinate and revaccinate all inhabitants. Up to 1881, the Board's statistics showed a steadily decreasing number of children (of registered births) who remained unvaccinated. Whereas in 1872, about 5.1 per cent of registered births were not accounted for in the vaccination program, the figures were reduced to 4.3 per cent in 1878 and 3.8 per cent in 1881, the tenth anniversary of the compulsory Vaccination Act of 1871.[42]

This happy picture began to change in the mid-eighties, in part due to revived and organized publicity aroused by the anti-vaccinationists. By 1894, the Board's Medical Officer noted that 13.4 per cent of the

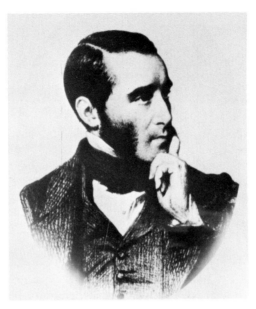

John Simon (1816-1904), at age 32.
Courtesy of the National Library of
Medicine

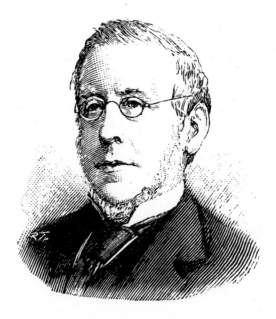

John Lambert (1815-92)

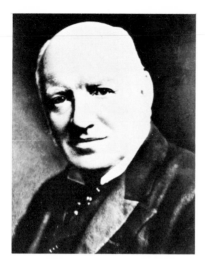

Dr. Edward Cator Seaton (1815-
80). Courtesy of the Wellcome
Historical Medical Museum

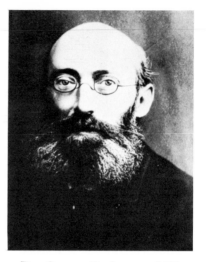

Dr. George Buchanan (1831-
95). Courtesy of the Wellcome
Historical Medical Museum

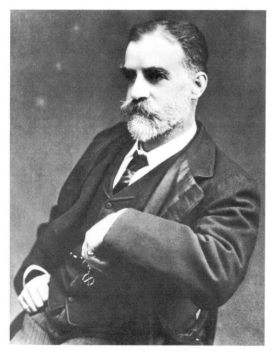

Dr. Richard Thorne Thorne (1841-99). Courtesy
of the Wellcome Historical Medical Museum

"A Case of True Cholera" — cartoon, 1832. Courtesy of the National Library of Medicine

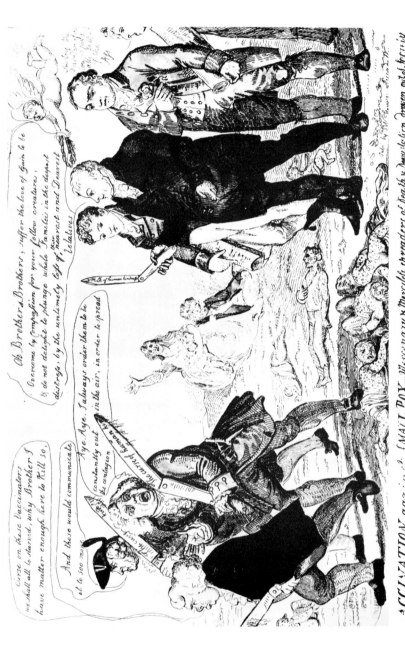

Early anti-vaccinationists—cartoon, 1808. Courtesy of the National Library of Medicine

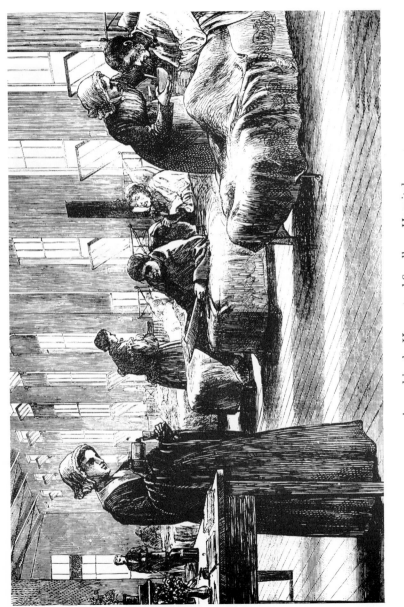

A ward in the Hampstead Smallpox Hospital

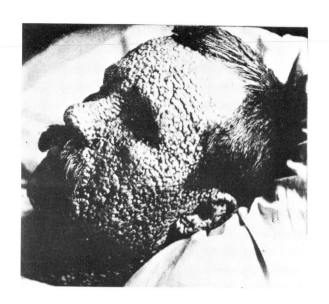

Smallpox cases in 1901

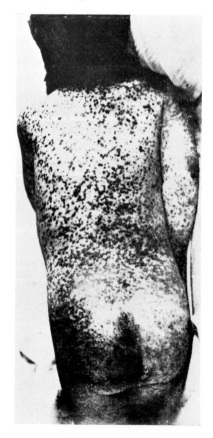

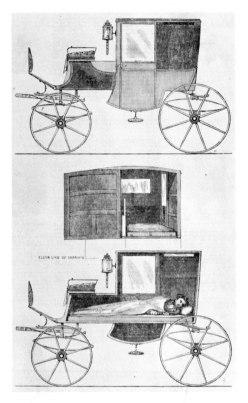

Hospital carriage for the conveyance of fever and smallpox patients, 1867

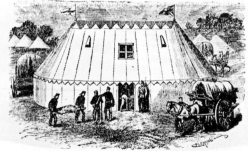
Advertisement for temporary isolation hospital marquees, 1894

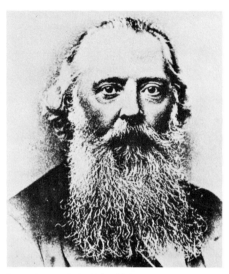

Dr. J. L. W. Thudichum (1829-1901). Courtesy of the National Library of Medicine

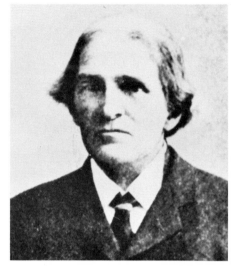

Sir John Burdon Sanderson (1828-1905). Courtesy of the National Library of Medicine

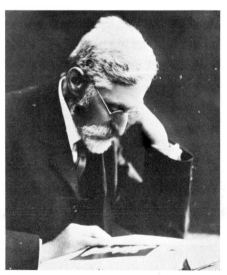

Dr. Edward E. Klein (1844-1925). Courtesy of the Wellcome Historical Medical Museum

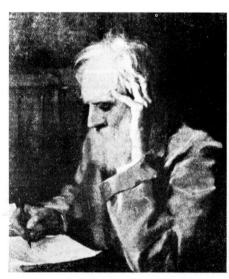

Dr. Edward Ballard (1820-97). Courtesy of the Wellcome Historical Medical Museum

children born in 1891 were still unvaccinated, and attributed this to increasing noncompliance with the Vaccination Laws.[43] The work of the anti-vaccinationists was directly reflected in this changing picture. The London Society for the Abolition of Compulsory Vaccination, headed by Mr. P. A. Taylor, M.P., had been turning out a monthly organ known at the *Vaccination Inquirer* throughout the eighties.[44]

Despite its unscientific tenets, the movement attracted the support of such vocal public figures as John Bright and George Bernard Shaw. The charge that medical men profited from vaccinations had great appeal for such confirmed enemies of the medical profession as Shaw. In actuality, attendance upon hundreds of patients afflicted with small-pox might have been far more remunerative to physicians. The anti-vaccinationists also charged that vaccination caused personal injuries, and alleged that syphilis and erysipelas were transmitted in the process of vaccination. The Board's medical staff had made it their business to inspect complaints of this nature, and, while occasional cases of technical mistakes in vaccinating were revealed in the earlier days of the process, later investigations proved that such allegations were without basis.[45]

The increasing noncompliance with the law for compulsory vaccination of infants, combined with the publicity aroused by the anti-vaccinationists, led to the appointment in 1889 of a Royal Commission on Vaccination. After holding 136 meetings and conducting several investigations of local smallpox outbreaks, the Commission decided that repeated penalties for refusing to obey vaccination laws were inadvisable. Their final report intoned: "A law severe in its terms, and enforced with great stringency, may be less effectual for its purpose than one of less severity and which is put in force less uncompromisingly." [46] The *British Medical Journal,* however, chafed at the decision, feeling that the compulsory factor of the vaccination law must be maintained if smallpox were to be eradicated.[47]

The Royal Commission's recommendations were transmuted into law in the Vaccination Act of 1898. Under this legislation, a parent, who satisfied the court within four months of the birth of a child that he conscientiously believed that vaccination was prejudicial to the health of the child, would be free of penalties. In no case were proceedings to be taken more than twice against a parent or child.[48] In an effort to enforce the program of vaccination, it was made obligatory on public vaccinators to visit the homes of unvaccinated children and to offer to vaccinate them.

This relaxation of compulsory vaccination had some support within the Local Government Board, whose administrators felt that inflicting an excessive number of penalties only created more sentiment against the Vaccination Laws. As a result, however, an increasing number of children escaped vaccination, and, by 1899, it was noted that 22.7 per cent of those born two years earlier were still unvaccinated.[49] It is probable that the conscientious-objection "escape clause" of the 1898 Act was not the sole cause. The fear of smallpox had abated considerably over the years, so that the earlier success of vaccination in reducing the incidence of smallpox contributed to its gradual disuse.

ISOLATION HOSPITALS

Preventive measures were only a part of the Local Government Board's work against smallpox. In fostering isolation hospitals throughout the country, whose services were available to all, the Board actually extended public responsibility in curative medicine.

Two smallpox hospitals had been established in the eighteenth century in London—one in Old Street Road and one in Cold Bath Fields. These were merely small houses and were replaced in 1794 by a single larger building at Battle Bridge (King's Cross). In 1848 a new smallpox hospital was opened in Highgate, and this building was to remain the only smallpox hospital in London until 1870.[50] The overwhelming numbers of smallpox victims during the 1870–1871 epidemic presented new problems, however. The medical staff of the Privy Council and, subsequently, of the Local Government Board, tried seriously to arouse the country to the need for isolation hospitals to prevent the further spread of smallpox. A memorandum was dispatched to local sanitary authorities urging them to fulfill their obligations under the Sanitary Act of 1866 in providing hospital accommodation for infected persons. The Board also issued instructions for the setting up of temporary hospitals and offered consultation service on building isolation hospitals.[51]

In London the Metropolitan Asylums Board, working in close cooperation with the Local Government Board staff, set up special isolation hospitals at Hampstead, Homerton, and Stockwell, and borrowed a ship (the *Dreadnought*) from the Admiralty to accommodate convalescent smallpox patients.[52]

The heavy smallpox casualties of the first years of the eighteen-seventies aroused the general public to the need for publicly supported isolation hospitals, not only for paupers, but for others afflicted with the disease. The Metropolitan Asylums Board in London found it impossible to admit only paupers to the isolation hospitals and, by 1879, obtained legal authority to contract with local authorities for the admission to isolation hospitals of any person suffering from a dangerous infectious disease. Several years later, a survey showed that the largest number of persons cared for in smallpox hospitals came from the wage-earning class. Some, treated in the larger and better constructed hospitals, had backgrounds in commerce, trade, and the professions.[53]

Meanwhile, acting under the provisions of the Public Health Act of 1875, local authorities elsewhere in the country moved sluggishly into action to provide isolation hospitals, prodded by the Local Government Board. In 1879, about 18 per cent of the sanitary authorities of England and Wales (apart from the metropolitan or port sanitary authorities) had set up some form of isolation care for victims of infectious diseases. By 1892, 36 per cent of the same sanitary authorities (representing 62.1 per cent of the population) had established accommodations for smallpox patients.[54]

The Board's medical staff, throughout the eighties and nineties, continued to work closely with local authorities, developing instructions for standardizing treatment in isolation hospitals. Even in non-epidemic years, the Board's medical inspectors kept a close watch on endemic smallpox cases and reported to the Principal Medical Officer, offering suggestions for issuing and reissuing warning circulars to local authorities. When, in 1893, the Government sponsored a bill to increase isolation hospital accommodations throughout the country, the Local Government Board's Medical Department supported the bill's provision for authorizing County Councils to establish such hospitals if the local authorities defaulted.[55]

By 1899 smallpox deaths in England and Wales were recorded at a low of 174 persons—in contrast to the 23,126 who succumbed in 1871 at the start of the Local Government Board's program.[56] But the close of the century did not see smallpox entirely eliminated from England. Indeed, the years 1901 to 1906 were epidemic years. But after 1906 there were only minor outbreaks of severe smallpox, and these were chiefly of imported origin.[57]

Unquestionably, the strong action taken by the Local Government Board's medical staff in inspections, and in encouraging local authorities to more active antismallpox measures, helped to reduce the incidence of the disease. The continuance of wide-scale vaccination measures and improvements in the administration of the program, in extended vaccination training facilities, and in better methods of utilization of lymph supplies were major factors in the reduction of epidemic smallpox by the end of the century. Although the compulsory feature of child vaccination was softened by the Vaccination Act of 1898, the over-all vaccination program, as such, was not relaxed by the central government authority. The Medical Department of the Board steadily urged local authorities to provide hospitalization for smallpox patients, and their efforts were speeded by the Isolation Hospitals Act of 1893. Technical medical advances in the administration of glycerinated calf lymph, and in better techniques for the recognition and early diagnosis of smallpox developed by Dr. Thomas Ricketts (1864–1918), also contributed to a reduction of the disease.[58]

Typhus

Typhus is a disease which flourishes under conditions of personal and environmental insanitation, overcrowding, and destitution. During the first half of the nineteenth century few physicians could distinguish between typhus and typhoid, the two major endemic fevers with high death rates. By the fifties, the writings of William Jenner, of the American, W. W. Gerhard, and others had established the separate identities of the two diseases; and in 1869 typhus was listed as a specific disease in the mortality returns of the Registrar-General. The same year, 1869, initiated a dramatic decrease in the number of typhus deaths throughout England and Wales (see Table 1).

This reduction in typhus cannot be attributed to any remarkable activity on the part of the Local Government Board's Medical Department. In fact, beyond occasional medical inspections of severe outbreaks and recommendations for isolation of typhus patients and disinfection of bedding, the Board paid relatively little attention to this disease, as such. The decreasing incidence, however, was directly linked to improved sanitary conditions developing throughout the country.

Earlier in the nineteenth century, the swarming new industrial cities with their unwholesome dwelling quarters had provided ideal habitats for the typhus louse vector. For many years Liverpool abounded with typhus. Immigrants who crossed to the city in the years following the Irish potato famine had swollen its already overcrowded slums, causing conditions of gross insanitation. European travelers, pouring through

TABLE 1. Typhus Deaths in England and Wales, 1869–1900 [59]

	Number of Deaths		Number of Deaths
1869	4,281	1885	318
1870	3,297	1886	245
1871	2,754	1887	211
1872	1,864	1888	160
1873	1,638	1889	137
1874	1,762	1890	151
1875	1,499	1891	137
1876	1,165	1892	85
1877	1,104	1893	137
1878	906	1894	115
1879	533	1895	58
1880	530	1896	71
1881	552	1897	49
1882	940	1898	47
1883	877	1899	29
1884	328	1900	29

the port city en route to the New World, also spread the disease. Despite large-scale condemnation of insanitary dwellings, Liverpool in the eighties still offered many congenial quarters for lice. Two cases, described by Dr. Stopford Taylor in dealing with typhus in Liverpool in 1884, reveal existing sanitary conditions in some sections of the city responsible for the continued prevalence of typhus and other diseases:

Matilda Crosby, age 35, 1/13 Eaton Street: The poor creature in this filthy abominable court has been five or six days ill. The room is so dark as to necessitate the use of wax matches to examine the patient. The room is foul and filthy, almost bare of furniture, and the other inmates are clothed with rags. Two or three half-naked children bear evidence of chronic starvation.

Melaney, 6/1 Hughson Street. The intense foetor of the room in which the sick people lay necessitated waiting outside until the window was opened. The occupants of the bed, which is about 3 feet by 6, were five in number, and all exceptionally filthy. The mother is a fish hawker, and the fish were in a basket under the bed. The family appeared to be suffering from chronic starvation, and two members had fever.[60]

Nevertheless, even in Liverpool the mortality from typhus declined markedly by the end of the century.[61]

The Local Government Board's role in the reduction of typhus consisted largely of contributions to the framing of sanitary bylaws for new buildings (as, for example, regulations to eliminate back-to-back housing), in sending medical inspectors to investigate and report on more severe outbreaks of typhus, and in encouraging the increased use of isolation hospitals. In 1886, a special inquiry was undertaken by an inspector from the Board's Medical Department, Dr. John Spear, who visited sixty-seven localities in England and Wales. Spear's findings confirmed the statistics of the Registrar-General, that nowhere in England and Wales did typhus exist in any such epidemic forms as it had twenty or thirty years earlier. It was not until 1909 that Charles Nicolle, Director of the Pasteur Institute of Tunis, identified the body louse as the typhus vector. As the Local Government Board's Medical Officer reviewed the situation in 1886, he saw little hope of eliminating typhus entirely from the country "until the time shall come when masses of population brought down nearly to starvation point, shall cease to inhabit foul courts into which no air can enter, and to huddle their miserable families into rooms that ought not to hold the half of them." [62]

Typhoid Fever

In the course of establishing differential diagnosis for typhus and typhoid, observers had noted that while typhus was primarily present among the poor, typhoid evidenced no such class discrimination. Typhoid bacilli were not identified until 1880. But by the time of the Local Government Board's establishment in 1871, it was beginning to be recognized that typhoid was spread through infection from the discharges of the diseased intestine. A number of epidemiologists in the mid-seventies still believed the disease was spread through atmospheric infection.

When he published his thoughtful study on typhoid fever in 1873, William Budd had pinpointed the danger of drinking water being contaminated through typhoid-infected sewers. English plumbing of the period featured broken drain-pipes, leaking cesspools, and contaminated wells. Budd also knew that the spread of this fever could be controlled by destroying the particles of infected discharges. In pleading for a community approach to eradicate the disease, Budd had warned, "he that was never yet connected with his poorer neighbor, by deeds of charity or love, may one day find, when it is too late, that he is connected with him by a bond which may bring them both, at once, to a common grave." [63]

The prevalence of typhoid was sufficiently high during the early years of the Local Government Board's operations, that its medical staff were as desirous as Dr. Budd that all men, rich and poor, should avoid the common grave of typhoid. The disease was not made notifiable until 1889. In 1869 the death toll from diseases that came under the broad designation "enteric and simple continued fever" was 13,967. From 1876 to 1880 the average annual deaths from typhoid were reduced to 8,657, and between 1881 and 1885, they fell to 6,671.[64]

The Board's Medical Department kept a continual surveillance upon outbreaks of enteric fever and regularly carried out investigations into the sources of the disease in stricken communities. Each investigation added more proof to existing knowledge of the means of transmitting typhoid. In the early seventies, following inspections of typhoid outbreaks, the Medical Department noted the necessity for improvements in privy and privy drainage.[65] In two cases milk supplies were found to be polluted. By 1874 a localized attack of enteric fever at Caius College, Cambridge, had been traced to contamination of college drinking water pipes. An outbreak at Lewes in the same year again pointed to infected water supplies and an intermittent water service. In 1875, a severe outbreak of typhoid occurred at Croydon; but here the Board's medical inspection staff could only indict atmospheric infection to account for the spread of the disease.

Nevertheless, as the years passed, more and more evidence was collected which pointed to the specifically infective properties of intestinal evacuations of those attacked by enteric fever. In 1879, an outbreak of 352 cases at Caterham and Redhill, were clearly traced to the use of water from a deep well which had been infected by an enteric patient.

The publication of these investigations in the Board's annual reports, however, had no wholesale, salubrious influence upon local sanitary authorities in eliminating conditions in which enteric fever could flourish. In 1891, a special investigation by Dr. F. W. Barry of the Board's Medical Department into enteric fever in the Tees Valley revealed large-scale pollution of the river and its banks by excremental filth and refuse. Similar conditions in the Tees Valley had been referred to in 1875 by a parliamentary committee. Again, in 1887, other expert testimony had indicated the distressing insanitary conditions of the Tees riverbanks. Dr. Barry attributed the 1891 outbreak to floods which carried large masses of filth downstream to the water intakes.[66]

Although the over-all incidence of typhoid was gradually reduced by the nineties, serious outbreaks still occurred intermittently. By 1898, in reflecting on the general reduction in typhoid, the Board's Medical Officer noted some sanitary improvements. But he observed also that in certain sections of England and Wales, enteric death rates failed to drop. This, he attributed, to the maintenance in those communities of conditions involving the organic pollution of the soil.[67]

Diphtheria

Unlike many of the other contagious diseases, fatal diphtheria increased, rather than decreased, in the years from 1870 to 1900. Diphtheria became seriously prevalent in England about 1857, when a waning French epidemic swept across the channel. From that year until 1895, when the use of an antitoxin, developed three years earlier, brought the disease under control, diphtheria broke out with regularity in the harsh winter months. Selecting its victims mainly from among children under ten and taking a heavier toll of males than of females, diphtheria, on an annual average, killed 261 per million of those living in 1871–1880, 286 per million in 1881–1890, and 314 per million in 1891–1900.[68]

It was recognized by 1871 that diphtheria was often spread by personal communication, although the identification of the *Corynebacterium diphtheriae* waited until 1883 for Klebs' description and until 1884 for Loeffler's proof of its causative relationship to the disease. Local Government Board inspections of diphtheria outbreaks in the late seventies indicated the role of school attendance in spreading the disease. After this was confirmed in an 1882 investigation, John Lambert and Dr. George Buchanan met with authorities of the Education Department to discuss provision for closing the schools when the local medical officer of health felt that the prevalence of infectious disease required it.[69]

Throughout the eighties, the Board's Medical Department continued its investigations of large scale diphtheria outbreaks, notifying the local authorities of their findings—at Shaftesbury in 1885 and York

Town and Camberley in 1886. Dr. (later Sir) William Power,* who served as a medical inspector with the Board from 1871 to 1887, explored the Camberley epidemic, tracing it directly to milk infection. Power noted that the heavier diphtheria casualties among the higher class of milk consumers of the area resulted from the upper class practices of storing milk after purchase, giving an opportunity for the development of bacterial infections.

The local investigations notwithstanding, diphtheria continued to increase, and from 1880 on became particularly marked in urban areas. It was not only the rising diphtheria death rates that caused anxiety, but the alarming permanent injuries in those who recovered from the disease—injuries to the nervous system, heart, and other tissues caused by the powerful toxin. By the nineties, the Board's scientific staff had embarked on other types of diphtheria research. Dr. Edward Klein, who was to serve with the Board from 1871 to 1907, conducted a series of pathological studies of diphtheria for a number of years. Klein experimented at length, inoculating cultures of the diphtheria bacillus in animals and observing the appearance of characteristic forms of the disease in rodents, cats, and milch cows. It was slow work, but more and more information was being amassed on the habits of the bacillus, and groundwork was being laid for a later development of the antitoxin.[70]

In 1891, Dr. Richard Thorne Thorne published a study on diphtheria, utilizing the knowledge that the Board's scientific staff had accumulated their investigations. Thorne Thorne noted that the steady rise in diphtheria mortality had been unaffected by the sanitary improvements in water supply, sewerage, and drainage. He concluded that the general geological features of a district bore no direct relation to the spread of the disease, but that the dampness of the site and exposure to cold wet winds seemed to foster fatalities from the disease, especially from September to November. He warned against milk contagion by the bacillus and advised the use only of milk which had been boiled. Early isolation of the infected, and the application of disinfectant measures, were advocated as immediate treatment.[71]

---

* Sir William Henry Power (1842–1916) qualified from St. Bartholomew's Hospital in 1864. He joined the Local Government Board's staff in 1871 and carried out a variety of original investigations of smallpox, diphtheria, and scarlet fever. He subsequently served as Principal Medical Officer of the Local Government Board from 1900 to 1908. Power was elected F.R.S. in 1895, became a C.B.E. in 1902, and, on retiring from office was awarded the K.C.B.

By 1895, diphtheria antitoxin, pioneered in France, Germany, and by sanitary authorities in New York City, began to come into general use, and case mortality declined.

Scarlet Fever (Scarlatina)

Another disease, whose agents (*Micrococcus scarlatina*) spread rapidly through transmission of mouth droplets of infected persons, was scarlet fever. Up to 1861, scarlet fever had been classed with diphtheria in the annual returns of the Registrar-General. In its more severe form it was then known as scarlatina, and the death rates had been climbing in the twenty year period before the establishment of the Local Government Board. During the decade 1861–1870, the average annual death rate was 97 per 100,000. But in succeeding years, the rate dropped, until by 1886 it averaged only 17 per 100,000. This decline in scarlet fever death rates was attributed to the prevalence of a milder form of the disease than had occurred in earlier years, and evidence from hospitals of the Metropolitan Asylums Board confirmed this.[72] The Royal Commission on Vaccination in 1896 assigned the fall of death rates to the greater frequency of isolating scarlet fever cases early.[73]

Epidemiological research and knowledge of the means of transmission of disease were equally important in the reduction of scarlet fever mortality.[74] In this area, the Medical Department of the Board contributed significantly by recognizing milk as a culture medium for the micrococcus.

The major scarlatina investigation by the Board was undertaken during the 1885 outbreak in St. Marylebone. Other North London areas soon began to be affected, and the infective source was traced to a dairy farm in Hendon by the Board's medical inspector, Dr. William H. Power. Dr. Power and Dr. Edward Klein, who studied the bacteriological aspects of the epidemic, concluded that the dairy herd was infected with the disease, which caused lesions on the cow's udders. In the process of milking, the lesions transmitted the infection to the milk supply, which then infected hundreds of children with scarlatina.[75] The specific contagious aspect of scarlatina was clearly established, and in later Local Government Board investigations Dr. Klein proved that the organism present in both cows and human beings was the same—*Micrococcus scarlatina*.

The Board's medical staff throughout the period 1871–1900 maintained a routine check on scarlet fever death statistics. Whenever outbreaks with large mortality figures occurred, a medical inspector from the Board visited the afflicted community. As with the other contagious diseases, the presence of this central inspector aided the local authorities in detecting sources of the outbreaks, and, in backward communities, spurred isolation treatment and disinfection methods.

From 1891 to 1900, the average annual scarlet fever death rate was 158 per million living (all ages, both sexes), or 49 per cent less than in the previous decade. The death rate from 1881 to 1900 had also shown a reduction of 52 per cent over the prior period of 1871–1880. The disease was most fatal to children under five, especially to those dwelling in urban areas.[76]

Influenza

There was little need for the medical staff of the Board to be concerned about influenza before 1890, as no epidemic outbreaks had occurred since the year 1885. The death rate from influenza averaged three per million of estimated population for the five years ending 1889. Late in 1889, however, influenza started to move from the Continent, and, from this time on, it clung to English soil, breaking out periodically in greater or lesser waves, well up to the present day. From 1891 to 1900, the influenza mortality was an average of 361 per million persons living. The worst epidemics occurred during the years 1889 to 1895; the total number of deaths from influenza was high—4,523 in 1890, 16,686 in 1891, and 15,737 in 1892.

In 1890 and 1892, Dr. H. Franklin Parsons (1846–1913), Assistant Medical Officer to the Board, conducted a special investigation into the new infectious disease which was taking such heavy death tolls. Parsons' report merely confirmed the "eminently infectious" nature of the disease and the rapidity of its spread through ordinary personal relations.[77] The Board's Medical Department recognized that there was little hope for successful preventive measures in this disease. The high infectivity, often manifested before the disease was diagnosed, the short incubation period, and absence of immunity based on previous attacks, all combined to make prevention very difficult.[78] Isolation and disinfection were all the Board could recommend, coupled with sound advice on general measures for maintaining good health.

In the absence of a successful vaccine, little else could have been expected of the Medical Department in handling a disease which, even today, when it arrives in epidemic form, presents similar problems.

Notification of Disease

Throughout its first thirty years, the Local Government Board was greatly handicapped by the absence of any national compulsory system of notification of infectious disease. It was not until 1899 that notification of disease became mandatory throughout all of England and Wales. Had the Board's administrative staff supported the views of its Principal Medical Officer, compulsory notification might have been enacted almost fifteen years earlier.

Medical men for many years had recognized the necessity for building up a body of national disease statistics to provide more accurate information with which to fight disease. By the early seventies, the British medical profession was generally agreed that a central authority should be notified of all cases of disease which were treated at public cost. Both the Poor Law Medical Officers Association in 1870 and the British Medical Association in 1873 and 1874 had petitioned the Local Government Board for returns of all cases of disease treated at public institutions.[79] In testifying before the Royal Sanitary Commission, John Simon had also advocated notification for all sickness treated at public expense, and the Commission itself recognized the need for such statistics as an important factor in preventing the spread of infectious disease.[80]

But the notification of diseases treated at public cost was not enough. There was a broader need for a national system of compulsory notification of all infectious disease. Medical and lay opinion was split on this point. Nineteenth-century concepts of private property rights constituted one obstacle. Should a man be forced to communicate to the public the fact that there was a case of infectious disease in his family? Some feared that such compulsion would restrain people from calling in the physician and thus result in a further spread of the disease.[81] Some medical men in private practice believed that compulsory notification of disease would violate the secrecy normally prevailing in relations between doctor and patient, thus making the doctor a "common informer," forced to betray his patient. There was also the question of who was to be required to do the notifying to the public authority—the householder in whose home the patient lay, the medical practitioner who attended the patient, or a relative? While many physicians concurred on the necessity for over-all notification, they felt that the responsibility should rest with the householder rather than with the attending doctor.[82] A lively correspondence on the whole subject of notification of disease filled page after page of the medical journals of the seventies and eighties.

Despite the varied objections, by 1879 many cities and towns throughout the country had adopted local systems of compulsory notification. The majority of these local acts, which were ratified by Parliament, set up a dual system of notification, making it obligatory both upon the medical practitioner and the householder.[83] Increasingly, regional associations of medical officers of health, sanitary associations, and other groups petitioned the Local Government Board to seek legislation requiring a national notification system.[84] Additional support for such a law came in 1882, both from the Royal Commission on Hospitals for Infectious Diseases and from a Select Committee of the House of Commons, which presented a report on sanitary regulations. By the following year, a total of 34 towns, with a total population of 2,653,565, had adopted compulsory notification.[85] The diseases included were usually smallpox, cholera, typhus, typhoid, scarlet fever, relapsing fever, continued and puerperal fevers, scarlatina, and diphtheria.

George Buchanan, who had become the Board's Medical Officer in 1879, observed the growing support for notification with much interest. In his annual report for 1879–1880, Buchanan pointed out that the Board now required poor law medical officers and medical officers of district schools to notify the local authority of any case of dangerous infectious disease arising among pauper patients or in schools. Buchanan acknowledged that he hesitated, without further experience of the effectiveness of the local compulsory notification regulations, to introduce any general measure on the subject.[86]

By February of 1885, however, Buchanan felt ready to move, and he forwarded a memorandum to the Board's President, Sir Charles Dilke, stating, "I think the time has come when a local sanitary authority desiring to have powers in respect of compulsory notification of disease, might acquire such powers by by-law to be conferred by this Board, and without ratification by Parliament." Dilke, however, replied in the same month that he was not prepared to propose legislation on this subject. When, the following year, Buchanan urged the same suggestion upon Dilke's successor, Joseph Chamberlain, Chamberlain answered: "I doubt if Parliament would give these powers. I should certainly not recommend any attempt at legislation by the Government until the opinion of the House had been taken by resolutions on a Bill brought by a private member." [87]

The local pressures for national legislation continued, and, in October of 1887, the Metropolitan Asylums Board wrote directly to the Secretary of the Local Government Board, Sir Hugh Owen, pressing him to obtain legislation from Parliament at the earliest possible moment. Two months later, the Local Government Board sent out a circular to local sanitary authorities in towns where compulsory notification was in force, asking for information on how the system worked. The returns were almost wholly in favor of the system.[88] By 1887, 48 towns, with over 4,000,000 people, were under compulsory notification acts—towns like Manchester, Nottingham, Bradford, Salford, Leicester, Aberdeen, Dundee, and Edinburgh. On the basis of the replies to the Board's circular, Dr. Buchanan, in January of 1888, again urged the Board to initiate general legislation.[89]

Finally, under Local Government Board sponsorship, an Act was passed on August 30, 1889, which made notification of infectious disease compulsory in London, and which permitted its adoption by other sanitary authorities merely by resolution. In less than three years, five-sixths of the population of the whole country had been brought under its provisions.[90]

By the time this Act had been passed and implemented by a Local Government Board Order, the matter was wholly out of the hands of the Medical Department. Indeed, a rather pathetic memorandum from Dr. Buchanan to Sir Hugh Owen dated September 19, 1889, appears in the files, stating:

> I see in *The Times* of yesterday an account of an Order made by the Board in the subject of the matter of Infectious Disease notification.
> 1. Ought not copies of such Order to have been sent to the Medical Department?
> 2. May I see the stages through which the Order passed before its issue?
>
> G.B.[91]

Most of the early opposition to notification had vanished by the nineties. Notification in England and Wales was not made wholly compulsory until 1899, after it had been accepted by most of the country in local acts or under the permissive feature of the Act of 1889. In order to implement the knowledge to be gained from national notification, the Local Government Board undertook to tabulate, print, and circulate returns sent to it from notification towns. Some years elapsed before the returns were sufficiently standardized to permit scientific study of the incidence of infectious disease in England and Wales.

At the outset, the Board's Medical Department had played a waiting role in the movement for notification. Rather than run the risk of failure by compulsive action too far in advance of public opinion, the Board delayed, letting the evidence and petitions in favor of the legislation pile up until a clear case could be made out for central action. When Buchanan finally moved in 1885, the administrative and political leaders of the Board dragged their heels, fearing public reaction. Finally, when the powerful Metropolitan Asylums Board demanded action, and favorable reports of the operation of local notification acts were received, the Board pushed through the 1889 London Act.

If the Board's medical staff had not taken a decisive role, the Medical Officer had at least kept careful watch in his annual reports on the state of notification in the country and had, finally, urged the Board's administrative staff to action.

If we base our judgment on a summary view of their work from 1871 to 1900 in controlling infectious disease, the medical staff of the Local Government Board can be said to have functioned quite ably. In guarding against cholera and smallpox, the most dreaded of the infectious diseases, the Medical Department maintained a continual alert. The prompt and efficient measures instituted in periods of threatened cholera invasion, the surveys to warn port sanitary authorities, the abandonment of quarantine as outmoded, and the institution of more satisfactory port security measures, eliminated cholera as a real menace by 1900. Equally forceful was the Medical Department's campaign against smallpox—its emphasis upon a careful vaccination program, development of revaccination as further prevention, and the encouragement of local authorities in the establishment and effective use of isolation hospitals. The Board's fostering of general sanitary measures throughout the country and its use of new bacterial knowledge in combating all infectious disease were undoubtedly responsible in part for the general reduction of disease by 1900. Both Dr. Power's observations on milk-borne scarlet fever and Edward Klein's findings on the scarlatina organism forwarded epidemiological understanding.

Although Dr. Klein's view was not immediately accepted by his contemporary bacteriologists, it was later confirmed and constituted an important advance in knowledge of the disease.

In proportion to the very high death rates for tuberculosis during the first thirty years of the Local Government Board's work, there was relatively little interest in controlling the spread of tuberculosis. The infectious properties of phthisis and other forms of tuberculosis were recognized during this period. Dr. Edward Klein and others had carried out for the Board several investigations of the etiology and differentiation of tuberculosis during the late seventies and mid-eighties. Although the Local Government Board showed some interest in the effects on health from the consumption of milk and meat from tubercular animals,[92] it was not until the twentieth century that the Board paid more attention to this major killer.

The Board's Medical Department also ignored venereal disease almost completely, except for occasional comments in annual reports on mortality returns. The attempt at "contagious disease" legislation in the sixties, which required compulsory examination of prostitutes in military areas had failed, and the Acts had been suspended by Parliament in 1883, and then repealed in 1886, following a public controversy led by Josephine Butler and James Stansfeld. The new diagnostic discoveries in syphilis were not presented until 1906. Within the confinements of the Victorian era's views on sex, it would have been difficult, if not wholly impossible, for the Local Government Board to commence an active program of controlling venereal disease in the civilian population of England and Wales. It was not until the First World War that venereal disease became a matter of serious concern to the government.

It cannot be maintained that the Medical Department was in advance of public or medical opinion in its attitude towards compulsory notification of infectious disease. But the medical staff kept the problem under surveillance and, finally, assisted by pressure from local authorities, moved the Board's administrative staff to action.

The Board's medical officers inherited a strong tradition of state intervention in preventing the spread of infectious disease. In their work from 1871 to 1900, the medical staff maintained and strengthened this tradition to meet the health needs of the growing population of England and Wales.

Chapter IV

The Local Government Board:
Medical Inspection and the
Auxiliary Scientific Investigations

THE Local Government Board carried out two other activities linked to the prevention of disease—central medical inspection and the support of auxiliary scientific investigations. The medical inspectorate was severely limited in number. Nevertheless, over the years, the small staff prepared a series of competent, often wide-scale, analytic reports, whose recommendations, if consistently implemented by the local authorities concerned, could have radically changed many communities of England. And, as Sir John Charles has observed, the auxiliary scientific investigations, initiated under Simon's brilliant leadership at the Privy Council, were for almost half a century the only government-sponsored medical research studies which had any continuity.[1]

Medical Inspection

At the outset, the Board's Medical Department was administratively barred from any systematic role in the supervision of local sanitary government. Periodic sanitary inspection, as such, was considered by Stansfeld and Lambert to be a nonmedical function. In the early years of the Board, it was only occasionally that the administrative staff saw fit to refer a sanitary complaint to the Medical Department.[2]

Much of the purely sanitary inspection was thus carried out by nonmedical, "general" inspectors. Many were well equipped by experience for their duties, although it was not until 1895 that they were required to hold qualifying certificates of "such bodies as the Board might appoint." [3]

As the years went by, the medical staff increasingly carried out medical inspections on their own initiative. Had the men employed as medical inspectors been political appointees of routine abilities, the work of the Department would have been far more pedestrian than it was in actuality. The reports of the medical staff who were sent on special sanitary investigations throughout England and Wales testify to the high caliber of the physicians employed.

Yet only a very small group was occupied in this work. The Privy Council had not employed permanent medical inspectors for sanitary purposes before 1869. Simon at first used outside medical specialists of considerable distinction in their respective fields for necessary special investigations. By 1865, permanent inspectorships were established in connection with vaccination supervision. Two permanent medical inspectorships for sanitary investigations were finally set up in 1869, and Dr. George Buchanan and Mr. John Netten Radcliffe were appointed to the posts. Gradually other staff was added, at first temporarily, and then on a permanent basis.[4] The limitations to any really comprehensive and regular system of medical inspection, however, can be seen by the fact that in 1874 there were only three medical sanitary inspectors to cover 1,558 sanitary localities. It was impossible in such a setting to mobilize the active central medical inspectorate Simon had desired.

Well before the days of the Local Government Board, Simon had commented on the difficulties raised by the shortage of inspectorial personnel. In 1870 he had pointed out that the inspectors were able to visit only a third of the districts where it was necessary to communicate with local authorities. The Medical Officers of the Board who succeeded Simon reiterated his complaint.

Nevertheless, despite the limitation on their number, the tradition of employing men of proven ability in their fields, which Simon had initiated, was retained and carried over into the medical staff of the Local Government Board. The essential function of inquiry and report, which had been built up as a fundamental of the Privy Council Medical Office, survived and was elaborated in the program of medical inquiries carried out by the Board. More and more, as time went on, local authorities were to welcome the type of expert, scientific guidance which the central medical inspector could offer them.

GROUNDS FOR MEDICAL INSPECTION

Medical inspections were initiated on five general grounds: complaints of local inhabitants about poor sanitary conditions; requests for inspection from district councils or other local authorities; information sought from local medical officers of health; insufficiency of reports of medical officers of health; and investigations of mortality returns of the Registrar-General. Although in many instances inspections were locally inspired, the Medical Department, increasingly throughout the years 1871 to 1900, initiated investigations on the basis of death statistics indicating some extraordinary prevalence of disease. More frequently, the role of the Medical Department in sanitary investigations was that of the Harley Street consultant whose opinion on a difficult case is solicited by the uneasy local doctor.

The philosophy underlying this was, of course, the primacy of local responsibility for public health. As noted in a Medical Department memorandum of 1880: "Under a properly organized system in which the sanitary authorities are furnished with an efficient staff of local Medical Officers of Health and Inspectors of Nuisances, the necessity for intervention of skilled experts from the Central Board will seldom arise." [5] Even John Lambert recognized that such a happy condition represented the millennium, and, in reply, noted that he "cannot but think that the reports of Medical Inspectors have operated as a wholesome and important stimulant in many cases." [6]

Many reports of the medical inspectors were inspired by the zeal of the enthusiastic sanitary reformer, the importance of whose mission makes all other considerations secondary. Senior medical staff of the Department, nevertheless, exercised a certain restraint in carrying out sanitary inspection, in obeisance to the theory that the central authority existed to service the local authority, not to impose force from above.

CONDITIONS REQUIRING INSPECTION

Widespread urban and rural sanitary improvements had been put into effect in England and Wales since the days of Chadwick and Southwood Smith. Yet, in the years which followed 1871, the reports submitted by the medical inspection staff abounded with recommendations for local reforms—with respect to overcrowding of houses, improved water supply, excrement disposal facilities, and the erection of local isolation hospitals for infectious disease. Much remained to be done before even minimal sanitary needs were met.

In 1874, the report of Dr. Edward Ballard * on conditions in the Upper Sedgley Urban Sanitary District presented recommendations fairly typical of those found in inspectors' reports throughout the Board's early years. Dr. Ballard advised that the local board should undertake the removal of excrement; that villages in the district should be provided with proper sewers; that there should be provision of a supply of wholesome water for the district's inhabitants; that an isolation hospital should be set up; that the sanitary board should meet at least every fortnight to execute the Nuisances Removal Acts; that the registrar of deaths should furnish weekly returns to the local medical officer of health; and that the local board should "at once set earnestly about its long neglected work of putting into active operation the abundant powers it possesses, under the Nuisance Removal Acts, of dealing with the unwholesome conditions or nuisances which defile the district from one end to another." Dr. Ballard's caustic summation was even more trenchant:

> It is well to state the fact plainly, for it is notorious that for some time past, party contention in the Local Board has run so high, and the time of the meetings has been so frittered away with squabbling upon matters of comparatively trivial importance, that while all parties concur in admitting the frightful sanitary state of the district, nothing effectual has yet been attempted to improve it. For all practical purposes, the Board is in a state of utter disorganization.[7]

Recommendations for improved housing occurred over and over again in the medical inspectors' returns. In 1873, Simon had pointed sharply to insanitary housing conditions, saying:

> There are houses, there are groups of houses, there are whole villages, there are considerable sections of towns, there are often even entire and not small towns, where general slovenliness in everything which relates to the removal of refuse-matter, slovenli-

---

* Edward Ballard (1820–1897), following apprenticeship to an Islington surgeon, received an M.B. from University College, London, in 1843. The author of several books on medicine and diagnosis, Ballard was appointed medical officer of health for Islington in 1868. He joined Simon as a medical inspector for the Privy Council in 1871 (and subsequently for the Board) and carried out investigations in such subjects as food adulteration and offensive trades.

ness which in very many cases amounts to utter bestiality of neglect, is the local habit. . . .[8]

A survey by Local Government Board inspectors in 1875 on the working of the Public Health Act of 1872 emphasized the need for struc-
tural improvements by landlords, as well as the enforcement of cleanliness on the part of tenants. But the co-operation between landlord and
tenant for more sanitary housing was a desideratum, the investigators
felt, to which both groups "may possibly be led, but they certainly
would never be driven." [9]

Year after year, the medical investigators of the Board recommended
housing improvements, but there was little way of enforcing the recommendation upon local authorities. Reviewing the continued lack of
improvement in the housing of the poor classes in 1899, the Board's
Medical Officer, Dr. Richard Thorne Thorne, repeated the gloomy
observations of one of the medical inspectors in 1885: "Wherever
individual interests have to be opposed, or seemingly opposed, sanitary
administration has been paralyzed." [10]

Despite this awareness of sordid housing conditions, the Board's
Medical Department never attempted to constitute itself a housing
reform agency, and the primary impetus for improved housing sprang
from outside the Local Government Board. The medical inspectors'
reports did bring conditions to the attention of the local authorities
concerned and constituted a reservoir of information for other reformers.

Insanitary housing inquiries were only a part of the routine work
carried on by the central medical investigators. Complaints of food
poisoning received regular attention, and tests were routinely, if un-
spectacularly, carried out on samples submitted under the Food Adulteration Acts. Dr. Edward Klein, in examining an 1887 outbreak of
meat poisoning in Nottinghamshire, identified a special bacillus con-
taminating pork pies.[11] The same year, Dr. W. H. Power and Major
General A. C. Scott of the Royal Engineers, investigated the presence
of eels in the water pipes of the East London Water Company. A widespread inquiry relating to the influence of noxious and offensive trades
was begun in 1875 by Dr. Edward Ballard and continued over a number of years. This study was carried out partly as a medical inspection,
and partly as an auxiliary scientific investigation. Another inquiry in
industrial health was carried out in 1873 in a study of the health of
women and children engaged in textile manufacture, with specific

reference to hours and ages of employment. Among the investigators'
recommendations was a plea for the reduction of the hours of labor for
all women and children from sixty to fifty-four hours a week, and the
exclusion of children under nine from employment in factories.[12]

The most noteworthy medical inquiries undertaken by the Board's
inspectors related to disease control. By the end of 1870, a new and
significant influence for the control of disease was in effect. Through
Simon's influence, the Office of the Registrar-General had begun to
issue quarterly reports of death returns for the whole of England.
These were available to the Local Government Board's Medical Department and were regularly utilized in the campaign against epidemic
disease in England and Wales. In addition, weekly returns in the 137
subdistricts of London provided even more timely subjects for medical
investigations.

The annual reports of the Board's Medical Officer list an annual
range of some fifteen to sixty medical inspections of outbreaks of disease during the period from 1871 to 1900. A considerable amount of
useful information was disclosed in the process. Many districts had
failed to provide isolation hospitals, and medical inspectors often gave
practical and scientific advice to the local authorities in planning infectious disease hospitals. Other inspections led to conferences with local
authorities on framing regulations regarding infectious disease outbreaks in schools.

The recommendations submitted by the medical inspectors were
quite in step with the demands of the most earnest lay sanitary reformers, and in advance of much of the current emphasis on the sanctity of
private property rights. Community action to build sewerage and
central water supply systems, to remove nuisances, and provide infectious disease hospitals was recommended again and again in the reports
of medical inspection. The indictment of local authorities continued
throughout the last thirty years of the nineteenth century. In 1888,
Dr. Francis Blaxall's report on a long-standing epidemic of scarlatina
"puts on record the story of a community utterly indifferent about its
health or disease and receiving no adequate guidance from those who
had assumed the function of directing its sanitary affairs." [13]

EFFECTIVENESS OF THE MEDICAL INSPECTIONS

It is difficult to evaluate the effect of the Board's medical inspections
in the cumbrous advance to better national health. Sir Malcolm Morris

concluded that "such medical inspection as was carried out was quite casual, and indeed could not have been otherwise without that enlargement of the Medical Staff which the wisdom of Mr. Stansfeld deemed a superfluity." [14] The inspections may have been casual in the sense of not being periodically systematic throughout the country. The inspectors' reports were not casual in their individual thoroughness or in their recommendations.

But the power to recommend was not the power to coerce, and the Medical Department, limited by administrative handicaps, paucity of staff, and an established policy of suggestion instead of compulsion, clearly did not execute any overnight public health revolution. The statement which appeared in 1875 in the *Reports of Local Government Board Inspectors on the Working of the Public Health Act of 1872* was almost equally applicable in 1900:

> The policy of the Local Government Board, and of its late President, by which the local authorities have been encouraged to determine for themselves the arrangements that appeared to them best suited to their own localities, or that squared with their inclinations, has secured for the whole question a cordiality of acceptance which would certainly not have been accorded to it, had the attempt been made to force upon the country any uniform scheme however symmetrically, or scientifically correct. [15]

In many instances this "cordiality of acceptance" of the central medical inspector's recommendations consisted of little else than filing the report. There is evidence, in some districts, of sanitary evils persisting year after year, despite frequent investigations and suggestions by the central authority. [16] Herbert Preston-Thomas, the Board's skilled lay inspector, pointed out that under the Privy Council, a complaint from one of the Council's medical inspectors had been sufficient ground for an order from the Home Secretary requiring the work to be done. After the medical inspectors were absorbed into the Local Government Board, it was held that an inspector's report to his official superiors no longer constituted sufficient ground, and in the absence of a local petition, the Board was powerless to act. [17]

John Simon was particularly caustic on the ineffectiveness of the Board's medical inspections after the temporary impetus of the cholera scare of the eighties had waned. Of the national system, as current in 1886, he wrote: "[It] seems far too much to suppose that a free consumption of stationery may serve instead of skilled visitation . . . that average local reports will in general be of such completeness and exactitude that the central skilled officer can readily advise on them without having first in person or by deputy examined the facts." [18]

The main fault was simply that those inspections which were made were wholly insufficient in number to admit of any truly national program. Periodically, when cholera threatened, the numbers of inspections were increased. But directly public attention was diverted and funds for temporary additional medical inspectors had expired, the Board reverted to its spot check system. Despite Simon's ill-treatment by the Board, his personal stature and scientific detachment do not permit of too much doubt that his sharp criticisms of the medical inspection system are in large measure true. By the close of the century, several more medical inspectors had been added to the Board's staff. There was still no basic change, however, either in the policy or scope of the investigations.

But this was not the whole picture. Again and again, the medical inspectors gave practical, scientific advice to local authorities, and reforms were instigated. In an official re-examination of 100 local visitations of medical staff of the Local Government Board conducted from 1871 to 1880, a majority of the cases showed wide improvements in conformity with the medical inspectors' suggestions.[19] Lapses of from one to two years between the original inspection and ultimate improvement often occurred. In other cases, there were merely records of "correspondence in progress" with the local sanitary authority.

The inspectors' reports were also distributed and read by many interested in sanitary reform. Although at first only made available informally to local authorities and medical journals,[20] the reports began to appear by the early eighties as H.M. Stationery Office publications "at the instance of some officers of health and others interested in sanitary knowledge." [21]

It may fairly be observed, as the British Association for the Advancement of Science observed in 1874, that the Medical Department, as then organized, was less effective in the prevention of disease than in inquiring into the causes of disease which had already had fatal consequences.[22] But the Board's medical inspections, as the years passed, helped to keep the whole problem of insanitation and disease control in a national focus, necessitating community action. Expanding scientific knowledge and its popularization were the pillars upon which a national health program was later to be built.

The Auxiliary Scientific Investigations

Administrative and policy restrictions were at a minimum in one of the Board's Medical Department activities—the auxiliary scientific investigations. It was in this area that the high professional caliber of the medical staff was most evident.

AUXILIARY SCIENTIFIC INVESTIGATIONS UNDER THE PRIVY COUNCIL

Simon, during his Privy Council days, had recognized the value of the medical staff's carrying out long-term scientific investigations auxiliary to the day-to-day work of the department. Although many of these studies related to the etiology of disease, Simon pointed out that the work had no pretensions "to immediate popular application, but addresses itself primarily to the deeper scientific requirements of the Medical Profession." [23]

The Privy Council had first authorized "Laboratory Investigations (of sorts not likely to be undertaken on sufficient scale by private persons)" [24] in 1865. Parliament voted the first of the £2,000 annual grants in support of the investigations in 1871. The research carried out under the annual grants was sometimes linked to the epidemiological surveys of the Privy Council's medical staff and sometimes was carried out as separate projects. As a whole, the auxiliary scientific investigations initiated under the Privy Council covered less public health territory than did the Council's great epidemiological field surveys. The field investigations ranged through many social and disease conditions responsible for excessive mortality—nutrition, housing, infant care, venereal disease, epidemics, and the effect of industry on health.[25] The Privy Council's auxiliary, or laboratory, investigations centered about the study of infective processes and of physiological chemistry.[26]

AUXILIARY SCIENTIFIC INVESTIGATIONS UNDER THE BOARD

The Local Government Board's Medical Department continued to sponsor auxiliary scientific studies in the period 1870–1900. Year after year, reports on these research projects appeared as appendices to the annual reports of the Board's Medical Officer. The Board's administrative staff rarely interfered with these activities, and the reports were favorably received by the medical profession.

Upon one occasion, in 1875, the proposed budget for the auxiliary studies was challenged in the House of Commons. The Member from Swansea contended that however valuable such "amateur investigations" might be, they were not within the province of a public department. Other Members pointed out if such investigations were to be supported, they did not see where the expenditures would stop. A House vote of 165 to 27, however, effectively silenced the objections, the majority feeling that the public was ultimately benefited by the research.[27]

The medical department's commitment to these auxiliary research studies, and the steady financial assistance made available, helped to develop the important function of central government support for basic as well as applied research. Before the era of generous private and commercial provision for pure science, far less opportunity existed for the English physician to devote himself to research for long stretches of time. But the medical staff members of the Board were authorized and subsidized year after year, although at relatively low levels of support, to carry out research in many areas of pure science and public health.

The majority of those who were assisted by funds from the scientific grant had other duties to perform for the Board, chiefly medical inspections. Some of the funds were awarded to those holding appointments to the staff only for the purpose of carrying out research, as in the instances of Dr. Johann Ludwig Wilhelm Thudichum, father of brain chemistry, and the young Victor Horsley, then Assistant to the Professor of Pathology in University College. Horsley,* who subsequently developed into one of the world's greatest brain surgeons, carried out a study for the Board in 1881 on septic bacteria and their physiological relations. Funds were also awarded for several years during the seventies to the Pathological Society of London for research on pyemia and allied diseases.

* Sir Victor A. H. Horsley (1857–1916), distinguished neurosurgeon and physiologist. Horsley trained at University College, London, qualifying in 1880. After serving as surgical registrar at University College Hospital, he became Professor-Superintendent of the Brown Institution 1884–1890; Assistant Surgeon, University College Hospital 1885; F.R.S. 1886; Professor of Pathology at University College and Surgeon to the National Hospital for the Paralyzed and Epileptic (Queen Square); knighted, 1902; President of the Medical Defense Union; General Medical Council, 1897; active in the British Medical Association as Chairman of Representative Meetings, 1903–1906 and as member of the Association Council, 1910–1912. Horsley died of heat stroke during World War I at Amarah.

Nature of the Auxiliary Investigations. The auxiliary scientific investigations ranged over a wide area during the first thirty years of the Board's work: organic chemistry, infectious diseases, industrial diseases and industrial nuisances, anatomy of the lymph system, the etiology of cancer, chemical analyses of water, and other fields. Many of the studies had little promise of quick application to preventive medicine. This makes it even more remarkable that there appears, from the internal memoranda of the Board, to have been no attempt by the powerful lay administrators to require that the studies be confined to research more directly applicable to public health.

From the early eighties, when the bacteria of disease were successively identified, the Board's auxiliary studies began to deal increasingly with microorganisms. Many of these investigations sought to map out the action of bacteria in such different media as soil, water, and milk. One study examined the "antagonisms of bacteria," and others, the actions of various disinfectants on bacteria. Studies of agents in food poisonings and on the transmission of influenza began to appear in the nineties. Each year, from three to eight reports on the various research projects were issued, some in the form of progress reports on continuing studies, some as reports of completed projects.

Thudichum and Brain Chemistry. The most notable of the auxiliary investigations sponsored by the Board were the series of studies on the chemistry of the brain undertaken by Dr. Johann Ludwig Wilhelm Thudichum (1829–1901). Thudichum, a student of the distinguished German chemist, Justus von Liebig, had taken an M.D. at the University of Giessen in 1851 and emigrated to England two years later. His research on the changes produced by disease on the chemical actions of the body attracted Simon's attention. But it was through an incidental interest in the role of parasites in meat that Thudichum was drawn into some investigations of the Privy Council Medical Office in 1864.[28] A man of considerable culture and personal charm, Thudichum soon joined the distinguished circle of men, including Ruskin, Rossetti, and Burne-Jones, who gathered at Simon's home.[29]

The work which was to earn Thudichum the title of "father of brain chemistry" was begun under Privy Council auspices in 1866, in an attempt to discover what successive chemical changes the body underwent in the course of cholera. From this, Thudichum's investigations moved to what was to be a sixteen-year examination of the normal chemical constitution of the brain.

The relationship of chemistry to pathology had hitherto been almost wholly unexplored, and Thudichum's mapping of the new pathways

was laborious and expensive. Without Simon's support and the financial assistance, first from the Privy Council and then the Local Government Board, it would have been almost impossible for Thudichum,
father of seven children, to have continued his research. Writing to
Simon in 1869 to request an increase in funds for the project, Thudichum noted that: "It is on account of expense that this branch of
research has been abandoned by almost every chemist with whom I
am acquainted." [30]

Thudichum's reports on his research appeared regularly in appendices to the annual reports of the Medical Officer of the Local Government Board, and occasionally in scientific periodicals. Both the lay
administrators and the medical officers of the Board took a somewhat
proprietary interest in the publication of results of research supported
by the Board. At one point, in November of 1879, John Lambert issued
a formal rebuke to Thudichum for separately publishing four scientific
essays based upon his research for the Board, stating: "No publication
of researches on which gentlemen have been engaged for the Board
ought to be made except with the express sanction of the Board in the
particular case." [31] It was, of course, quite natural for Thudichum to
wish his results to reach the scientific world sooner than they would
through the ponderous official publication channels of the Board's
annual reports.

The considerable number of years during which Thudichum received support for this basic research on brain chemistry from the
Local Government Board would be notable even in the present days
of generous government grants—and Thudichum had no tiresome
grant application forms to prepare! But even he was not wholly free,
and the finger of authority kept prodding the scientific investigator for
an accounting of his time, for estimates, and results. In August of 1880,
the Medical Officer, Dr. Buchanan, drafted a letter to Thudichum, for
the signature of the President of the Board, in which Dr. Thudichum's
re-employment was confirmed for another year at £500 annually, plus
£420 for assistance and expenses. However, the letter noted that as the
researches had started in 1873 (under the Board), completion should
be expected by now "with certain pathological applications." Dr.
Thudichum was further directed to concentrate wholly on this study
of the normal brain for the following year.[32] In September of 1881,
replying to another letter from Buchanan asking for a report on the
researches, Dr. Thudichum set forth the scientist's unwillingness to

estimate the termination date of his researches: "With the clear consciousness of the validity of all my researches, I humbly submit that they have served the purpose for which they were undertaken, namely the advancement of the science to which they refer or are applicable." [33]

The Medical Department of the Local Government Board continued support to Thudichum until March, 1883. The collected results of his research for the Board were published in 1884 under the title, *A Treatise on the Chemical Constitution of the Brain.*[34] In the preface to this book, Thudichum gratefully acknowledged the support Simon and the government had given to the research.

During his lifetime, Thudichum's pioneer studies on brain chemistry went largely unrecognized. Indeed, scientific embroilments with such powerful physiological chemists as Arthur Gamgee and Oscar Liebreich cast doubt upon many of his findings. His obituary in the *British Medical Journal* observed:

> It is possible that Thudichum attempted in these researches too much—more, that is to say, than the state of physiological chemistry had rendered it possible to achieve; at any rate, the results were not generally considered to correspond adequately to the time and money which they cost, and his views have not, we believe, been generally accepted by other workers in this field of chemistry.[35]

It is in recent decades, and largely through the support of such outstanding biochemists as David Drabkin in the United States and Henry McIlwain in England, that Thudichum's work has been recognized as a monumental achievement.

Industrial Health. Among the other auxiliary scientific investigations supported by the Local Government Board in the period up to 1900 were a number related to industrial disease and industrial nuisances. The major investigations of industrial disease and occupational risks to health were, however, to be carried out at a later period under the Medical Inspector of Factories and the Industrial Health Research Board.

During 1875, Dr. Edward Ballard of the Board's medical staff started an extensive, three-year inquiry into industrial effluvium nuisances and their effect on the health of industrial workers, as well as on the community at large. In the course of his research, Dr. Ballard visited 850 trade establishments throughout the country, representing 70 types of business. Rather surprisingly, he reported that he found a "willing and cooperative attitude" on the part of the manufacturers. The result of Ballard's investigations was to demonstrate that by utilizing their contemporary knowledge of preventive methods, almost all businesses could reduce their offensive aspects to a degree which would make them "tolerable or even trivial." [36] Ballard pointed out in detail methods to reduce nuisances in the various trades. Lacking adequate statistics of disease, it was not then possible for him to specify the direct relation between the offense, the trades, and the production of disease and shortening of life. The study was a valuable one for the period, and undoubtedly Dr. Ballard's visits to factory owners had some effect in the reduction of industrial nuisances. Simon acknowledged Ballard's study to be without equal in its field but noted in 1890 that the valuable body of information in the reports, published in the form of appendices to annual reports, was not readily accessible to manufacturers.[37]

Other special research studies were undertaken in 1880 on the prevalence of anthrax among wool sorters in Bradford and, in 1887, on lead poisoning in Sheffield's water supplies.

Infectious Disease. The majority of the auxiliary scientific investigations carried out by the Local Government Board's medical staff were disease-oriented. Much of the tradition of the Board's repeated investigations into the microbic origins of infectious disease stemmed from work done under the Privy Council, particularly the work of the distinguished pathologist, Sir John Burdon Sanderson.* It was Dr. Burdon Sanderson who has been credited with commencing the experimental study of infectious disease in England. The teacher of William Osler and Victor Horsley, Burdon Sanderson throughout his life was intensely interested in pathology. His studies, carried out first for the Privy Council and subsequently for the Local Government Board, ranged over such subjects as contagion, infection of wounds, and the pathology of blood poisoning. Not only did Burdon Sanderson link acute septicemia and chronic pyemic conditions as manifestations of blood poisoning, but he identified bacteria as the causal agents.[38]

Certainly one of the most notable of the disease investigations was

---

* Sir John Scott Burdon Sanderson (1828–1905); Medical Officer of Health of Paddington, 1856–1867; part-time Privy Council medical inspector; F.R.S. 1867; Professor of Physiology and Histology, University College, London, 1871; Waynflete Professor of Physiology, Oxford, 1882; Regius Professor of Medicine, Oxford, 1895–1903. (*Dictionary of National Biography*, Supplement II, Vol. I, 267.)

the study made by Dr. Edward Klein * into the etiology of scarlet fever. In 1885, Dr. Klein identified the scarlatina microphyte, and the Hendon epidemic of 1886 provided fertile territory for further observation of the behavior of the organism. This lengthy report was considered by the *British Medical Journal* to be one of the most important in the series of auxiliary scientific investigations.[39] Dr. Klein's researches into the nature of infective diseases led him to describe the micrococcus of the foot and mouth disease in 1885 and, later, to make detailed observations on the activities of the typhoid bacillus outside the animal body.[40]

The reports of the auxiliary scientific investigations into infectious disease are numerous, and year after year as they appeared in appendices to the annual reports of the Board's Medical Officer, the body of knowledge grew. Included were: Dr. Klein's report of 1874 on intimate anatomical changes associated with enteric fever; Dr. Buchanan's report of the Croydon epidemic of the following year; Dr. W. H. Power's findings on smallpox in 1880, showing that the disease was capable of infecting the air quite apart from human contact; and Dr. Edward Ballard's researches into epidemic diarrhea and food poisoning. Dr. Sidney Martin, M.D., F.R.C.P., F.R.S., who was employed in chemical pathological investigations of the Board from 1889 to 1901, also made notable pioneer contributions in the chemical pathology of anthrax, diphtheria, and tetanus. Martin demonstrated in experiment that diphtheria toxin produced diphtheritic palsy.[41]

During the eighties, a large-scale investigation was begun into the effectiveness of various types of disinfectants. A paper by Dr. Burdon Sanderson on the products of putrefaction in relation to the prevention of disease set forth, as the Medical Officer stated, "the chemical facts which serve as the points of departure for important researches on disinfectants." [42]

While the Local Government Board was slow in attacking the problem of tuberculosis, some start was made during the period 1871–1900 in auxiliary scientific investigations on tubercle. In 1878, Dr. Edward Klein was exploring the anatomy of the lymphatic system of the serous membrane of the lung with reference to tuberculosis. The pathology of tubercle also was under continual investigation during the early eighties by the indefatigable Dr. Klein and Dr. Alfred Lingard. In

* Edward E. Klein (1844–1925), M.D., carried out pathological and bacterial inquiries for the Local Government Board, 1871–1907. The author of several textbooks on histology and bacteriology, Klein also lectured on advanced bacteriology at the medical school of St. Bartholomew's Hospital.

1888, Dr. Lingard examined the relationship of scrofula, lupus, and tuberculosis.

CONTEMPORARY RECEPTION OF THE AUXILIARY SCIENTIFIC INVESTIGATIONS

The professional reception given to the auxiliary scientific studies was never effulgent. The medical profession in all nations has been historically disinclined to greet new pieces of scientific research with wide and instant acclaim. But the accounts, issued as appendices to the annual reports of the Board's Medical Officer were noted in conjunction with the rest of the Department's work and commended by the medical journals.

The Lancet cheered the reappearance in 1875 of the reports of the auxiliary scientific investigations after a lapse in publication of three years, noting:

> The sanitary workers preceding the new sanitary era had been accustomed to looking to Mr. Simon's reports as the great source of information concerning sanitary medicine . . . and when the Gwydyr House epoch was initiated with the suppression of these reports and the relegation of Mr. Simon to some departmental limbo, the apparent official demise of that gentleman was not unnaturally regarded as the demise of scientific official medicine in this country. . . . [However] it would appear that the sanitary and scientific work of his department went on as heretofore, and that during the suppression of the reports the stuff was accumulating out of which the reports were accustomed to be made.[43]

The *British Medical Journal,* while urging in 1887 the allotment of increased funds to the Board's Medical Department, commented on the continued excellent research carried out under the Department's auspices: "The valuable scientific researches of Professor Burdon Sanderson, Dr. Klein and a host of other able investigators, reflect credit on the department under which they have been mainly carried out in spite of many disadvantages." [44]

The auxiliary scientific investigations into what Simon termed "branches of science collateral to our province of duty," formed a distinct and unique contribution both to the advancement of pure science and the cause of public health. The Board's medical inspectors who followed Simon extended the program and enlarged the province of the research investigations to fields of contemporary interest. By the nature of their specialization, the auxiliary investigations were largely free from administrative interference. Sustained by a steady, if limited, annual subsidy, the studies carried out for the Board were ably planned and competently executed. Far from some of the pedestrian "nose-counting" activities, which in today's climate at times pass for "research," many of the studies reflected the originality and high integrative skill of men of the caliber of Thudichum and Burdon Sanderson. The medical men who carried out the "auxiliary investigations" for the Board made a distinguished contribution to the role of the state in support of scientific research.

Summary: The Medical Department of the Local Government Board

It was the view of Sir Richard Thorne Thorne, Medical Officer of the Local Government Board in 1895, that "concentrated medical officialism is not a desirable thing in this Country." [45] This was a doctrine thoroughly compatible with the operations of the Local Government Board and its Medical Department. A religious adherence to the negative implications of this doctrine constituted one of the reasons for the Medical Department's weakness. Yet, the same view had been advocated outside government circles for decades. Even the liberal Dr. Henry Acland, in a widely reported address to the National Association for the Promotion of Social Science, noted:

> So far as England is concerned, our Government has just said: You may trust the general guidance of a Central Office, combined with the local management by town councils, guardians and their officers. I believe the Government is right.
>
> In saying this I know I am putting myself in opposition to some in this Congress whom I much respect, but I say it because I believe the conclusion is founded on a fundamental principle of modern civilization . . . Who are to manage this country in the future, despots or the people? Are you going to make these people take care of themselves, or are you going to treat them like children? [46]

This distinguished Oxford physician defined the government's role in public health as striving "to ascertain what hindrances there are in the way of the people's health and to remove those they cannot remove for themselves." [47] The onus for action was placed on the local authority. As long as such thinking was rooted in a large section of the articulate public mind, the Local Government Board's Medical Department was justified, in a democratic state, in proceeding in accordance with the will of those it was established to serve.

The period 1870 to 1900, however, was an era of transition, and sanitary reformers were then promulgating a much wider view of the role of the state in health. It was only very slowly that this broader view permeated the minds of the Local Government Board authorities.

The basic reason for the Medical Department's failure to develop a major central health program lay in the reactionary attitude of the Board's administration. Even as late as 1910, Beatrice and Sidney Webb, the Fabian reformers, noted that the Chief Medical Officer of the Board had no regular share in advising the Board's president on health matters.[48] Because of its inherently weak administrative position, the Medical Department was only sporadically able to influence the Board's policy making. Those innovations which the Department introduced were outgrowths of previously established, routine functions, and were consolidating, rather than policy-initiating steps.

The Medical Department was also handicapped by the separation of health functions throughout the Government. The Board's researches into industrial disease, for example, could not be co-ordinated, in the same department, with the findings of the Factory Inspectors.

The lack of a strong, forward-looking central medical authority undoubtedly delayed the expansion of government into the personal health services. The Local Government Board was slow in its approaches to the problems of tuberculosis and of maternal and child welfare, both of which, by the nineties, were recognized by the lay and medical press as requiring public aid. As one physician commented in 1878, "The local authorities followed at a humble distance the example of the Local Government Board, which declines to supervise or to coerce them." [49]

If the Board's medical staff did not create out of their new office a dynamic, central organization to stimulate and supervise national health, their operations from 1871 to 1900 should not be brushed aside. Budget restrictions limited their program, and they were shut out from the drafting of over-all policy. Yet, even without the leadership of John Simon, the traditions of the Privy Council Medical Office carried on. The Board's Medical Department maintained and widened the concept of State intervention for the control of disease. Although the medical inspection program under the Board was limited, those inspections which were carried out were thorough and competent. The Department kept step with the new bacteriological discoveries,

TABLE 2. Annual Deaths per Million Persons Living of Both Sexes in
England and Wales, 1881–1900

Causes of Death	1881–90 [a]	1891–1900	Difference in 1891–1900 Annual Decrease	Annual Increase
Smallpox	44	13	31	—
Measles	406	414	—	8
Scarlet fever	312	158	154	—
Influenza	20	361	—	341
Whooping cough	414	377	37	—
Diphtheria	153	263	—	110
Croup (not membranous)	133	51	82	—
Enteric fever	198	174	24	—
Diarrheal diseases	631	738	—	107
Puerperal fever and childbirth	161	152	9	—
Pneumonia	1,041	1,227	—	188
Tuberculosis (all forms)	2,429	2,010	419	—
Phthisis	1,775	1,391	384	—
Tuberculosis meningitis	234	216	18	—
Tuberculosis peritonitis, tabes mesenterica	257	217	40	—
Tuberculous diseases (other forms)	163	186	—	23
Rheumatic fever (rheumatism of heart)	94	85	9	—
Cancer	602	758	—	156
Diabetes mellitus	58	75	—	17
Laryngitis	52	45	7	—
Bronchitis	2,081	1,811	270	—
Pleurisy	56	54	2	—
Bright's disease	286	337	—	51
Other causes	9,563	9,091	472	—
All causes	18,734	18,194	1,516	976
Net decrease			540	

[a] The death rates for 1881–1890 are based on the sex and age constitution of the mean population of England and Wales in 1891–1900.

and the auxiliary scientific investigations formed a significant contribution to science.

Writing in 1919, Sir George Newman, the last "Principal Medical Officer of the Board," and the first Chief Medical Officer of the Ministry of Health, in discussing his predecessors, commented that "no one I think can examine its [the Medical Department's] work without finding abundant evidence of its open-mindedness, its extraordinary diligence, its loyalty to great scientific ideals, its reliability and integrity and its splendid record of work done." [50] Sir George was paying no mere courteous compliment to the past. The personal abilities, qualities, and merits of the Board's medical staff were readily apparent. So, too, was their sincerity in desiring to advance public health on a pragmatic basis. The spirit of the Medical Officer of the Local Government Board was typified in the statement with which Dr. Thorne Thorne concluded his survey of the progress of preventive medicine in the Victorian era:

> It has, indeed, been contended that there are limits beyond which the saving of human life is not consistent with the public welfare, and that the present tendency is towards an undue multiplication of the human race, and to a corresponding increase of poverty and misery. But I venture to assert that, so long as the work we are engaged in goes, as it has gone hitherto, to the lessening of death, so long must it ensure the diminution of sickness, and a corresponding promotion of a higher vitality, and a greater capacity for remunerative work amongst the living. [51]

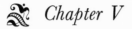

Chapter V

The Poor Law Medical Officers, 1871-1900

THE GOVERNMENT's medical representative whose duties brought him closest to the daily life of the English people was the poor law medical officer, or "parish doctor." Overworked and underpaid, he could rarely satisfy both the medical needs of his patients and the shilling-pinching demands of his tough-minded employers, the local Boards of Guardians. In the years up to 1871, the poor law medical officers as a professional group had become inreasingly vocal on the need for reform in poor law medical care.

The Zeitgeist of Poor Law Medicine by the Eighteen-seventies

State responsibility for caring adequately for the sick poor was grudgingly accepted by modern society. By the middle of the nineteenth century, a variety of forces had moved England away from the policy of supplying only minimum relief to the poor. Changes in the patterns of urban living created by industrialization, the evangelical revival with its accompanying humanitarianism towards the poor, the sweeping cholera epidemics before which all levels of society were equally vulnerable—these and other influences had softened the harsh policies of the Poor Law Amendment Act of 1834 which forced the indigent into workhouses in order to obtain assistance. But the gap between legal provision for medical care to the poor and provision for adequate care (even by nineteenth-century standards) was still wide in 1871 when the Poor Law Board was merged into the new Local Government Board. Early reforming physicians like Neil Arnott, James

Kay-Shuttleworth, Thomas Southwood Smith and Henry Wyldbore
Rumsey, with the support of *The Lancet* and the Workhouse Infirmary
Association, had successfully broadened the concept of public responsibility to the sick poor. Nevertheless, medical care to the poor was still
marked by a chilling and pervasive atmosphere of deterrence.

This dichotomy was reflected in the respective attitudes of the central poor law authorities and the local Boards of Guardians. The Poor
Law Board from 1847 to 1871 began to bring administrative pressure
to bear upon Guardians to improve medical services to the poor. Time
and again, however, the Boards of Guardians blandly resisted these
overtures and continued to curtail medical relief to protect the rate-
payer's pocket. The Guardians' actions stemmed from the nineteenth-
(and in part the twentieth-) century view of the pauper, even the sick
pauper, as primarily a malingerer, who drained the resources of substantial members of the community and was therefore to be discouraged
from applying for any public assistance.

Actively opposing the concept of "deterrence" in poor law medical
treatment were the leaders of the humanitarian movement, among
them the idealistic champion of the oppressed, Dr. Joseph Rogers
(1821–1889). The descendant of three generations of medical men,
Rogers devoted his life to the reform of medical relief. He had earlier
agitated, on sanitary grounds, for the prohibition of intramural inter-
ment in crowded London and for the repeal of the odious tax on
windows. As the founder and president of the Poor Law Medical Officers Association, Rogers, in the sixties and seventies, repeatedly denounced the evils of deterrence in medical care of the poor. Even
before Rogers began his crusade, Thomas Wakley,* founder of the
medical journal *The Lancet,* had called for improvements in poor
law care.

In describing the spirit of the mid-Victorian Age, Beatrice Webb,
that charming and spiritual pragmatist, suggested that it was a period

* Thomas Wakley (1795–1862) founded *The Lancet* in 1823, after a number
of years in medical practice, to expose abuses in hospital administration and
to report medical lectures. A close friend of William Cobbett, Wakley was
one of the leaders in the medical reform movement of the first half of the
century. He became a medical authority in Parliament, where he represented
Finsbury from 1835 to 1852. Wakley spearheaded *The Lancet* campaign to
eradicate the common practice of adulteration of foods and drugs, and took
part in the movement to improve poor law medical service, shortly before
his death. See Samuel Squire Sprigge, *The Life and Times of Thomas Wakley*
(London: Longmans, Green & Co., 1897), *passim.*

when "the impulse of self-subordinating service was transferred consciously and overtly, from God to man." [1] Certainly public attention to the sick poor was only one part of the new humanitarianism driving members of the English middle class to look outside themselves for a greater personal fulfillment. Organizations like the Society for the Relief of Distress and the London Society for Organizing Charitable Relief and Repressing Mendacity selected their memberships from a charitable and religious middle-class group, anxious of ridding themselves of the fundamental conflict between the Christian ethic and the struggle for survival. Despite this, the spirit of the greatest of utilitarians, Jeremy Bentham, was still strong, and Joseph Rogers wisely used utilitarian as well as humanitarian arguments to emphasize the advantages of a more generous attitude toward the sick poor, saying:

> that a more liberal administration of poor relief meant true economy to the rate-payers, because if they cut short the sickness of the poor, and if they diminished the amount of deaths that took place among the bread-winners, they would, as the ultimate result, economize expenditure and out-relief.[2]

The severe winters of 1860 and 1861, together with a general trade depression culminating in the Lancashire cotton famine, had flooded the workhouses. Meanwhile, the apparent inability of the Poor Law Board to cope with the crisis had led to the appointment of a Select Committee of the House of Commons. After three years of investigations, the Committee had cleared the poor law system of the public charges of wholesale inadequacy. Among other recommendations, however, the Select Committee had stressed the need to provide wards for the sick poor, particularly in London. By 1867, the Metropolitan Poor Act, otherwise known after its sponsor as the Gathorne Hardy Act, had brought about some reform of the care of the sick poor in London. This Act had provided for the establishment of district asylums, formed by combined parish action, for the sick, infirm, or insane. A Metropolitan Asylums Board was set up to superintend the new facilities and the administration of the Metropolitan Common Poor Fund. The Act also provided for the erection of dispensaries in London to cope with the growing problem of "outdoor" medical relief (medical care for the sick poor outside the workhouses).

The late sixties continued, nevertheless, to be a period of depressed trade conditions, and an average of 4.6 per cent of the total population of England and Wales, slightly over one million persons, was forced to

apply for poor relief during the years 1866–1871.[3] Economic recovery
was slow, especially in London. The national expenditure for poor
relief, as recorded by the Local Government Board, advanced steadily
from £6,439,517 in 1865–1866, to £7,673,100 in 1868–1869 and rose to
£8,007,403 in 1871–1872.[4]

It was in this *Zeitgeist,* whose philosophic and economic threads can
only be traced briefly here, that some four thousand poor law medical
officers carried out their duties in hundreds of parishes throughout
England and Wales.[5]

Qualifications of the Poor Law Doctor

By 1870 poor law medical officers, who earlier in the century had
been chosen "without regard to merit or qualification, and mainly for
their willingness to accept the lowest rate of pay," [6] were being appointed more selectively. Following passage of the Medical (Registration) Act of 1858, the Poor Law Board demanded that all poor law
medical officers should be registered and should possess a legal qualification to practice both medicine and surgery in England and Wales.[7]
This double qualification required that the poor law medical officers
obtain better professional training than some of their medical colleagues in private practice, who might take only one qualification.
This is not to say, of course, that all parish doctors ranked with Harley
Street men. But their status within their profession and in the eyes of
the public had increased remarkably.[8] For the most part they were
engaged on a fairly permanent basis and in many large cities employed
full-time as medical officers for the workhouses. Salaries, set by local
Boards of Guardians, varied greatly and were the cause for frequent
complaint. Despite this, at the close of the nineteenth century, the posts
were sought after competitively, as they carried many advantages, and
often provided the holders with a "publicly guaranteed introduction
to the neighborhood." [9]

As early as 1868 the Poor Law Board had also expressed itself firmly
on the use of unqualified assistants to poor law medical officers, saying:
"The Board feel it necessary to request the cooperation of Boards of
Guardians in discouraging the employment of unqualified assistants." [10]
Poor law medical scandals, frequent in the forties, were markedly
reduced by the eighteen-sixties. When, in 1869, the Poor Law Board
began to include in its annual reports the number of dismissals of

medical officers, the number was negligible.[11] The Poor Law Medical Officers Association had worked industriously to raise the professional standards of its members throughout the country. Nevertheless, much remained to be done in the years after 1870 before the higher standards of professional competence were uniformly applied by Boards of Guardians throughout the country.

Poor Law Medical Officers and Central Supervision

Between 1847 and 1871, the relief of England's poor had been centrally supervised by a Board which never met—the Poor Law Board, successor to the old Poor Law Commissioners. Its President was the Lord President of the Privy Council, and the duties of the ex officio Board were carried out under the President as in an ordinary government department.[12]

The new Local Government Board, set up in 1871 under the domination of administrative personnel of the defunct Poor Law Board, controlled the administration of grants to local authorities and sent out directives and circulars regarding administrative procedures and the medical treatment of the poor. The Local Government Board also maintained a central inspectorate for poor law purposes.

Supervision of poor law medical care was not given to the Medical Office of the Local Government Board at any time after the merger. And there was no adequate central medical supervisory staff to whom the poor law medical officers could report.

The anomaly of maintaining an active medical administrative staff in the Medical Department of the Local Government Board, and then failing to use it for that large area of poor law medical care for which the Board was responsible was not unperceived in official circles. John Simon had felt that poor law medical questions should have been submitted to him as Medical Officer of the Board. But he refused to concede to Lambert's wish, at one point, that the Medical Department assume responsibility for poor law medical care, if no additional medical staff were provided. Some consideration to a possible merger of poor law medical responsibilities with the work of the Medical Department took place, later, in 1892. At this time, Sir Hugh Owen, Permanent Secretary to the Board, was ready to accede to the step. The Medical Officer, Dr. Richard Thorne Thorne, however, had second thoughts about accepting such a responsibility—apparently because of preoccupation with the needs of preventive medicine and possible personnel complications.[13]

CENTRAL INSPECTION

Like the old Poor Law Board inspectors, Local Government Board inspectors were laymen, not physicians. Yet they were empowered to survey and report regularly upon the quality of medical treatment to the sick poor.

The lack of medical supervision had earlier in the century been brought to the attention of an investigating committee in 1854 when a majority of the doctors giving evidence advocated a medical supervisory staff in the Poor Law Board. Dr. Henry Rumsey, in his *Essays on State Medicine* of 1856, had remarked of the lay inspectors of the Poor Law Board, that, although they

> unanimously deprecated the appointment of *medical* authorities, they nevertheless admitted there were no securities for the proper treatment of the sick beyond the legal or nominal standard of qualification possessed by the medical officers and . . . that there was no supervision of practice, except a cursory perusal by the Board of Guardians of the weekly sick lists presented to them.[14]

Some small attempt at central medical inspection had been made by the appointment of Dr. Edward Smith as a poor law inspector in 1865, with special reference to medical relief. Dr. Smith was in no sense, however, a general or administrative supervisor of the local poor law medical officers. His early duties dealt with an investigation into workhouse hospitals in the "metropolis and provinces" and with the improvement of poor law dietaries.[15]

There were later added to the Local Government Board two medical inspectors, Dr. Andrew Fuller for provincial England and Dr. (later Sir) Arthur Downes for the London area. The number was far too limited to provide any real medical supervision.[16] Dr. Fuller's visits in the provinces were customarily made only at the general request of the district lay inspector. Sir Arthur Downes, who served as Medical Inspector of the Board from 1889 to 1918 was to be instrumental in improving London poor law hospital treatment of pulmonary tuberculosis.[17] During the period 1871–1900, however, these two medical inspectors had relatively little effect on the over-all pattern of poor law medical care.

The staff of general inspectors who supervised the work of poor law medical officers from 1871 to 1900 was well imbued with poor law principles. For many years there were only a dozen of them to cover all of England and Wales, but by 1888 the small group had been strengthened until it numbered fifteen, and by 1894 it totaled eighteen. Inspectors were charged with interpreting the Local Government Board policy to the local Boards of Guardians, and with supervising the administration of central policy in the local districts. To implement these charges inspectors attended meetings of each Board of Guardians at least once or twice a year, making semiannual visitations to all poor law establishments in each district and preparing annual reports on conditions.

A German investigator of the eighties, Paul Aschrott, commented that "the social position of the inspector is such that there can be no suspicion of personal interest in the advice which he gives as to local administration." [18]   Indeed, when he queried the qualifications of the inspectors, Aschrott was told by the Local Government Board that "they must, above all, be gentlemen, who, on account of their previous occupation and their position in life, enjoy consideration and are accustomed to exercise authority.   Stress is laid upon a certain talent for organization, and they must already have shown some interest in the welfare of the poor." [19]

From the quality of their reports, it is clear that at least a good proportion of the general inspectors were able and well-motivated men. But there was little in either the inspector's duties or social position which qualified him to judge the professional adequacy of the poor law medical officer.

CENTRAL DIRECTIVES

The central control imposed on the parish doctor (other than that exerted by the district inspector) lay in the general orders and circulars on policy statements which the Local Government Board issued from time to time. An examination of these sporadic directives together with ancillary material in the otherwise invaluable correspondence files of the Local Government Board gives a very limited picture of the relationship between central policy and the extension of the poor law medical service.

Critics of the poor law system claimed that such regulations as existed were largely in the nature of suggestions offered, or permissions granted,

and could hardly be used to compel local Boards of Guardians to provide adequate medical care for their poor. Even when certain directives were called to the attention of local Boards, they might be ignored.[20] In the main, the over-all outline of duties seems not substantially to have changed during the period 1871–1900. New orders for
district medical officers had been issued in April, 1871, revising the
orders of 1847, to make provision for the new establishment of infirmaries. The 1871 orders instructed district medical officers to attend
the workhouse dispensary every day except Sundays for a minimum of
one hour, or for a longer period as directed by the Guardians. Provision was also made in the same orders for the medical officer to visit "at
the home of the poor person on whose behalf application is made, or
elsewhere as the case may require, and [to] supply all requisite medical
or surgical advice and assistance to every pauper in the District placed
under his charge." [21]

Additional regulations provided for the maintenance of a medical
relief register, for notification (to the Boards of Guardians) of paupers
named semiannually to a permanent medical relief list, and for attendance at meetings of the Dispensary Visiting Committee when required.

Duties prescribed in 1896 for medical officers attached to the workhouse were very similar: personal attendance upon "as far as may be
practicable the poor persons entrusted to his care," reporting to the
Guardians as required upon the conditions of paupers, attendance
at the workhouse at fixed periods, examining the state of paupers on
their admission, maintenance of records, giving directions for the
classification and treatment of sick paupers, children, and nursing
mothers.[22]

With a more adequate professional inspection service the quality
of medical care provided to the poor under these over-all regulations
might have been better. Without the presence, either of adequate enforcing authority or of any national standard of performance, such
general and permissive regulation made for not only considerable
variation in performance but outright abuse.

Limitations Inherent in Poor Law Medical Care

The actual and potential role of medical officers treating the poor
was severely limited by more than general regulations and ineffective

inspections. The basic dichotomy of poor law medical service was as present in 1871 as when it was expressed by Beatrice Webb in 1909:

> What many members of the Poor Law Medical Service feel most is not the miserable pay they get, not the lack of official appreciation, or encouragement nor even the absence of honours and dignity, but the *extraordinarily narrow scope* that, under the necessary limitations of the Poor Law they find for useful work. It is not encouraging, for instance, to have pass through one's hands (as the Poor Law Medical Officer does) one third of all the deaths from phthisis; and yet, as several Poor Law doctors told us, never to have seen among them a single curable case. It breaks the spirit of a man who cares anything at all about his professional work to have to go on year after year merely pretending to deal with cases, which have come to him only when destitution has set in, and therefore usually too late for any permanently remedial treatment under structural and other conditions which he knows will prevent cure, but which he, as a mere Poor Law Doctor, has no power to prevent.[23]

Measured against the curative potential of medicine today, late nineteenth century medical and surgical care was obviously very limited, and poor law treatment even more constricted. At its best poor law care was palliative treatment, most often with limited resources, and without chance of prevention.

One aspect of this fundamental problem was reflected in the provision of "medical extras." The significance of strengthening foods, often a high protein diet for the recovery of the sick, was well recognized by 1871. Yet the final decision as to whether a seriously ill workhouse patient was entitled to such "medical extras" as meat broth or stimulants rested not with the poor law medical officer, but with the Boards of Guardians. In February 1871, the *British Medical Journal* reported the case of a Shropshire medical officer, Dr. W. P. Brooks, who complained to the Poor Law Board when an Assistant Overseer of the workhouse counteracted his order for two pounds of meat to make broth for a patient suffering from inflammation of the womb. The Poor Law Board, however, replied that they "consider that a certificate given by a Medical Officer for the allowance of nourishment or stimulants to any of his pauper patients can only be regarded as a recommendation or expression of his opinion as to what is required for such patient," and that the final decision rested with the relieving officer or with the Guardians. The *British Medical Journal* commented gravely: "we think that the discretion of the medical officer to order nourishment necessary on medical grounds should be so far absolute as not to be interfered with by subordinate officers, whose means of judgment must be inferior to his own." [24]

The objective of the Poor Law Board, and later the Local Government Board, in leaving the final decision to the lay authorities was, of course, the pursuit of "less eligibility," and the fear that the poor law medical officer, given free reign over medical extras, would send the costs of medical relief soaring. The problem of medical extras arose repeatedly in the period 1871–1900, and the Poor Law Medical Officers Association discussed it on a number of occasions.

Repeated conflicts between poor law medical officers and Boards of Guardians revolved about the unwillingness of the local Boards either to pay for sanatoria facilities and expensive medicines, or to provide adequate salaries or special fees to poor law medical men. Yet these same Boards of Guardians with whom the poor law medical officers were so often at loggerheads included many persons who might most have been expected to understand the plight of the poor. As Aschrott described them in 1888: "In rural districts they are usually tenant farmers of repute, in towns they are respectable tradesmen who sympathize with their poorer neighbours, partly young and energetic men who desire to take part in public life." [25]

As the years passed after 1871, concomitant with the gradual evolution in the concept of public responsibility for curative treatment, there developed a gradual relaxation in the application of "less eligibility," particularly in the larger cities. By the late eighties, medical recommendations for "extras" were usually followed. Nevertheless, the overall situation made for tension between medical officers and guardians or relieving officers, and continued to foster resentment among the poor law medical men.[26]

Extension of and Improvement in Poor Law Medical Facilities

One area of treatment for the sick poor underwent a marked change between 1871 and 1890—namely, the improvement of hospital and dispensary facilities. Early efforts of the Poor Law Medical Officers Association, in conjunction with the vigorous campaign carried out by

The Lancet in 1864–1865, successfully aroused public opinion to the need for a reform of poor law hospital and infirmary conditions. Even before the establishment of the Local Government Board, the Poor Law Board had fully accepted the need for an improved infirmary service, and in the late sixties new institutions for the care of the sick poor began to be constructed in populous areas throughout England and Wales. Outbreaks of smallpox and the building of public infectious disease hospitals in the seventies stimulated the building of separate poor law infirmaries to replace the old sick wards in workhouses.

The greatest improvements in furnishing hospital service to the poor took place in London, where the existence of the Metropolitan Common Poor Fund facilitated the erection of the new buildings. The Metropolitan Poor Act of 1867 had been beneficial to London poor law districts in standardizing poor law medical facilities and, for the first time, bringing to the poorer districts measures of assistance which would not have been possible for them alone. In the first nine years of the operation of the Act in London, twenty-two separate infirmaries for the sick poor were opened. By 1877, only six London parishes still housed their sick poor in mixed workhouses.[27]

Extension of hospitalization for the destitute poor was accompanied by a similar provision for the class just above the destitute. Under the stimulus of the humanitarian reform movements of the sixties and seventies, the Local Government Board encouraged hospital care for the poor who could not be technically classified as destitute.[28] This new approach was originally justified on grounds of protecting the public against persons suffering from infectious diseases, whose homes did not offer adequate isolation facilities.

In 1875 it became the official policy of the Local Government Board to admit to poor law hospitals, without an order, anyone afflicted with fever or smallpox, if refusal to admit such patients involved danger of infection. Under the Poor Law Act of 1889, the managers of the Metropolitan District Asylums were legally empowered to admit patients suffering from fever, who were other than paupers.[29] The Public Health of London Act of 1891 permanently removed the possible disqualification for admittance to a pauper hospital.

It is both curious and significant that the whole process of extending poor law medical treatment to other than the destitute or to those suffering from infectious disease evolved through central administrative encouragement, from an administration still heavily weighted with "deterrence" in other respects.

Improvements in staffing and equipment of poor law infirmaries also developed in the seventies and eighties, most notably in London and gradually in other large cities. By 1879 the Local Government Board related with satisfaction the disappearance from London inspectors' reports of such criticisms as "no day rooms for the sick or separate kitchen, bad ventilation, inadequate lavatories, no paid nurses or nurses for sick children, no hot water supply, no infectious wards, poorly constructed sick wards." [30] The amount of space per patient, which in 1866 had been 500 to 600 cubic feet (exclusive of day room), had been improved by 1883 to 850 cubic feet. This did not equal the usual allotment of a general hospital, but was "regarded as sufficient for diseases of the chronic class treated in poor law infirmaries." [31] The ratio of poor law medical officers to patients had not been increased by 1883, but in London a majority of the medical officers served full-time, and were no longer engaged in private practice.

New standards of treatment also gradually found their way into poor law treatment, despite an undoubted time lag. Asepsis, anesthesia, better technical equipment, and the new emphasis on skilled nursing which sprang from the Nightingale tradition were all adopted as the official policy of the Local Government Board, usually some time later than their general use in the large London hospitals. From time to time the lay inspectorate of the Board drew the attention of Boards of Guardians to advances in medical and hospital care, commenting on the presence or absence of the new facilities. By 1893, Robert Hedley, poor law inspector in London, stated (albeit somewhat complacently) before the Royal Commission on the Aged Poor:

> The infirmaries of the metropolis are equal, I think, in their treatment of the poor to anything the poor will get in what are called the large hospitals of the metropolis . . . They are all built on the best principles of ventilation and they are all provided with medical officers . . . The Poor Law infirmaries of the metropolis now furnish between 12,000 and 13,000 beds, whereas what are called the hospitals of the metropolis, the large hospitals, St. Thomas', Bartholomew's, and Guy's, I believe only provide about 5,000.[32]

The improvements in some large cities did not extend to rural areas, where poor law infirmaries were considerably less than satisfactory at the end of the century. And even in some large cities, local Boards of Guardians kept up resistance to the central policy of lessening deterrence and expanding the curative principle.[33] Outside of the big cities the lag was marked. Poor law reformers in 1909 were to comment dismally that apart from the populous cities:

> the sick are still in General Mixed Workhouses—the maternity cases, the cancerous, the venereal, the chronically infirm, and even the infectious, all together in one building, often in the same ward where they cannot be treated. For the phthisical, for instance, there is (except in a few unions) no proper provision at all.[34]

Local Government Board officials were well aware of this lag and of the financial problem of providing separate infirmaries throughout England and Wales. In the 1894–95 annual report the following statement appears:

> It must . . . be borne in mind that the workhouses in the country districts of Wales are for the most part very small, the inmates very few, accustomed to an exceedingly simple and primitive style of life; and it takes a long time to convince the Guardians of such unions of any necessity for marching with the times so far as providing trained nurses and modern hospital appliances. Still, matters are improving steadily, if slowly.[35]

Poor Law Nursing Service

Nursing services available under the poor law had also improved by the close of the century. Abuses in pauper nursing care had been manifold and attracted considerable publicity in the sixties and seventies. Dickens' Sairey Gamp had caricatured an uncomfortable reality. The foundation of the Workhouse Nurses' Association in 1879 to develop a program for training nurses in the care of the sick poor was to be a landmark in the history of poor law nursing. Louisa Twining and her associates helped to set standards and also recommended accredited nurses to Boards of Guardians. By 1889 the Association, while still lamenting degrees of imperfection in nurses' training, reported to the Local Government Board on the "neat and becommingly dressed young women in suitable uniform, in place of the wretched old creatures who, in pauper dress and black caps, prowled about the beds of our sick poor." [36]

Dr. Arthur Downes, in 1865, had been successful in persuading the Poor Law Board to recommend to local Guardians that they "as far as possible discontinue the practice of appointing pauper inmates of the workhouse to act as Assistant nurses in the infirmary and sick wards." [37] Considerable improvements were made between 1865 and 1895 in the introduction and extension of a paid nursing service. But the Local Government Board's policy was still used as an excuse by many Guardians to continue the employment of paupers as attendants to the sick.

By the end of the century it was officially recognized that the nursing of sick paupers left much to be desired. Although Guardians might be forbidden to employ paupers as nurses, it was still very difficult to find qualified women willing to serve in workhouse infirmaries.[38] Even in London, George Lansbury's testimony before the Royal Commission on the Aged Poor stated:

> The wards in the workhouse [of the Poplar Union] are very much understaffed; there are not enough nurses, and we have to rely a very great deal—very considerably—on the inmates to assist in the work of nursing and attending to the aged, infirm and sick.[39]

More especially in rural areas, Guardians were reluctant to provide in infirmaries and workhouses a degree of trained nursing service which, in time of sickness, "neither they themselves, or their families or the independent labouring classes could afford." [40]

Outdoor Medical Care

"Outdoor" medical care for the poor not confined to hospitals or infirmaries also underwent several changes from 1871 to 1900, including the building of dispensary facilities and a restriction in the extent of outdoor relief (in favor of indoor treatment).

During the period 1847–1871, outdoor medical attendance had been encouraged by the Poor Law Board, with no attempt to force the sick into workhouses. During the middle sixties central inspectors, together with the Poor Law Medical Officers Association, began to urge the building of dispensaries at which the swelling numbers of pauper sick could regularly be treated by poor law medical officers.

The Poor Law Board in 1867 called the attention of all Boards of Guardians in London to sections of the Metropolitan Poor Act of that year which related to the provision of dispensaries in London.[41] By 1871 six poor law dispensaries had been started in London; the following year nine appeared in the provinces, and inspectors urged the use of the dispensary system in other urban and rural districts of England and Wales. Outside London, however, building of dispensaries proceeded slowly in the following years.

In part the lag was associated with a new policy initiated in 1871 by poor law authorities of the Local Government Board, aimed at reducing outdoor relief and forcing the sick poor into the newly erected infirmaries. This policy, so close to a reversion to the principles of 1834, was carried out during the period when admission of other than the purely destitute to poor law infirmaries was being extended. The policy of restricting outdoor relief was enforced through the Board's inspectorate rather than by any specific circulars of the Local Government Board.[42] In actuality, infirmary treatment was often a considerable improvement on the normal housing conditions of the poorer classes.

Gradually, however, more and more dispensaries began to make their appearance. By 1886 forty-four serviced the London poor, and the Local Government Board noted that the original objections of some London Guardians to establishing dispensaries on the grounds of expense had disappeared by 1888. However, there was no significant change in the numbers of paupers who received outdoor medical care from the mid-eighties until the end of the century,[43] and testimony before the Royal Commission on the Aged Poor in 1895 confirmed the prevalence of a policy which still restricted outdoor care in favor of indoor treatment.[44]

The poor law medical officer who was engaged in outdoor medical relief outside of London worked at a considerable disadvantage. In some instances he was still forced to supply his own drugs out of a meager salary, was often without a dispensary or the services of a dispenser, and had minimal district nursing service to call upon.

The Poor Law Medical Officers Association and Reform

It was among these changing trends in poor law administration that the parish doctor carried out his daily routine. Shifts in policy affected individual poor law medical officers at different times, depending on the attitudes of local Boards of Guardians. The poor law medical officer, of course, was not merely the passive instrument of authority in all this, he was also a participant in the evolution of a broader, more humanitarian administration of the service.

The relation of the parish doctor to the growth of society's obligation to the sick poor cannot be evaluated by any precise scientific measurement. Like all pressures in a complex industrialized society, it was only a part of the kaleidoscope pattern of a rapidly changing world. It is impossible under traditional methods of historical research to utilize the individual annual reports of over 4,000 poor law medical men serving in England and Wales for this thirty-year period. Many, indeed, have been destroyed, or exist only in local files. Nor (if such tasks could be performed with the relentless efficiency of IBM methods) is there any evidence which could determine the reactions of the Guardians to these reports. We thus must view the poor law medical officer primarily through the activities of his group association.

THE ASSOCIATION

By 1871, there was in existence an articulate professional organization, headed by the redoubtable Dr. Joseph Rogers, which represented the poor law medical officers of England and Wales. Stemming originally from the membership of the Poor Law Committee of the Provincial Medical and Surgical Association, the group had passed through several stages. In 1868 the organization known as the Metropolitan Association of Poor Law Medical Officers reconstituted itself as the Poor Law Medical Officers Association, and its Council was revised to include an equal representation of metropolitan and provincial members.[45] The Association had attracted considerable support as well as publicity by its efforts in the late sixties to bring about reforms in poor law care. Together with *The Lancet* and the Association for the Improvement of Workhouse Infirmaries, the Poor Law Medical Officers Association had been instrumental in securing passage of the Metropolitan Poor Relief Act of 1867.

Joseph Rogers, following a bitter personal struggle with the Guardians of the Strand Union, embarked upon a new program of strengthening the Association at the close of the sixties. Touring Ireland, he observed that the all-embracing program of medical relief there seemed to offer considerable improvement on the English system. Rogers also visited the principal cities of England and induced a number of cities to adopt legislation similar to the Metropolitan Act.[46]

Meanwhile, other supporters of reform of relief to the sick poor had joined in the fray. J. H. Stallard, M.D., published a study of London pauperism, offering plans to revise the structure of poor law administration in favor of more efficient, central control. Dr. Thomas Hawksley, Physician to the Infirmary for Consumption and Diseases of the Chest, spoke (to the Association for the Prevention of Pauperism and Crime in London) on the plague "constantly raging in our midst . . . more dangerous because overlooked in forms of poverty that from familiarity with them we come to view as inevitable." [47] The medical journals maintained a continuous clamor in support of the poor law medical officers,[48] and reports of poor law inspectors provided grist for reformers' mills.[49]

DEMANDS FOR REFORM IN THE SEVENTIES

During this decade, the Poor Law Medical Officers Association was to reach a new high in repeated demands both for improved working conditions for members and improvements in the quality of medical care for the poor.

By February of 1871, the Association had drawn up a nine-point reform program which was circulated in the leading medical journals.[50] Six of the points were aimed at improving the status of the poor law medical men, but three called for reform in the medical care—namely, establishing of additional dispensers and dispensaries, providing for consultation service, and placing midwifery cases under the authority of the medical officers. Commenting on these demands with sound utilitarian sentiments, the *British Medical Journal* observed:

> All of us who have considered the question and the medical officers of the Poor-law service especially, have long since aimed at the conclusion that a very large amount of pauperism which weighs upon the resources of the nation, arises from sickness of preventable character; and that under a better organized system of Poor-law relief, and especially by attributing to the medical officers of the Poor-law preventive as well as curative functions, much of this pauperizing sickness would be prevented, and where it is unavoidable, it might be more promptly and effectively cured.[51]

The following February (1872), a deputation hopefully called upon James Stansfeld, the new President of the Local Government Board. The deputation was headed by Frederick Corrance, M.P. and Rogers, and was accompanied by Dr. Ernest Hart, voluble editor of the *British Medical Journal* and Chairman of the Poor Law Committee of the

British Medical Association. They asked Stansfeld for a thorough over-hauling and reorganization of the poor law medical service, appoint-ment of more medical officers, payment of drugs by funds from the rates instead of by poor law medical officers, and a greater degree of independence for medical officers in their relations with Boards of Guardians. Moreover, they urged that medical officers of health strengthen enforcement of sanitary measures.[52] These were, on the whole, less self-interested demands—aimed at a more general reform than were the previous year's list. Stansfeld, following an old pattern, promised consideration of the matter, but no sweeping administrative changes followed.

Two years later in 1874 the Association made another attempt, this time through passage of a resolution with only one aim—extension of dispensary facilities.[53] Building of dispensaries was underway in the metropolis, but rural Boards of Guardians needed more than a reso-lution to solve the problem.

Another mammoth push for reform came in February, 1878, when, acting together with *The Lancet,* the Poor Law Medical Officers As-sociation rounded up eight thousand signatures to a new, comprehen-sive memorial addressed to the Local Government Board. In good Benthamite language this document emphasized that the petitioners' "claim to a hearing must be understood to be based upon the strictly utilitarian and economizing view of the subject on which we speak." [54] Once again some of the old complaints were put forward: local poor law medical officers should be responsible to the Local Government Board (not to the Guardians); better pay was needed; medical officers should not be responsible for the supply and dispensing of drugs. The "memorial" also urged that medical treatment of the poor should be separate from the workhouse, that medical officers should have direct control over the supply of "necessaries" (medical extras) for the sick poor, that paid nurses be available for home nursing, and that a de-partmental or legislative commission be appointed to investigate these matters.

The Local Government Board took a leisurely approach to answer-ing the memorial. Six months after it had been received, John Lambert, the Board's Permanent Secretary, responded casually stating that the pressure of business had heretofore prevented consideration and he hoped, shortly, to be able to communicate the Board's views on this subject.[55] On November 13, 1878, the Board finally dispatched a formal reply to the memorial, stating coolly:

1. The proposal for greater responsibility of the Poor Law Medical Officer to the Local Government Board is at variance with the policy of Poor Law Amendment Act, 4 & 5 William IV, which left the main control in the hands of the Guardians.

2. From time to time, the Board attempts to improve the salaries of the Poor Law Medical Officer.

3. The Board cannot agree, especially in rural districts, to a separation of drugs and provision of dispensers.

4. The Board cannot see anything in the nature of medical relief which requires it to be regarded as a matter distinct from the Workhouse.

5. The Board feels that leaving the supply of necessaries to the Medical Officer instead of the Relieving Officer would 'unquestionably increase the expenditure for the relief of the sick poor and diminish the control of the Guardians.'

6. With reference to paid nurses, there was nothing to prevent the Guardians from providing such assistance.[56]

The reply concluded that the Board saw no grounds which necessitated further investigation.

Such a reply would have dashed the hopes of any reformer. Part of the Board's rigidity was undoubtedly due to the authoritarian personality of John Lambert, a man who tended to regard all change as suspect. But a more underlying factor than Lambert's reactions, or the acceptance by the central authority of the recalcitrance of the Boards of Guardians, motivated the reply: namely, the basic assumption that final procedural responsibility rested with the local authorities.

Following this 1878 setback an extended lull fell over the efforts of the poor law medical officers to change central policy. Much of the Association's energy during the eighties and the early nineties was concentrated upon the defense of particular medical officers who fell afoul of their Boards of Guardians, as well as in efforts to obtain superannuation, payment of medical witnesses, and improvements in salary scales.[57] The medical journals and files of the Board's correspondence do not record major petitions again being placed before the Board for a number of years. The annual meetings of the Association continued to discuss the familiar poor law medical problems, as did the poor law district conferences which had been held annually since 1868. The district conferences, which had been founded by Mr. Barwick Baker in the West Midlands, aimed at an exchange of views of "men of practical experience in poor law administration with regard to the measures adopted in particular districts and their results." [58] Both the district conferences and the annual central conferences of poor law authorities, which were convened from 1871 on, kept alive discussion of the many problems in treatment of the sick poor.

Poor Law Medical Reform
in the Nineties

By the early nineties a variety of new agents were at work unearthing fresh evidence of drawbacks in the whole poor law system. Charles Booth's studies on *The Life and Labour of the People in London*, carried out with a team of early "research investigators," began to appear in 1892; Booth's *Aged Poor in England and Wales* appeared in 1894. Fabian researchers were active on the subject. The growth of the trade union movement had also brought into articulate being united forces living close to the lives of the destitute, and acutely aware of their needs.

In 1888 a select committee of the House of Lords was appointed to investigate the powers held by the Guardians and their adequacy to cope with distress which might occur in London or other heavily populated cities. The Lords' investigation was not an exhaustive one and it did not take testimony from local poor law medical officers or from the Association. Some of the gains in poor law medical care were pointed out by Sir Hugh Owen, Lambert's successor as Permanent Secretary to the Board—particularly the increase in numbers of full-time medical superintendents of poor law infirmaries and the improved dispensary system in London. It was officially admitted, however, that the medical staff serving under the poor law had not been sufficiently increased to cope adequately with the medical needs of the poor.[59]

The report of the 1888 select committee, insofar as it related to medical relief of the poor, was quite favorable. It observed that because of the excellence of treatment in London poor law infirmaries there was even a tendency to "regard them as a kind of state hospital, entrance into which does not imply that the patient is a pauper." [60]

By the early nineties the public and central government's attitude towards medical care to the poor had altered considerably, and in 1893 the Poor Law Medical Officers Association decided on another major push for further reforms. In March a deputation headed by the Association's Council members called upon the President of the Local Government Board, Sir Walter Foster, and presented a list of reforms on which the Council felt the time had arrived for legislation. Five points were stressed: first, the advisability of extending the successful London dispensary system to all large towns throughout England and Wales. Second, the parish doctors urged again that the practice of forcing them to pay for medicines should be eliminated. Next came the old question of superannuation; fourth, a reminder of the insufficiency of pauper nursing; and finally the Board was reminded that no official provision had been made for the use of anesthetics in poor law work.[61] Although for the past thirty-five years anesthetics had been in general use in medical practice, the Association's delegates stated that in many unions "operations were performed where private patients would undoubtedly have anaesthetics, whereas the pauper had to suffer without them." [62]

The Association delegates were accorded a far more favorable reception by the President of the Local Government Board in 1893 than they had had from John Lambert in 1878. Sir Walter Foster assured the group of his "strong sympathy" with respect to the extension of the infirmary system throughout the country, as far as it might be feasible. The encouragement of infirmary building was, he emphasized, the official policy of the Board. The Board had discouraged the system of making medical men buy drugs and would continue to do so. With respect to anesthetics, Sir Walter assured the delegation of his entire willingness to provide anesthetics. The Board had already sent out a circular about providing trained nurses, and had discouraged pauper nursing insofar as possible. Sir Walter recommended further, with respect to superannuation, that the Association draw up a workable scheme.[63] Shortly after the March visit of the deputation, the Local Government Board issued an order for providing anesthetics in pauper treatment.

This was heartening news for the Association. The changed, cooperative attitude of the Board and the widened public humanitarianism toward the poor was also evident in central orders permitting a weekly screw of tobacco for paupers in 1892 and, later, considerable improvements in the diet under a General Order of 1900.[64]

The same humanitarian outlook was to inspire the appointment of a Royal Commission in 1895 to investigate the condition of the aged poor. At this time almost a third of the old people in England and Wales received poor relief. Nevertheless, neither the Royal Commission of 1895 nor a Select Committee on the Aging Deserving Poor three years later made any major recommendations for improvement in the care of the aged sick poor. The Poor Law Medical Officers Association, however, in 1896 passed a resolution stating that "the time has arrived when Boards of Guardians should take into their serious and earnest consideration the necessity of providing for the aged and infirm inmates of workhouses accommodation which will be more suitable to their infirmities and other requirements than now exists." [65]

This resolution had little or no effect within the next few years. An important step in improving the position of the poor law medical officer occurred in 1895 when Walter Long, former Parliamentary Secretary to the Local Government Board, introduced an Association-supported bill to provide superannuation allowance for poor law medical men. The bill was successful and the cause of many years of strife was finally resolved. Although superannuation had been one of the major planks in the formation of the Association, the Council meeting in March 1897 unanimously resolved that the passing of the Poor Law Officers Superannuation Act "had by no means rendered the further existence of this society unnecessary." [66]

The Position of the Poor Law Medical Officer in 1900

The years from 1870 to 1900 unquestionably had brought improvements in public care for the sick poor. New infirmaries, particularly in the large cities, stood as tangible evidence of loosened purse strings of formerly unwilling Guardians. Society had quite fully accepted Dr. Henry Rumsey's midcentury statement that "the simple refusal of medical relief, will neither cure their destitution nor prevent their improvidence." [67]

As the great Poor Law Commission of 1909 was to reveal a few years later, however, the defects of medical service to the poor were still manifold in 1900 and the Poor Law Medical Officers Association had been unable to bring about a major material betterment. Public opinion continued for many years to be tolerant of abuses in treatment. While some large cities by 1900 had established fairly advanced programs,[68] other areas were slack, even callous, in their administration of the program. Not all parish doctors were men of the stamp of Joseph Rogers. George Lansbury, indeed, in discussing the London poor law medical service had claimed that "workhouse doctors do neglect their duty." [69] The actual efficiency or inefficiency of the poor law medical officers cannot be measured. Those in the best position to testify, the sick poor, were historically voiceless.

Out of this changing pattern, however, there had clearly emerged a greater affirmation of the principle of curative treatment for all. Clearly recognizable were the stirrings of a new public attitude, characterized by Thomas Mackay: "The subject is now approaching a critical stage. There is a strong momentum bearing down all opposition and leading to an almost gratuitous treatment of sickness." [70] Legislation in the first decade of the twentieth century was to make these words prophetic.

Insofar as he was able, the poor law medical officer had testified to the abuses of the system in which he worked, had at times been baffled by the spectacle of central acceptance but local deviation in the application of reforms, and had been supported by the new forces of social reform in the community. By 1900 he was still awaiting that sweeping investigation of the massive problem of poor relief—which was to come nine years hence—and as a result of which England was to enter into a new age of social responsibility.

Chapter VI

Local Medical Officers of Health and State Intervention

THE USE of a medical practitioner, trained in public health, to act as a full-time guardian to the health of England's local communities did not become common practice until late in the nineteenth century. Liverpool, as early as 1847, under the pressure of a new immigrant population, had appointed the country's first medical officer of health, Dr. William Henry Duncan.* London, by the Metropolis Management Act of 1855, had provided for the compulsory appointment of medical officers of health in all districts of that metropolis. Although about fifty local bodies outside of London employed medical officers of health prior to 1872, until the passage of the Public Health Act of that year there was no country-wide requirement for their appointment.[1]

After 1872, however, medical officers of health constituted a new trained force in the sanitary scene. And the influence which they brought to bear on sanitary conditions was to be considerable, despite early public indifference to their work. In 1860, Sidney Herbert, close friend and supporter of Florence Nightingale, had commented on the occasion of the opening of the Army Medical School in Chatham: "with the exception of the army and navy medical officer, it may perhaps be said that there are no medical men who could gain a living

---

* William H. Duncan, M.D. (1805–1863), son of a Liverpool merchant, received his medical training at Edinburgh and established himself in practice in Liverpool before his appointment as medical officer of health there in January, 1847. He worked with Edwin Chadwick on the famous Report of 1848 and was a man warmly sympathetic to the suffering of the poor. Together with James Newlands, the civil engineer who worked with him, Duncan laid the foundations of Liverpool's sanitary improvements. See William M. Frazer, *Duncan of Liverpool* (London: Hamish Hamilton Medical Books, 1947), *passim.*

not by curing but by preventing sickness." Fifteen years later, Dr. François de Chaumont, the army hygienist, pointed out in recounting the incident: "we have, in 1875, the spectacle of hundreds of educated gentlemen, who, as officers of health or public analysts, are profitably devoting the whole of their time to that very duty which fifteen years ago his lordship thought so unpromising a branch of our art." [2]

From 1872, when the Local Government Act was passed, to 1890, there was a steady growth in the numbers of medical officers of health employed under the Act. By 1876, 825 medical officers had been appointed; by 1881, 1,088; by 1885, 1,146; by 1894, 1,376; and by 1898–1899, the Local Government Board was receiving 1,771 annual reports from medical officers of health throughout England and Wales.[3]

Qualifications and Conditions of
Medical Officers of Health

Medical officers of health, claimed a leading article in *The Lancet* in 1872, are "not much better informed than other persons on questions relating to the public health," and, furthermore, having a "desire to make matters perfect all at once" were liable to "excessive zeal." [4] From a journal in the forefront of reform, this was an interesting comment.

How much better informed than other persons was the medical officer of health? The Local Government Board, in prescribing the regulations for their employment required that medical officers of health be registered under the Medical Registration Act of 1858. Upon application of the sanitary authority, however, the appointment could be made if the medical officer were registered in either medicine or surgery.

There was, nevertheless, more than a germ of truth in *The Lancet* statement; formal training in public health methods had not advanced very far by 1872. The University of Dublin, influenced by Dr. William Stokes, had become, in 1870, the first body to grant a Diploma in State Medicine. It was not until 1892 that appointment as a medical officer of health was predicated upon the possession of a legal qualification in public health per se.[5]

The most frequent qualifications held by early medical officers of health were: M.R.C.S. (Member Royal College of Surgeons, England) with the L.S.A. (Licentiate Society of Apothecaries); or the L.R.C.P.

(Licentiate Royal College of Physicians, Edinburgh) and the L.R.C.S. (Licentiate Royal College of Surgeons, Edinburgh). Those who were trained at Edinburgh, some under Dr. William Pulteney Alison, Professor of the Practice of Medicine, were perhaps better qualified in sanitary science.[6] As Dr. C. Fraser Brockington pointed out in his study of some of the early medical officers of health, many were men of exceptional capacity and excellent medical training.[7] Other research, on the qualifications of some of the later provincial medical officers of health, suggested that their medical degrees as a whole were not such as could have obtained the appointments on staffs of the leading hospitals.[8]

During the period 1872–1900, a marked growth of specialized training in public health took place. As early as 1877, the Society of Medical Officers of Health commented on improvement in the teaching of hygiene given in such great London medical training centers as St. Thomas', St. Bartholomew's, Guy's, and Charing Cross Hospitals.[9]

For the medical diploma of the late seventies, preventive medicine was an optional not an obligatory subject. And during these years, it was quite possible for a man unfamiliar with techniques of public hygiene and preventive medicine to serve as a local medical officer of health. One effort to remedy this lack of training occurred in the publication of a semiofficial *Manual for Medical Officers of Health,* written by Dr. Edward Smith, Assistant Medical Officer of the Local Government Board.[10] This convenient little book, first published in 1873, went through several editions. Obviously, though, it could not replace systematic training in public health.

By 1895, the General Council of Medical Education and Registration (also known as the General Medical Council) had appointed a committee headed by Dr. Richard Thorne Thorne to investigate the examinations in sanitary science held by the respective universities and licensing bodies. The committee recommended a variety of improvements, subsequently put into effect in new regulations issued by the General Medical Council in 1900. It was the committee's opinion that too many licensing bodies had been set up in sanitary science to maintain standards of a "distinctively high scientific and practical efficiency."[11]

The Act of 1872, while it created a new force of medical officers of health, erred seriously in not specifying whether such officers were to serve full- or part-time. In many instances, sanitary districts complied with the law in name only, by appointing a part-time medical officer of health whose salary was so ridiculously low as to prevent his spending any substantial time in sanitary duties. Such a situation makes understandable the *British Medical Journal's* prototype of the medical officer of health as an "amateur" without training in sanitary science, devoting to public health duties only "such scraps of time as he can spare from his private practice," serving limited-term appointments without tenure, and overly dependent upon his masters, the local sanitary body.[12] Often the sheer size of the sanitary areas assigned to medical officers of health precluded any effective performance.

Duties and Functions of Medical Officers of Health

A detailed circular of the Local Government Board (No. 27 of 1872), attempted to specify duties of medical officers of health who received the central government's grant. This list of eighteen responsibilities ordered the medical officer of health systematically to inspect and record the sanitary condition of the district, to give advice to the sanitary authority, search out causes of disease through personal visits to the affected areas, inspect food supplies for adulteration or unfitness and inquire into offensive trades. In relation to the Local Government Board, the medical officer of health was required to submit annual reports and to supply immediate information on the outbreak of dangerous infectious disease.[13]

Most of these duties were very similar to those prescribed locally by communities which had established positions for medical officers of health prior to 1872. Liverpool had, in addition, specified that its medical officer of health should "point out the most efficient means for ventilation of churches, chapels, schools, registered lodging-houses and other public edifices." [14] Merthyr Tydfil had added compulsory, statistical, quarterly reports.[15] Other local areas included such special functions as those of port sanitary officer or analyst.

All too often, complained the Local Government Board, in 1877, medical officers of health concerned themselves chiefly with outbreaks of infectious disease, neglecting their other sanitary functions. To remedy this, the Board issued specific instructions emphasizing the importance they attached to systematic inspection and a full reporting upon general sanitary conditions in each district.

Relatively little difference existed between the prescribed duties issued in 1872 and those appearing in a simplified reissue by the Board in March of 1891. New clauses related to the local adoption of the Infectious Diseases (Prevention) Act, 1890, extended the list of articles to be inspected, and listed new requirements regarding the sanitation of dairies, cowsheds, and milk shops.[16]

Whether or not a medical officer of health should also serve as a poor law medical officer was a subject of considerable controversy. Many poor law medical officers favored the combination of offices in one person, and in 1872, the Council of their professional association sent a resolution to the Local Government Board to this effect.[17] Joseph Rogers, however, opposed the practice on the realistic grounds that poor law medical officers, in their capacity as medical officers of health, would hesitate to offend their Boards of Guardians, among whose property-owning members might well be found cardinal offenders against the sanitary acts.[18]

In a large proportion of those appointments made after 1872, the poor law medical officer was, in fact, named medical officer of health "serving *quasi ex officio* in the second capacity." [19] The Local Government Board after 1880 urged sanitary authorities to discontinue such arrangements, and reported that in numerous instances their suggestion was adopted.[20] But the difficulties inherent in part-time appointments continued for many years after.

Administrative Relations with the Local Government Board

The relationship between the local medical officer of health and the Local Government Board, which subsidized his appointment, was tenuous. Technically, the Board had to approve the appointment of the medical officer of health chosen by the local authority. Technically, the medical officer of health was required to submit an annual report on the sanitary condition of his district to the Local Government Board, and to advise the Board of local outbreaks of infectious disease. But, like the poor law medical man, the medical officer of health had in reality no central medical authority whom he might consult. On a national scale, the result of this loose relationship between the Board and the medical officers of health was a wide diversity in standards of performance throughout England and Wales.

Commenting on the disorganized atmosphere in which medical of-

ficers of health performed their duties in 1874, Lyon Playfair complained: "I am perfectly certain that the utter confusion could not
have resulted had the Local Government Board consulted the experienced State medical officers who belonged to them." [21] But here, too,
John Simon and his colleagues were hopelessly outflanked by Lambert
and the lay administration.

In later years, the Board's Medical Department regularly reviewed
reports sent in by the medical officers of health, and issued corrections
and suggestions where necessary—not always without rebuttal. Following submission of an annual report from Dr. Francis Bond,* medical officer of health for the Gloucester Union of Sanitary Authorities,
the Board wrote Bond in 1877, inquiring what precautions had been
taken against infectious disease in his district. The irritated Dr. Bond,
questioning the Board's authority, replied flippantly: "Experience
leads me to the belief that in the present state of sanitary matters, to
restrict preventive action to what is indubitably contained within the
four corners of the Public Health Act, is to do nothing at all." [22] Edward Seaton, by then Medical Officer of the Board, forwarded Bond's
reply to John Lambert, noting that the letter was a very improper
and impertinent one, and statingly defensively: "All Medical Officers
of Health are not Dr. Bonds (God Forbid!), and many most useful
notices and cautions are prepared and circulated to Medical Officers
of Health which are quite within the terms of the law."

From time to time, the Medical Officer of the Board commented in
his annual reports on reviewing the hundreds of reports each year
from medical officers of health. In 1880, Buchanan noted he still received reports "which show very imperfect appreciation of sanitary
science and which are easily recognizable as the production of medical
practitioners who find themselves under the necessity of writing an
essay on a subject to which they have devoted no special study." [23]
Many other reports, however, Buchanan continued, testified to efficient
work on the part of the medical officer. And three years later, he again
noted further improvement in the quality of the reports submitted.

---

* Francis T. Bond (1833–1911) was, in fact, a well-educated (A.B., M.B.,
M.R.C.S., M.D., F.R.C.S.) physician and surgeon. He was Professor of Chemistry, and, subsequently of Clinical Medicine at Queen's College, Birmingham,
where he had served as Dean of the Faculty. He was to be President of the
West of England and South Wales Branch of the Society of Medical Officers
of Health from 1896 to 1897 and, again, from 1905 to 1906, and was the
author of a number of papers on sanitary subjects.

The Role of the Society of
Medical Officers of Health

While any sampling of the thousands of annual reports filed by medical officers of health from 1872 to 1900 can provide ample evidence of their concern with broader state intervention in public health, their attitudes are most clearly evidenced in the work of their professional organization. The Society's interests spanned a wide range of public health problems. An attempt to trace the whole history of the Society of Medical Officers of Health and its regional branches is, therefore, unfeasible in the present context.[24] A survey of the pressures exerted by the organization does give an impression of a group of pragmatic yet farsighted medical practitioners, who recognized a need for broad government action to improve the health and living conditions of the people of England and Wales.

BACKGROUND OF THE SOCIETY

In 1856, one year after passage of an act requiring appointment of medical officers of health in all London districts, eight of the new medical appointees organized a Metropolitan Association of Medical Officers of Health. The aim of the new association, subsequently renamed the Society of Medical Officers of Health,[25] was announced as "mutual assistance and the advancement of sanitary science." John Simon served as its president for the first five years. By 1873, the year following passage of the Public Health Act of 1872, the Society's membership had jumped to 115, of whom 33 practiced outside London.[26]

In addition to the London Society, several provincial organizations of medical officers of health had been formed in 1875: the Northwestern Association, the Yorkshire Association, and the Birmingham and Midland Association. These three groups were amalgamated with the London Society in 1888 as its branches.[27] Membership of the united branches, which in 1888 totalled 369, had grown to 650 members by 1894–1895, and by 1898–1899, had reached 762.[28] At the end of the century, the membership could count over half the total number of full-time and part-time medical officers of health appointed in England and Wales.

At its start, the Society's public health interests were heavily oriented towards disease control and improved sanitation. Research papers presented by the members at periodic meetings in the sixties included many on infectious disease, improved water supply in London, and the need for increased use of morbidity statistics. The Society tried unsuccessfully in 1867 to persuade the President of the Poor Law Board to publish weekly statistics of "sickness" among the poor. Seven years later, the Local Government Board instructed clerks to the Boards of Guardians to report all new cases of illness to medical officers of health.[29]

By the early seventies, the Society was a small, but well-organized body, whose voice had been raised on many aspects of preventive medicine. The group was already an acknowledged force in the growing demand for an extension of the public sanitary services.

PRESSURES FOR BROADER AUTHORITY AND
CENTRALIZATION IN PUBLIC HEALTH

It is not surprising that in their general attitudes towards greater centralization and state enforcement of health measures, the Society of Medical Officers of Health was considerably in advance of many of their contemporaries. Much of their "advanced" thinking during the sixties and seventies revolved about the extent to which the individual should voluntarily surrender "personal liberty" in order to live, in health, in a healthful community.

The Local Government Board perceived its role as advisory, and central enforcing powers were kept to a minimum in accordance with the general premise that the public would not, and should not, be coerced against its will. Despite much good work by the Local Government Board's medical staff, the Board's secretariat unquestionably still tended toward that earlier description of the "official attitude" which Edwin Chadwick's sharp pen had phrased:

> The object of the more consummate of these official and practical statesmen would seem to be not to commit themselves . . . and cover with pomp or a bland routine the *dolce far niente* of office; averting their heads from calamities so long as they are unnoticed, and letting evil principles work themselves out on the community unless they are forced into notice by clamour.[30]

The local medical officer of health lived in day-to-day contact with the results of such central diffidence. In many areas, of necessity, he had become a leader in the fight against disease and poor sanitation.

When the Society in 1874 sent out a circular letter to medical officers of health querying the state of death returns in their respective districts, many of those who replied used the opportunity to comment on the indifference and apathy of the local authority. Repeatedly, sanitary reforms were urged by medical officers of health in their annual reports. But the principle of the greatest good for the greatest number carried little weight in areas where local authorities were often themselves the owners of property which constituted a nuisance to the public health. The issue was posed eloquently in 1872 by the Medical Officer of Health for the Parish of St. Mary, Lambeth:

> A property has its duty as well as its rights; it cannot be a diffi-cult matter to require that such places should be put into and kept in decent order. I will put to one side the moral and social obli-gation which devolves upon such owners, and appeal to them on the grounds of self-interest, for in this age of retrenchment and economy there is no argument goes further to do that which they do not otherwise feel disposed for other than the £s.d. argument. It is little wonder that we are sickly, but it is a great wonder that so many of us have escaped disease.[31]

The only national answer to the indifference and intransigence met by the medical officers of health lay in extended compulsory statute authorities and greater unity through centralization. In his presiden-tial address before the Society of Medical Officers of Health in 1883, Dr. T. Orme Dudfield pointed out that even in London public health was entrusted to some forty separate authorities, each practically in-dependent and rarely holding communication with one another.[32] Dudfield's answer for London was a central legislative and executive board. A decade earlier Ernest Hart,* editor of the *British Medical Journal,* had also recognized the need for consolidated local authori-ties, as well as additional central government staff to advise the med-ical officer of health.[33]

Support by the medical officers of health for the extension of com-pulsory legislation cuts through the whole field of public health reform from 1872 to 1900. Primarily their campaign for wider state interven-

---

* Ernest Abraham Hart (1835–1898), the fiery, voluble opthalmic surgeon, who edited the *British Medical Journal* from 1866 to his death in January, 1898, devoted his life to sanitary reform and improving the physician's status. He served as chairman of the powerful Parliamentary Bills Committee of the British Medical Association from 1872 to 1897 and was the founder, in 1883, of the Medical Sickness Annuity and Life Assurance Society for physicians. The record of his public work covered almost the whole field of sanitary leg-islation of the period.

tion was a slow and unco-ordinated one, aimed at specific needs as they were perceived. The Society, nevertheless, carefully reviewed prospective consolidation of public health legislation, and on several occasions succeeded in obtaining strengthening clauses prior to the passage of the acts. The Society's role in state intervention for public health becomes clearer, however, through a consideration of some of the specific subjects which engaged their attention from 1870 to 1900.

REGISTRATION AND NOTIFICATION OF DISEASE

Medical officers of health quite early in their history recognized the widespread need for accurate statistics on both sickness and causes of death. Many local acts throughout England requiring compulsory notification of disease originated under pressures from local medical officers of health. It was not until 1899 that notification of disease was finally made compulsory throughout England and Wales. Many years before this concluding step, however, medical officers of health had urged such legislation.

Together with several other medical groups, the Metropolitan Association of Medical Officers of Health petitioned the Poor Law Board in 1869 to publish sickness returns on a systematic basis.[34] Responding to a circular letter in 1874, some 300 medical officers of health again went on record as considering that the lack of periodic sickness returns constituted "a serious obstacle to the proper performance of sanitary duties."

The problem was raised repeatedly by members of the society in succeeding years at group meetings and in public addresses.[35] Dr. John Tatham (1844–1924), Medical Officer of Health for Salford in 1873 and subsequently for Manchester, was in the forefront of those who recognized the national importance of sickness statistics. Tatham was to join the General Register Office as Superintendent of Statistics in 1893.

Meanwhile, the Society of Medical Officers of Health as a group continued, unsuccessfully, to press the Local Government Board and Parliament for action.[36] The argument for compulsory notification simmered on through the eighties, confused by the diversity of opinion as to whether notification did not constitute a break in the confidential relationship between doctor and patient, as well as a lack of agreement on who had primary responsibility for notification—doctor, householder, or relative of the patient.

With the introduction of the Infectious Disease (Notification) Bill of 1889, which, if adopted by local authorities made notification by the attending medical practitioner compulsory, the Society took heart. Resolutions were passed urging that the Act require compulsory adoption by the local authorities. The Act was passed, however, without the compulsory requirement. Three years later the Society again called on the Local Government Board to extend the measure (which had then been adopted for five-sixths of the population of England and Wales) by a general act to cover the whole country. Dr. John F. J. Sykes, Secretary of the Society, in the same year urged the inclusion of additional diseases as notifiable.[37]

One of the most active physicians in the fight to make notification compulsory was Dr. Arthur Newsholme, then serving as Medical Officer of Health for Brighton. Newsholme had been interested in this subject for many years. In December 1895, in a presentation to the Royal Statistical Society, he called for a wide extension of the schedule of diseases already notifiable, the publication of weekly returns of sickness by the Registrar-General's Office, the inclusion of returns of accidents, and the periodic notification of all cases of sickness treated at the expense of public funds, charity, or Friendly Societies. "The only obstacles," concluded Newsholme, "are the *vis inertiae* of the responsible heads of Government departments and the expense that would be incurred." [38]

Notification of disease was finally made compulsory throughout England in 1899 with the passage of an Act amending the 1889 legislation. The Society of Medical Officers of Health had been in the forefront of the movement from the outset.

HOSPITAL AND ISOLATION FACILITIES

Notification of infectious illness was only one avenue of attack on a problem which disturbed most medical men in the seventies and eighties—how best to control the spread of disease. Most medical officers of health of the period were convinced that only through hospital services provided by the state could infected persons be isolated. And the medical officers of health helped to change the public attitude to the stigma of pauperization which hung over all entry into publicly supported infectious disease hospitals. They also repeatedly brought pressure upon local and central authorities to extend and improve hospital facilities for infectious disease patients.

In 1878 the Society forwarded a resolution to the Local Government Board urging that "the assistance afforded to the sick in Hospitals for

Infectious Disease and aid given for other sanitary purposes ought not to be considered pauper relief." [39] John Lambert, in replying, advised the Society that assistance given to patients in hospitals established by sanitary authorities did not constitute pauper relief, but that he could offer little hope that this provision would be extended by Parliament to those cared for in poor law hospital facilities. A bill, introduced the same year by Sir Charles Dilke, to remove disqualification or loss of voting rights through the acceptance of medical relief for infectious disease, failed to pass the House of Commons.

The subject continued to be a lively topic and frequently cropped up in annual reports of medical officers of health in the eighties. When, in 1881, the Royal Commission on Hospitals asked for the Society's views on hospital accommodation, the medical officers of health once again pressed the need for more public hospitalization for infectious disease and for its separation from poor relief. The Society also joined in a deputation to the Local Government Board in May of the same year to emphasize the necessity for removing the social stigma on those treated in infectious disease hospitals.[40]

The Diseases Prevention Act of 1883, annually renewed, together with the Medical Relief Disqualification Removal Act of 1885, supported by the Society, did away with the disqualification (for those who received only medical relief) for voting for Parliament and county and town councils. The Public Health of London Act of 1891 aimed to eliminate any further possible disqualifications, and to remove provisions for making a charge for care in isolation facilities. As late as 1910, however, Beatrice and Sidney Webb pointed out the many local variations in applying these laws.[41]

During the eighties and nineties, local medical officers of health in their annual reports continued to stress the need for extended hospital facilities. Meanwhile, the three main branches of the Society of Medical Officers of Health followed the problem carefully, reporting on the provision and effects of hospital care for infectious disease as it was required in successive local acts. Throughout the period, medical officers of health reached a high degree of unanimity on the necessity for isolation hospital facilities provided by the state.

Housing

Few facets of the drive towards state action in sanitary improvement were more controversial than the housing movement. Underlying the long campaign for better housing was the dichotomy of the old tenet that the Englishman's home was his castle, opposed to the wider, complex needs of the new industrialized society. The doughty Edwin Chadwick, still pouring forth pamphlets at the age of 85, attacked the emotion-hung "castle" argument, saying:

> The cry may be expected to be raised by the landlords of inferior tenements against such indoor inspection, that "every house is the Englishman's castle." It may be so, but it is a castle without defences against raids and slaughter greater than those of any wars by invisible enemies, the foul air diseases, against which the guards of the palace are proved to be of as little protection as any now given to the cottages, where from twenty to thirty thousand are now annually slain in the Metropolis.[42]

This was, however, an answer that took long to convince many house owners, particularly those whose "castles" were rented out to the poor at very profitable rates.

Medical officers of health encountered one of their most difficult problems in the conflict of private property rights and the menace to public health caused by improper housing facilities. Slum property brought high income, as George Bernard Shaw testified in his *Widower's Houses,* where Lickcheese, the slum agent talks of:

> Tenement houses, let from week to week by the room or half room: aye, or quarter room. It pays when you know how to work it. Nothing like it. Its been calculated on the cubic foot of space, sir, that you can get higher rents letting by the room than you can for a mansion in Park Lane.[43]

The causes of bad housing were not difficult to trace. One of the leading medical officers of health of the period, Dr. John F. J. Sykes, of St. Pancras, in delivering the Milroy Lectures on public health and housing to the Royal College of Surgeons, saw slums as the result of the extreme pressure of population, particularly in sections in the centers of the great cities. Here, the growth of commerce attracted more workers and made competition for housing sharp. The effect, said Dr. Sykes, was to drive the destitute into workhouses, the "dissolute and the necessitous into the badly built, decaying, and out-of-date areas," and "respectable" workers into tenements or rooming houses which better-class occupants had vacated. Sykes urged public demolition and reconstruction, and the building of new suburban housing with adequate transportation to urban centers.[44]

In his felicitous *Trends of Opinion About the Public Health,*

1901–51, Professor James Mackintosh, formerly Professor of Public
Health at the University of London, describes taking a short cut to the
park as a boy, on the first day of the twentieth century. His shocked
stepmother, on learning of the expedition, warned him: "These are
the slums, you must never go through them." And, continued Dr.
Mackintosh, for years afterward, he thought of the slums as a special
quarter "voluntarily inhabited by a race different from ourselves." [45]
Contemporary English novels echoed this assumption. Today, the
National Health Service, improved nutrition, and land redevelopment
are beginning to erase, in new generations, the short stature and poor
physique of England's slum dwellers. Only the accent remains as an
immediate mark of differentiation.

In the late nineteenth century, however, slum dwelling and poor
health went hand in hand. Successive investigations by the Registrar-
General's office, as well as by medical officers of health, had demonstrated that the population of city center districts was frequently subject to the highest mortality rates and to lowered resistance to disease.
Children's diseases spread quickly under conditions of overcrowding.
While modern research has confirmed the nineteenth century belief
in the correlation between adverse housing and adverse health, it also
emphasizes the extent of the psychological effects of poor housing, as
well as the inextricability of poverty, sickness, and poor housing.[46]

That there was a constant housing problem in the years 1871–1900
and that it was a continuing menace to public health was unquestion-
able. The increasingly prosperous Victorian towns and cities drew
more and more inhabitants to their already distended living quarters,
while country districts suffered from dilapidated cottages with bad
drainage and ventilation.

At best it would have been difficult for the supply of housing to
meet the demand. Builders throughout the nineteenth century faced
high costs; many went bankrupt and few made fortunes. The rents
which workingmen could afford to pay were low. Consequently, those
working-class houses which were erected were not infrequently jerry-
built. Even in the last decade of the nineteenth century, when very
considerable building took place in England, the supply of housing
could not provide for the greatly increased city populations.[47]

That the state should intervene to solve the housing problem in the
nineteenth century was very debatable. Even regulations which local
and central government authorities had established were sidestepped
or ignored in innumerable instances. Some medical officers of health

undoubtedly acquiesced to such situations. Dr. Cornelius Fox (1839–
1922), an Essex medical officer of health, in 1884, quoted a colleague,
with whom he had discussed the requirements under the Public Health
Act of 1875 for closing cottages unfit for human habitation. "I am not
such a fool," said Fox's brother medical officer of health. "Why, every
cottage in my district belongs to the Squire, who, with his family are
my best patients, and whom I could not afford to offend!" [48]

Despite such economic hazards, which were particularly significant
for part-time medical officers of health, many, in their annual reports,
repeatedly included recommendations for the improvement of housing.
Dr. William Duncan of Liverpool inveighed again and again at the
evils of cellar dwellings. George Buchanan, as Medical Officer of
Health for St. Giles, London, commented as early as 1857 on the problem of the housing of the poor:

> When I look at which the effect would be of erecting such insti-
> tutions on a sufficient scale adapted to the wants of all classes, and
> becoming popular even amongst the lowest; when I am convinced
> that the houses might be made to pay well, and that disease and
> pauperism would decline with their prosperity; when I know that
> the laws against overcrowding could then be exercised without
> scruple, and that from that moment some hundreds of lives would
> be annually preserved—with all these convictions, I feel it my duty
> to raise the question at whatever risk of being thought wild and
> utopian. [49]

Three obvious factors underlay the continuing housing problem:
first, that houses decay and require repair and modification to meet
changing standards; second, that a certain amount of demolition and
replanning is necessary; and third, that new houses must be built to
meet the needs of growing populations. [50] The government had acted
to meet some of these needs well before 1870. Under the benevolent
inspiration of Lord Shaftesbury, the first legislation in 1851 authorized
local authorities to erect dwellings for the working classes. The Torrens
Act of 1868 was designed for the demolition of condemned dwellings.
It gave local authorities power to take possession (with compensation)
of such buildings and made provision for improving dwellings of artisans and laborers. The comprehensive Richard Assheton Cross Acts of
1875 and 1879 armed municipal authorities with powers to demolish
and reconstruct large insanitary areas, and to own and rent their newly
constructed houses.

Despite these positive steps, by the eighteen-seventies great latitude still existed in local building regulations, and even new housing was often poorly constructed, ventilated, and drained. The Local Government Board's feeble inspection powers had little effect on the correction of housing evils. Even with the additional information available in the annual reports of medical officers of health, the Board lacked the power to force local authorities to correct housing defects.

In this setting, what role in housing reform did the Society of Medical Officers of Health assume? They were unanimous on the need for better construction of new houses in London and surrounding areas. Together with the Charity Organization Society, they formally urged the Home Office, through an 1870 memorandum, to take steps to ensure better construction of new houses. "Whole streets," the Society pointed out, "have been built on a foundation composed of street sweepings, refuse from factories, old buildings and many objectional matters." To add to the problem, materials used had sometimes been saturated with the effluvia of slaughterhouses and cesspools, while the construction of the buildings interfered with good light and ventilation.[51]

It was another matter, however, to take a united stand on the thorny question of government coercion to improve existing houses or to build new ones for the poorer classes. And the Society could not agree on a united course of action on this subject. At one meeting, where the suggestion was advanced that the government should buy from landlords, at a fair price, unfit working class homes and then make them habitable, a Holborn Medical Officer of Health denounced the idea as a step toward Communism![52] Even such competent medical officers of health as John Tatham of Salford and James Vinen of Bermondsey showed reluctance to urge too much state intervention to improve the housing of the poor lest "unlimited assistance" to the lower classes relieve them from practicing habits of thrift and industry. Wrote Dr. Tatham in 1876:

> Insofar as by imposing upon property owners the necessity of providing decent and healthy habitations for their tenants, we place health and comfort within reach of the poor—we as a sanitary authority do well. But when we go further than this, and compel landlords to atone for the filth and slothfulness of their tenants, we, *pro tanto,* encourage habits of indolence and filth in a class of people previously prone to such faults by nature.[53]

By 1877, improvement schemes under the authority of the Artizans and Labourers Dwellings Improvement Act had been commenced in

Liverpool, Nottingham, Swansea, and Birmingham. The advances under this and earlier acts, together with the housing improvement schemes subsidized by private philanthropy, offered just that measure of improvement to enable opponents of further state intervention to suggest that no further advances were necessary.[54] Vigorously rebutting such arguments the following year, G. W. Child, M.D., Medical Officer of Health for Oxfordshire, demanded further government action with the words: "The *deus ex machina* which must intervene is the Legislature of the Country" to cure the "social cancer" of bad housing.[55]

Despite the diversity of views on the extent of the central government's role in the improvement of housing, the Society of Medical Officers of Health maintained a fairly constant official interest in the over-all problem. In April 1879, they drew up and dispatched to the Local Government Board a draft code of sanitary regulations for lodging houses.[56] The Society also, that year, supported the Artizans-Dwellings Act Extension Bill, simultaneously proposing some amendments of which the Bill's parliamentary sponsor, William Torrens, approved. However, the Society's records make no mention of any group action with respect to the significant Housing of the Working Classes Act of 1885, which empowered rural sanitary authorities to provide housing for rural laborers and to adopt the Labouring Classes Lodging Houses Acts. A number of members of the Society testified that year before the Royal Commission on the Housing of the Working Classes, and a majority pointed out to the Commission that existing legislative enactments to improve housing were insufficiently applied in their respective districts.[57] Among the Royal Commission's recommendations were two directly related to medical officers of health— that they be required to serve full-time and to be resident within a mile of the district to which they were appointed.

The establishment of the Society's official organ, *Public Health,* in May 1888 furnished a new medium for reporting their proceedings and for articles and editorials on the various legislative bills affecting the public health. By September, this journal was commenting favorably on a Local Government Board investigation on back-to-back housing.[58]

By the late eighties and nineties, quite broad-scale housing improvements had been undertaken, both in urban and rural areas. In 1890, Parliament passed another Housing of the Working Classes Act, an important piece of amending and consolidating legislation directed primarily against urban slums. This Act strengthened the authority of medical officers of health by making it mandatory for the local authority to take action after the medical officer advised them that any property was unfit for human habitation.

The Society's Council watched the passage of this legislation closely, and submitted to the bill's sponsors a number of amendments designed to make the Act more practical. Following adoption of the Act, regional branches of the Society met to discuss interpretations of their responsibilities under the legislation.

At its Annual Provincial Meeting in October, 1891, the Society decided to petition the Local Government Board for new housing legislation which would prohibit the erection of back-to-back houses, require a separate backyard and water closet for every new house, and prescribe a minimum width for front and back streets.[59] In Manchester alone, in 1885, there were still 10,000 such dwellings.[60]

Throughout the nineties, the Society (now the Incorporated Society) continued to observe various aspects of the housing problem, reflecting an interest which individual medical officers throughout the country were manifesting in their annual reports and in letters to the major medical journals. *Public Health* frequently carried lead editorials on working-class housing, and at least two presidential addresses to the Society's branches dealt with this problem.[61]

In April of 1900 an editorial in *Public Health* attacked the Housing of the Working Classes Bill of that year. This Bill proposed compulsory acquisition of land by a local authority at a price pegged to the tax assessment, and *Public Health* viewed it as "an admirable example of what may be expected when those who have nothing to lose gain the power to legislate in their own class at the expense of those who are blessed with worldly possessions." [62]

Sorting through the thirty-year chronicle of activities on housing, it is patent that medical officers of health were alive to the general need for housing improvements, and that both individually and in group association they raised the question in its many-sided forms for public attention. Although there was no consensus within the Society that central government financing for demolition and building was the best approach, a number of medical officers of health favored such measures. The Society recurringly attempted to bring to the government's notice the need for better building regulations. As a professional group, medical officers of health did not play a major political part in the passage of some of the earlier housing acts. Individual members of the Society, expert in the field, testified, however, before investigating commissions in favor of legislative action. The Society's first concern was in the improvement of urban slum housing, but in the nineties they also agitated for improvements in rural housing.[63]

By 1900 much additional public and private action to improve housing was still called for, and medical officers of health could safely concur with the words of their President, Dr. J. S. Tew: "we are still a long way from a simple and satisfactory solution of the query, how to provide at rents in proportion to the rate of earnings decent accommodation for the working classes. . . ." [64]

INDUSTRIAL HEALTH AND HYGIENE

The spectacular growth of industries in nineteen-century England spawned a variety of new health hazards, both for the worker and the community. Early foundations of industrial hygiene had been developed late in the seventeeenth century by the Italian physician, Bernardino Ramazzini (1633–1714), and published in his famed *Treatise on the Diseases of Artisans*.[65] Throughout the eighteenth century, Ramazzini's successors gradually extended the store of information on dangers to workers employed in industrial trades.

England's first factory act passed in 1802, The Health and Morals of Apprentices Act, started a long series of laws extending government regulatory protection to special groups of industrial workers: to children and young persons (1802 and 1819), to women (1844), and to workers in special industries. At first, such protection was limited to textile workers, but was gradually extended to workers in other trades.[66]

Meanwhile, a series of scientific investigations into dangerous trades had been carried on by the Medical Office of the Privy Council. Under John Simon's direction, Dr. Edward Greenhow * and others had made important studies which widened the existing knowledge on the subject and provided excellent fodder for the social reformers. The Factories and Workshops Act (1867) consolidated and extended the protection available to workers, including those in establishments employing under fifty people.

By 1870, a considerable area of central government intervention existed in statutes for regulating hours of work, sanitary conditions

---

* Dr. Edward H. Greenhow (1814–1888), M.D., Aberdeen; Lecturer on Public Health St. Thomas' Hospital, 1855; Physician to the Middlesex Hospital, 1870; served on several Royal Commissions and prepared a number of parliamentary reports including, "On the Prevalence and Causes of Diarrhoea in Certain Towns," and "The Excessive Mortality of Young Children Among Manufacturing Populations." (*Dictionary of National Biography*, XXIII, 81.)

of work, and numbers permitted to work in a specific area, and for setting forth special requirements in dangerous trades.

Enforcing such legislation throughout the country was another matter. Not until 1833 had any provision been made for the appointment of paid, full-time factory inspectors. The first four factory inspectors appointed by the Home Office, together with their assistants were, with one exception, laymen not medical men. By 1872, some 110,424 workplaces were being regularly surveyed by the factory inspection staff.[67] But the supervision of cleanliness, ventilation, and prevention of disease in factories was generally left to the local authority or the medical officer of health.

Where industries were strongly localized, the medical officer of health at times could identify the relation between the industry and its effect upon the workers' health.[68] Dr. Sidney Barwise and his successor as Blackburn's Medical Officer of Health, Dr. James Wheatley, pointed out the effects on health of temperature, humidity, and dust from cotton and size in the weaving sheds. Sanitary improvements in Blackburn's factories subsequently helped to make death rates among weavers up to age 55 considerably lower than those of any other cotton group.[69] Sheffield's Medical Officer of Health focused on the hazards to health among handfile-cutters and in the grinding trades.

Those reports of local medical officers of health published as addenda to the Local Government Board's annual reports over the period 1872 to 1900, however, contain relatively few references to the health of the industrial worker. Some attention was given to the need for eradicating industrial nuisances, such as noxious gases and pollution of streams, which affected the health of the whole community. But in Durham's white lead smelting factories where, until prohibited in 1898, the hazardous filling and emptying of stoves was performed by young women who succumbed by the hundreds to lead poisoning,[70] the medical officer of health in the nineties either ignored all industrial health, or merely noted that no reports were included on conditions in factories and workshops.[71] It is undoubtedly true that many of the abuses suffered by industrial workers were not personally observed by many local medical officers of health, because inspection of the larger congregations of workers was simply left to the nonmedical factory inspectors.

As a group, it was only sporadically in the seventies and eighties that the Society of Medical Officers of Health devoted any attention to problems of industrial hygiene. Dr. John Syer Bristowe, M.D., F.R.S., former Medical Officer of Health for Camberwell, spoke on industrial diseases at the International Health Exhibition of 1884, discussing at length the effects of lead, copper, and arsenic poisoning, on phthisis in connection with sedentary work, on defective ventilation, and on the spread of infectious fevers in connection with certain industries. He did not, however, advance any suggestions for broader state regulatory mechanisms. The major paper on "Health in the Workshop," which did recommend extended controls, was presented not by a physician but by Mr. J. B. Lakeman, Her Majesty's Senior Metropolitan Inspector of Factories.

Similarly, the Society did not concern itself with the passage of some of the major legislation extending protection to the health of workers in industry—the Act of 1878, the Act of 1889 (Regulation of Cotton Cloth Factories), and the Factories and Workshops Act of 1891.

After the passage of the 1891 Act, *Public Health* reported some discussion at the Birmingham and Midlands Branch, on whether the legislation would increase the workload of the medical officer of health. The members noted that it was impossible, with the press of other duties, for the medical officers of health to inspect every workshop in a city like Birmingham. And the President of the Branch observed that, although Parliament's intention in giving power to two authorities was that one should check the other, the usual result was for neither to act, while if both set to work a row might ensue.[72]

As the nineties progressed, however, medical officers of health were increasingly drawn into problems of industrial health. The rising political power of the trade unions made the industrial worker a figure of greater importance in the community, and his problems of more widespread interest. A House of Lords Committee on the Sweating System publicized some working-class difficulties, and the important research studies of the Fabian Society, using new tools of social science, drew increasingly wider audience. The curricula of the recently founded College of State Medicine, and other teaching bodies dealing with public health, began to include industrial medicine and hygiene.

The Factories and Workshops Act (1895), which tightened regulations concerning temperature and overcrowding of workrooms and required notification by attending physicians to the Chief Inspector of Factories of cases of anthrax, and of lead, arsenic, and phosphorus poisoning, was a significant advance. The Society of Medical Officers of Health submitted a number of amendments to the Home Secretary, after the bill had been introduced in Parliament, including a clause to provide for a thorough ventilation of workshops during time allowed for employees' meals. After final passage of the Act, however, the Medical Officer of Health for the Strand District, Dr. Francis J. Allan, complained bitterly about its complications and the unsatisfactory double authority to be exerted by factory inspector and sanitary official alike.[73]

The appointment in 1896 of a medical officer of health, Dr. Benjamin A. Whitelegge,* as Chief Inspector of Factories, led the Society's journal to publish a leading article which reviewed, with satisfaction, the recent growth of powers of medical officers of health in respect to factory supervision.[74]

As the new century approached, the Society displayed an ever increasing interest in the regulation of industrial hygiene. It expressed satisfaction with the Report of the Departmental Committee Appointed to Enquire Into the Conditions of Work in Wool Sorting and Kindred Trades (1897). It bestowed compliments on the valuable and detailed work of the new Lady Inspectors of Factories and on notices of new regulations for the protection of factory workers as they were issued by the Home Office, and, in 1898, reminded sanitary authorities of their duties with respect to providing sufficient and suitable sanitary conveniences in factories and workshops. In 1900, when the final report of the four-year Departmental Committee Appointed to Inquire Into and Report Upon Certain Miscellaneous Dangerous Trades was issued, *Public Health* acclaimed the Committee's work.[75]

Although a few medical officers of health involved themselves as individuals in problems of industrial health and hygiene, the field was only beginning to concern the Society as a whole in the final years of the nineteenth century. The kindling of public interest in the fate of the industrial worker, together with an extension and clarification of duties of medical officers of health under the Factories and Workshops Act (1895), opened for the Society new perspectives on factory hygiene as it affected the worker's health. The Society did not, however, play any major role in influencing special legislation on industrial hygiene being passed towards the end of the century.

* Sir Benjamin Arthur Whitelegge, M.D., D.P.H., M.R.C.S., F.R.C.P., (1852–1933), Medical Superintendent of the St. Pancras Smallpox Sanitorium and the Sheffield Fever Hospital, M.O.H. for Nottingham (1884–1899), and for the West Riding of Yorkshire (1889–1896); Chief Inspector of Factories, Home Office, 1896; Member, Royal Commission on Arsenical Poisoning, 1901; author of *Hygiene and Public Health* (1890); C.B.E. 1902; K.C.B. 1911. (*Lives of the Fellows of the Royal College of Physicians of London, Munk's Roll,* IV (1955) 407–408.)

INDUSTRIAL NUISANCES

In the wake of the industrial revolution there had trailed over England a new, self-generating stream of nuisances—noxious effluvia from manufacturing processes, streams and rivers polluted by industrial waste products, and air corrupted by acrid clouds of smoke. As the country became aware of these increasing afflictions, local authorities and, finally, Parliament enacted a variety of nuisance removal acts.

The early medical officers of health frequently pleaded for greater control of such nuisances. In the late fifties a committee of the newly established Metropolitan Association of Medical Officers of Health explored some of the current nuisances arising from trade, together with their effect on health. And by 1870, much had been legally accomplished to bring industrial nuisances under state control—through nuisance statutes, smoke abatement acts, and general sanitary statutes. The broad-scale Public Health Act of 1875 was also one of the pillars of smoke control.

The Society of Medical Officers of Health during the period 1870 to 1900 did not as a national group exercise any significant influence in the elimination of industrial nuisances. Examples can be found of the occasional continuing interest of individual medical officers of health in the field. Dr. Henry Letheby * presented a paper on the subject before the Society in 1875. The Medical Officer of Health for Leeds, Dr. George Goldie, noted in his annual report for 1876 that: "A great amount of labour is yearly incurred in looking after the many public complaints coming to us, respecting the effluvium arising from many of those [offensive] trades, and it is by such public report that we are enabled to prevail upon the owners of works to adopt every possible practicable means to abate the nuisance." [76]

The Northwestern Association of Medical Officers of Health in January 1879, petitioned the Local Government Board to amend and extend the Alkali Acts "for the further mitigation of the injury to health and other evils resulting from noxious vapours." [77] Again, in 1884 and 1885, the Council of the Society petitioned the Metropolitan Board of Works for public protection against offensive effluvia from brick-burning. No reply was recorded, however, upon either occasion.[78]

* Henry Letheby (1816–1876), M.B. (London), Ph.D., Technological Chemist; Lecturer in Chemistry at the London Hospital; Chief Examiner of Gas for London under the Board of Trade; principal treatise: *Food, Its Varieties, Chemical Composition,* etc. (London, 1870).

While industrial nuisances were, nevertheless, gradually coming under control, even in the nineties there were still many complaints, particularly about smoke nuisances, which local authorities often ignored.[79] As individuals, medical officers of health were often involved in the problem. Indeed in 1896, Dr. William Graham, medical officer of health for the Borough of Middleton, suggested to the Society's Northwestern Branch that smoke nuisance duties of the medical officers of health had grown so heavy that they should be shifted to the factory inspectors or other authority.[80]

Much had been done to eliminate offensive industrial smells, however, by the close of the century. Dr. John Dixon, Medical Officer of Health for Bermondsey (at that time a district with a reputation for displeasing odors), delivered a presidential address on the subject to the Metropolitan Branch in 1899. Recalling the climate fifty years earlier, Dr. Dixon spoke with pride of the reduction of smells arising from such industrial processes as those involving bone-boiling, the leather trade, the production of artificial manure, fur-pulling, and jam-making.

Although *Public Health* in the nineties commented from time to time on industrial nuisances, the Society of Medical Officers of Health did not rouse itself to any vigorous action against industrial nuisances. In part, the problem was one of enforcement of legislation existing during the period 1870 to 1900, rather than one requiring major new statutes. That England by the close of the century had not found any final answer to successful enforcement of industrial nuisance statutes comes as no surprise to the dweller in a mid-twentieth century city. His air polluted by acrid fumes from factories and car exhausts, his rivers clogging with detergents, his soil and soil produce endangered by fertilizers and DDT, he may even view his nineteenth-century predecessor as fortunate.

THE SANITARY CONTROL OF FOOD AND DRUGS

Adulteration of food and drugs for profit was not uncommon in the last half of the nineteenth century, despite central and local regulations and sporadic prosecution of offenders. The Adulteration of Food Act of 1860 set up penalties for adulteration, and authorized the appointment of public analysts by local authorities. The Adulteration of Foods, Drinks and Drugs Act of 1872 made the appointment of local public analysts and inspectors compulsory.

While the prevention of adulteration fell within the general province of the medical officer of health, the sanitary inspectors and public analysts usually had more direct responsibility. In November of 1872, Dr. Henry Letheby, on behalf of the Association of Medical Officers of Health, forwarded to James Stansfeld at the Local Government Board a list of suggestions for the effective working of the Adulteration Act of 1872, together with the hope that provisions of the Act would be "strictly enforced" by the Board.[81] But after this one, fruitless effort, the Society during the rest of the seventies and eighties paid little attention to the subject. Indeed, their minutes are almost devoid of any mention of adulteration.

In 1889, the Society's journal, in commenting on the nineteenth annual report of the Local Government Board, noted that as a whole the acts governing the sale of food and drugs were not well administered throughout England. The fines were usually most inadequate, and butter and milk were frequently adulterated.[82]

The energetic Dr. Alfred Bostock Hill, Professor of Hygiene and Public Health at Birmingham University and several times a medical officer of health, was one of the few members of the Society in the nineties seriously concerned with adulteration. In September, 1893, Bostock Hill gave a major address before the Society, entitled "Food Adulteration and its Influence on Health." He pointed out that medical officers of health had neglected the subject, and that there was a great need for their using their influence against adulteration. The discussion which ensued endorsed Bostock Hill's views.[83] But in the years immediately following, the Society took little action on the subject beyond the routine reporting in the pages of *Public Health* of prosecutions of violators of the Food and Drug Act. In May 1897, *Public Health* reviewed, but took no stand on, a parliamentary bill based on a recommendation of the Report of the Select Committee Appointed to Inquire into the Workings of the Margarine Act (1887) and the Sale of Food and Drugs Act (1875).[84]

Dr. Bostock Hill, several times during 1899, drew the Society's attention to the hazards of adulteration and persuaded them in May of that year to support before Parliament a series of strengthening amendments to the Sale of Food and Drugs Bill then pending.[85]

Meanwhile, from time to time, the Society had been concerned with other sanitary aspects of food, particularly the supply of milk. They supported legislation in 1876 for the regulation of London's dairies and cowsheds.[86] Again in 1878, 1880, and 1881, they urged the Local

Government Board to bring legislation before Parliament permitting local sanitary authorities to make bylaws for the regulation of milk supply.[87] By 1886, the Society's Council, after lengthy correspondence with members throughout the country, had drafted a code for the regulation of dairies, cowsheds, and milk shops in nonmetropolitan districts. In the nineties, in keeping with the growing concern with tuberculosis, tubercular meat began to attract the attention of the Society. Its Northwestern Branch in 1892 and 1893 advocated condemnation of all meat in which tubercle could be discerned.[88]

From an over-all viewpoint, however, the Society of Medical Officers of Health paid relatively little attention to the sanitary control of food and drugs from the seventies to the nineties. Largely under the influence of Dr. Alfred Bostock Hill, the Society then showed a little more interest in this field, and finally bestirred itself to action on the major Act of 1899.

Expanding Concepts of Public Health and Extended Co-operation with Government Departments

While the broad range of subjects falling under the term "public health" makes enumeration of all the Society's activities from 1870 to 1900 unfeasible, it is possible to perceive a change and widening of its program in the nineties. The research papers presented at meetings of the Society and its branches in the seventies emphasized general community sanitation, the question of pollution of water supplies, and the reduction of epidemic disease. As the nineteenth century drew near its close, medical officers of health became more concerned with the curative aspects of medicine, with the new science of bacteriology, and with the development of the personal health services.

The Society investigated the possibility of setting up a national laboratory for the study of bacteriology and other experimental methods of investigation.[89] Infant mortality and the reduction of deaths of mothers were repeatedly discussed at branch meetings in relation to the duties of medical officers of health and the potential role of government facilities.[90] The Society's Council petitioned the Local Government Board to amend the Public Health of London Act of 1891 so as to include puerperal fever, and sought to strengthen the Midwives Registration Bill of 1900 to afford greater protection against unqualified midwives.

The prevention of tuberculosis also began to occupy medical officers of health, starting from an interest in the infective properties of tubercle in meat. The work of the two Royal Commissions on Tuberculosis in the nineties was aided by testimony from a series of medical officers of health, and two outstanding medical officers of health, Dr. Shirley Murphy and Dr. Thomas Legge served with the Commissions. Dr. Legge, who in 1898 was to be appointed her Majesty's first Medical Inspector of Factories, served as Secretary of the Royal Commission on Tuberculosis from 1896 to 1898. Another leader in the campaign against phthisis was Dr. James Niven, medical officer of health for Manchester.

A Committee on Tuberculosis of the Society of Medical Officers of Health sat from 1898 to 1899, and their report was subsequently adopted by the Society. This committee recommended that the decision to make phthisis notifiable should be left to local option. But they favored giving powers to local authorities to pay fees for voluntary notification of phthisis cases. The committee also suggested that all sanitary legislation which had an important bearing on the prevention of phthisis should be brought up to date.

The Society also extended its activities relating to the health of school children. Alfred Bostock Hill devoted an 1888 presidential address to this subject, suggesting the need for frequent medical inspection of both the children and the sanitary arrangements in schools.[91] School inspection was to become a lively topic in the nineties, and some medical officers of health commented that they increasingly were carrying out personal inspections of school children on a regular basis, sometimes in the schools, sometimes even house-to-house.[92] In May 1898, the Society's Metropolitan Branch drew up a memorandum to the London School Board urging that the Board co-operate with medical officers of health in preventing the spread of infectious diseases in schools.

One phase of personal health with which the Society was not heavily involved from 1870 to 1900 was venereal disease. True, in the early seventies, the Metropolitan Association of Medical Officers of Health had supported the very advanced idea of extending the Contagious Diseases Acts to the civilian population. Even John Simon recognized that insurmountable difficulties would ensue if such compulsory medical examinations of women, albeit prostitutes, were carried out throughout the whole country. Following their early resolutions of 1870 and 1872, medical officers of health dropped the thorny subject, and it appeared only very infrequently in the Society's minutes.[93]

The Contagious Diseases Acts were suspended in 1883 and finally repealed in 1886 as a result of the national campaign led by James Stansfeld and Mrs. Josephine Butler. Meanwhile, syphilis and its frightful consequences continued to spread unchecked, with no method of treatment except the dangerous mercury products. Wasserman's diagnostic method of 1906 and Erlich's discovery of Salvarsan in 1910 for the first time in history were to offer some hope for overcoming this insidious destroyer of lives.

In May of 1897, however, Dr. Reginald Dudfield, Editor of the Society's monthly journal, *Public Health,* penned an alarmed editorial entitled, "Shall Syphilis Become Pandemic?" The occasion was the publication of the report of a departmental Committee On the Prevalence of Venereal Disease among the British Troops in India. The figures in the Committee's report were indeed shocking. Of 70,642 men serving in India in July 1894, only 37 per cent had *not* been treated for venereal disease. Some 28 per cent had been hospitalized for syphilis. *Public Health*'s editor urged that compulsory inspections of all soldiers and of prostitutes and women loitering for the purposes of solicitation be reinstituted.[94]

Obviously, only a fraction of the work of the hundreds upon hundreds of medical men who served local communities as full-time or part-time medical officers of health is traceable in the records of their professional organization. It is clear that as a group medical officers of health in England did not advocate any wholesale, indiscriminate state intervention but attempted to meet specific public health problems as they arose.

The Society of Medical Officers of Health supported the strengthening of general sanitary legislation in the Public Health Acts of 1872 and 1875. Medical officers of health also saw the importance of compulsory notification of infectious disease, government provision of isolation facilities, and a strong public vaccination program.

While recognizing the need for better construction of dwellings, the Society of Medical Officers of Health did not agree on the need for government financing of working-class housing. Its members did advocate legislation for a national building code for housing and strongly opposed the construction of back-to-back housing.

Until the nineties the Society showed only sporadic interest in industrial health. And while expressing some concern with both industrial nuisances and the adulteration of foods and drugs, medical officers of health did not initiate any major moves to eradicate these problems.

Toward the close of the century the Society, moving with the times, began to give new emphasis to maternal and infant mortality, to school health services, and the control of tuberculosis. Members also began to consider seriously in the eighties and nineties the application to public health of the new science of bacteriology.

The Society's role may fairly be summed up as a constructive voice in the extension of government health services. Never a radical reforming organ, the Society was rather a pragmatic professional body which, in some of the more important phases of its work, attempted to extend the degree of control exercised by the central government, in order to attain a broader definition of "Public Health."

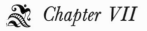 *Chapter VII*

Auxiliary Central Government Medical Organization

IN ADDITION to those medical officers who practiced within the general framework of local government, there existed certain other groups of government-employed medical men, notably Army, Navy, and Colonial Service doctors, Certifying Factory Surgeons, and medical appointees on the General Medical Council. Their work was carried out apart from the mainstream of public health within England and Wales, and was not primarily related to the growth of state intervention. A survey of the role of the government-employed physician, however, would not be complete without some mention of these medical services. In some respects their functions paralleled developments in other branches of public health.

The Army, Navy, and Colonial Service Medical Departments

British military medical services made many contributions to civilian medicine. As Sir Henry Acland reminded students of the Army Medical School in 1887, Army hospital construction and administration, Army sanitation, and Army medical experience "under every sun" had been shared with civil England.[1]

Those great reforms within Army medical care, which had followed upon the public exposure of the tragic conditions of medical treatment in the Crimean War, were a turning point in sanitary history. It had been a bitter lesson for the British public to learn that the majority of deaths in the Crimea resulted not from battle but from preventable disease, and the facts were skillfully driven home by the sanitary reformers led by Florence Nightingale and Sidney Herbert.[2] From 1855, with the issue of the *Report upon the State of the Hospitals of the British Army in the Crimea and Scutari,* until 1867, with the *Memorandum of Measures Adopted for Sanitary Improvements of India,* a steady stream of government publications on the sanitary state of the Army issued from Her Majesty's Stationery Office. The private writings of Miss Nightingale and her colleagues had added new demands for military and colonial sanitary reform.

Prior to the Crimean War, the Army's medical department was almost entirely composed of a regimental organization and was without a general hospital system. The changes instituted as a result of the Crimean War improved the organization of the medical department, raised the pay of medical officers, established an Army hospital system within England for the training of Army medical officers, and set up Army medical schools at Netley and Woolwich.

During the period 1870 to 1900, annual reports of the Army Medical Service recorded relatively few changes in established routine. Periodic breakdowns of sickness and mortality statistics of Army personnel were issued, as well as health statistics on troops serving overseas and in India. From time to time special reports on hygiene were included as appendices to the annual reports, prepared by such leading military sanitarians as Dr. Edmund Parkes (1819–1876) and Dr. François de Chaumont, Professor of Hygiene at the Army Medical School. Neither the annual reports nor their appendices, however, make any substantial recommendations for expanding the British medical services in the last thirty years of the nineteenth century.

Toward the end of the century, Army Medical Service statistical tables giving reasons for rejection for military service began to be recognized as useful indices to the health of the British male. The largest number of rejections in 1898, for example, was caused by defective physical development (in height, weight, and chest measurements).[3] In commenting upon the large numbers turned away for physical unfitness, the Director-General of the Army Medical Service noted that the bulk of Englands' soldiers were drawn from the unskilled laboring class, living close to poverty all their lives.[4]

The official rate of Army rejections in the period 1893 to 1902 was one out of every three examined by the recruiting officer. At least one Army General, Sir J. Frederick Maurice, estimated that 60 per cent of men who volunteered were unfit for military service. One result of the rising interest created by the Boer War in the health of the British common man as a potential fighting unit was the appointment of an Interdepartmental Committee on Physical Deterioration. The Committee's grave report, issued in 1904, alarmed the nation's leaders over the poor health of England's population.[5]

Administrative developments within the military medical services, however, bore only indirect relation to the extension of state medical care at home. Those investigating committees which reported on Army medicine during the period were primarily concerned with the pay and conditions of service of military medical men. General correspondence in the medical journals reflects the same theme. Medical officers of the Army distinguished themselves on several occasions for their heroism during the Zulu War against Cetewayo in 1879, in the Egyptian and Sudan Wars in the eighties, in the revolt of the Transvaal Boers, 1880 to 1881, and in the Afghan Wars. An Army Medical Warrant improved the pay of Army surgeons slightly and made some reform in the system of examination for entrance as a medical officer.[6] A War Office Committee appointed to inquire into the pay, status, and conditions of service of the Army and Navy medical services reported in 1889, but made no major recommendations for the reform of the military medical services.

However, Army doctors, the War Office Committee had noted in passing, appeared to be dissatisfied with their position. They did not, as medical officers, hold full military status, promotion was slow, pay was still poor. Following the campaign in Egypt, peacetime government economies slashed hospital and medical staff budgets. Complaints of Army medical men multiplied, and it proved almost impossible to obtain new recruits from the major medical schools in England.[7]

In 1891, the President of the Royal College of Physicians, Sir Andrew Clark, M.D., F.R.S., with warm backing from the Parliamentary Bills Committee of the British Medical Association, exchanged a series of letters with the Secretary of State for War on behalf of the unhappy Army medical men. Sir Andrew, however, obtained little satisfaction from the War Office.[8]

It was not until seven years later that the War Office met some of the demands when it established a Royal Army Medical Corps, whose officers, although they could command only within the Corps, bore the same military rank and titles as other Army officers.

Army medicine in the closing years of the century still lagged behind the best civilian medicine. No dentists or specialist anesthetists were employed. Jolting horse-drawn wagons, causing great pain to the injured, were used to evacuate patients, and basic principles of sanitary practice were often ignored by the troops.[9]

The Army paid the price for its neglect during the South African campaign. Only 22,000 men were treated for injuries and accidents in the 30-month struggle, but some 74,000 were struck down by preventable enteric fever and dysentery. Constant dust, broiling sun, and flies covered the battlefields. Few facilities for purifying water were available, and the men filled their water bottles from muddy, contaminated pools and streams. Nevertheless, conditions were better than at Scutari, 40 years before, in part owing to the excellent work of the 1,800 nurses who were sent out to the base and field hospitals.[10]

The South African War forced a re-evaluation of Army medical services. Repeated complaints in news dispatches alarmed the public and led to the appointment of a Royal Commission to investigate care of the ill in the campaign. The Commission reported that the complaints on the treatment of the sick and wounded were well-founded, but that there had not been any general breakdown of medical or hospital care. They nevertheless recommended appointment of a departmental committee of experts to survey internal problems of medical service organization.[11]

The expert committee reported in 1901, recommending a comprehensive reorganization of medical training for those medical officers who were to continue in the Army, stepped-up recruitment of better qualified medical men, and further expert scrutiny of the Army's medical services.[12] The Royal Army Medical Corps was then reorganized, a School of Sanitation was opened at Aldershot, and the Army Medical School at Netley was transferred to London as the Royal Army Medical College, with improved facilities and curriculum.

British Navy medical men, on the whole, experienced fewer difficulties in the same period. Their lack of training facilities was in part met by the establishment of the first Royal Naval Medical School at Haslar Hospital in 1881. For some years to come it did not provide training comparable to that available in the Royal Army Medical Corps.[13] By 1900, the curriculum was improved, however, by the addition of courses in bacteriology, pathology, and tropical diseases, subjects in which navy surgeons had considerable clinical experience. An 1884 investigation into the training and organization of the "Sick Berth and Nursing Staff" of the Navy also led to improvements in Navy nursing training.[14] The War Office Committee of 1889 glowed happily at the "satisfactory and contented condition" of the Navy's medical service.[15]

Senior naval medical men may have been complacent about the quality of their professional standards, but few major health problems disturbed Navy medical routine. The most prevalent naval complaint in the nineteenth century was venereal disease. Until the introduction of Salvarsan, mercury was the treatment of choice and was not uniformly effective. In 1898, a primary syphilis rate of 42.41 per 1,000 prevailed among naval personnel, and 27.69 per 1,000 for secondary syphilis. This represented a decrease in primary syphilis over preceding years, but an increase in secondary syphilis. Gonorrhea prevailed at a rate of 73.87 per 1,000, and, like syphilis, was most frequently found among naval personnel stationed in China, the Southeast coast of America, and Australia.[16]

Medical officers who served the state in the colonies faced many of the problems of the medical officer of health at home—often in magnified form. Gross insanitation and infectious disease were two of the main difficulties. Widely varying conditions from area to area, however, make it almost impossible to generalize on colonial service medicine. Venereal disease was increasing rapidly in many colonies towards the end of the century, and the administration of the Contagious Diseases Acts posed many problems for colonial surgeons.[17]

The dynamic Joseph Chamberlain, as Colonial Secretary during the years 1895 to 1903, infused a new spirit into colonial medicine. Chamberlain, a Liberal reformer, had helped to clean up Birmingham as its mayor from 1873 to 1875. Now, with the assistance, from 1897 on, of Dr. Patrick Manson (1844–1922) as Medical Advisor to the Colonial Office, he encouraged the investigation of the etiology of tropical disease. Manson's brilliant student, Dr. Ronald Ross (1857–1932) linked malaria to the anopheles mosquito and subsequently traced the transmission of the disease. Manson had already shown that filariasis could be vectored by a mosquito. Now, spurred by Ross's investigations, he persuaded Chamberlain to obtain government backing to open a School of Tropical Medicine in London. Chamberlain also secured government support for a Tropical Disease Research Fund to be administered by the Royal Society.[18]

While the control of tropical disease was never to be a major problem within England and Wales, Chamberlain and Manson opened the way to a new life in England's tropical dependencies. The dramatic story of the role of many heroic colonial doctors has yet to be written.

There is relatively little in the official record of the military medical services to show that military medical personnel advocated any position with respect to the general responsibility of the state in public

health. Military settings are rarely the habitat of social reformers. Some
military sanitary work paralleled health problems which were being
encountered by the civilian populace from 1870 to 1900. The closest
point of contact between civil and military medical services came at
the end of the century in the clear-cut public recognition that the ill
health of the English people was mirrored in the physical condition of
Army volunteers. If England was to continue as a major power, the
physical well-being of the fighting man was inseparable from his
civilian background.

The General Medical Council (General Council of Medical Education and Registration)

The Medical (Registration)Act of 1858 created a new, if small, group
of medical practitioners who were to hold government status as appointees to the General Medical Council. The members of this Council, which functioned administratively as a subordinate body of the
Privy Council, included medical representatives of the medical corporations of England, Ireland, and Scotland, six nominees of the Crown,
and a President.[19] The Medical Act of 1886 was to raise the number
of Council members from 24 to 30, by adding medical men elected
directly by the registered practitioners of the United Kingdom.

The General Medical Council had been established to regulate the
qualifications of practitioners in medicine and surgery, to maintain a
Medical Register of qualified practitioners, and to publish a British
Pharmacopoeia. It also secured reciprocity of medical practice in all
parts of the United Kingdom.

Insofar as the Council was a government body for regulating the
standards of the medical profession for the protection of the public,
it was an extension of state intervention in public health. At the time
of the Council's creation, government regulation for control of medical
standards was still unacceptable to the average Englishman, and what
was brought into being by the Act of 1858 was another advisory body.[20]
In actuality, therefore, the General Medical Council made slow progress
from 1870 to 1900 in attempting to persuade medical licensing bodies
to improve their standards.[21]

Legally, if the General Medical Council did not approve of the
standard of training of one of the recognized licensing bodies, it could
appeal to the Privy Council to suspend the licensing body's right of

registration. In practice, the Council did not exercise this right of appeal. Nevertheless, contemporary observers felt that the General Medical Council did have some impact on the licensing bodies. Dr. Walter Rivington, in his expanded study of the British medical profession, pointed out that the Council through visits and recommendations greatly improved professional examinations.[22]

The Council also carefully considered all parliamentary bills which affected the professional status of medical men. It took an active share in the passage of the Medical (Amendment) Act of 1886, which strengthened Government protection for its citizens' health by making a triple qualification (in medicine, surgery, and midwifery) requisite for registration in the *Medical Register*.

The General Medical Council did not engage in much political activity with respect to other areas of state intervention in public health. From time to time, the Council passed a resolution as, for example, the one sent to the Home Secretary in 1872 urging some amendment to the laws relating to death registry.[23] In an 1889 resolution to the government, the Council stressed the need for a measure relating to the education and registration of midwives. However, when the Parliamentary Committee on the Midwives Registration Bill of 1890 requested their advice in the framing of the Bill, the General Medical Council coolly replied that this was the Government's task, not theirs.[24]

For the most part, the Council was concerned with activities within its own frame of reference (medical education and qualification) and did not take stands on general public health legislation passed by Parliament from 1870 to 1900.

Certifying Factory Surgeons and the Medical Inspectors of Factories

The office of factory surgeon was created by the Factory Act of 1844, the surgeons being appointed by the factory inspectors. From 1858, "Certifying Factory Surgeons" were required to be medical practitioners, possessing some licensing qualification which would register them under the General Medical Council.[25] The factory surgeons were not vocal as a professional group in the last half of the nineteenth century. Their work, nevertheless, made some contribution to the extension of government regulation of industry for protection of the workers' health.

Primarily serving in part-time appointments, factory surgeons' duties were limited to reporting serious accidents to the factory inspectors, examining children and young persons for fitness to work, and periodically inspecting persons employed in dangerous trades. Their fees, paid usually on a contract from the factory owner, were small; often, the medical examination was perfunctory. Reports on accidents were paid for by the Home Office on a set scale. The factory surgeon was further handicapped by the lack of any authority to order re-examination.[26]

Certifying factory surgeons, nevertheless, exercised some general influence for the better health of the industrial worker. Robert Baker, the one early factory inspector who had had training as a surgeon, praised their work on several occasions. In 1868, he went so far as to say that "as a body they are unequalled by any other association of medical men for public purposes." [27] Baker spoke of the splendid cooperation the certifying surgeons had given him in various inquiries.

The work of some certifying surgeons must have been more than perfunctory, even in the sixties. *The Lancet,* in 1869, commented on two letters which appeared in the *Birmingham Daily Post* protesting the use of certifying surgeons in factories. The letters were no surprise, said *The Lancet's* editor, for "the manufacturing interest is so well-known to resent all interference with its supposed vested rights in human life and health. Fortunately, for humanity," *The Lancet* concluded, "the 'strength and healthy appearance' of every child under thirteen employed in a factory must be certified by a medical man." [28]

Relatively little space was given in the annual reports of the Chief Inspector of Factories to the work of some 2,000 certifying surgeons.[29] Occasionally, in referring to some specific problem of industrial health, the Chief Inspector would cite the opinion of a certifying surgeon.

Tables of accidents reported by certifying surgeons were also prepared for the Chief Inspector's report. In the nineties, the Chief Inspector began to issue over-all medical records of the numbers of children and young persons examined for employment by certifying surgeons, and, more significantly, to list the causes for rejection. In 1895 and 1896, 1.39 per cent of the applicants were rejected; in 1897, the figure was 1.27 per cent. The chief causes of failure to pass the factory surgeons' examinations were insufficient age, defective eyesight, imperfect growth, anemia, want of cleanliness, and "other medical reasons." [30]

It was not until the appointment of Dr. (later Sir) Thomas Legge *

---

* Thomas Morison Legge (1863–1932); Trinity College, Oxford; St. Bartholomew's Hospital; M.D., B. Ch. (Oxford); D.P.H.; C.B.E., 1918; knighted

as the first Medical Inspector of Factories in July 1898 that the work of the certifying surgeons was to be given more prominence. Legge's appointment followed two years after that of his brother medical man, Sir Arthur Whitelegge, K.C.B., M.D., who is credited with really integrating factory medical service with England's public health service.[31]

Dr. Legge, a man of personal charm and a deep sense of social responsibility,[32] did much to improve the health of the industrial worker. His appointment came at a time when all England was becoming aware of industrial health hazards. Under Whitelegge and Legge, a series of inquiries were initiated on lead poisoning, arsenic, phosphorous, and mercury poisonings, anthrax, and other hazards created by industrial processes. New Home Office regulations followed.

The new medical inspector rescued the reports of factory surgeons from the files, and began to quote sections in his annual report. Legge kept in close touch with the factory surgeons and channeled their findings to Whitelegge.

At the close of the nineteenth century, industrial medicine was entering a new era. The year 1899 saw the issue of the Final Report of the Departmental Committee Appointed to Inquire Into and Report Upon Certain Dangerous Trades, with its far-reaching recommendations for the protection of workers in twenty-six industries. In the same year, at the request of the Secretary of State, Professor T. E. Thorpe (F.R.S., Principal of the Government Laboratory) and Professor Thomas Oliver (M.D., F.R.S., Physician to the Royal Infirmary at Newcastle upon Tyne) had undertaken a special inquiry into the use of lead in pottery processes, and a code of rules for the health of pottery workers was drawn up. This was followed by similar inquiries into other trades. The result was a material improvement in the health of industrial workers in England and Wales.

1925. Dr. Legge's life was devoted to the advancement of preventive medicine. He served as Secretary of the Royal Commission on Tuberculosis, 1896–1898, and as Medical Inspector of Factories, 1898–1926. He published *Public Health in European Capitals,* 1896, and *Cattle Tuberculosis,* 1898, and conducted researches into the prevention of occupational lead poisoning and the prevention of industrial anthrax. See Preface to Thomas Legge, *Industrial Maladies,* ed. S. A. Henry (London: Oxford University Press, 1934), pp. vii-xiii.

Chapter VIII

The Private Practitioner and
the Role of the State, 1870-1900

OBSERVING THE attitudes of private medical practitioners to the changing role of the state in public health presents some obvious complexities. Busy with his practice, the average doctor had less time for such abstract questions than the government medical officer with his more routinely scheduled day. The private practitioner was not required to prepare periodic reports on the health of his community, nor was he always in as strategic a position to survey community needs as the government officer. He, nevertheless, had one clear advantage over the full-time state doctor: he saw daily a cross section of the British public in sickness and health and was a community source of reference for all matters pertaining to preventive and curative illness.

A portion of the private practitioner's views have been recorded in occasional essays and studies; a portion, where he was a teaching physician, in university lectures. From time to time, the private medical practitioner expressed himself for posterity at sanitary conferences, and in health and improvement societies. His thinking was in part represented (and influenced by) the medical journals of the period, and by that major professional organization, the British Medical Association. From these sources, a portion of the private practitioner's views on state intervention in matters of health may be gathered. Historically, it is not possible to ascertain how representative this material is of the body of thinking of private doctors from 1870 to 1900.

The Identity of the Private Practitioner

The varied social and professional backgrounds, from which the 20,000 to 35,000 registered medical men who practiced in the United Kingdom between 1870 and 1900 were drawn, could have fostered a variety of viewpoints on almost any issue. In 1869, a Chesterfieldian editorial in the *British Medical Journal* had concluded a summary of the aims of a young physician's training with the following advice:

> Remember that you will need for success in practice a double qualification; you must not only be a skillful doctor, but a trained gentleman. Has your early education been neglected? Improve it now. Are you conscious of any defect in manners or bearing? If possible get rid of it. Read the best books, and cultivate the society of the best companions you can get. Study the nutrition of your mind as you do that of your body, and with the most scrupulous care avoid all kinds of poison. Your character will be the outcome of what you *are,* and the possession of a sound, clear moral sense in the future will be your reward for self-restraint now.[1]

There was need, in some instances, for such advice, as the social background from which the private practitioner was drawn varied, as in any of the professions. Some, of course, were descended from a long tradition of family practice in medicine. In 1881, a popular article on the profession observed that the majority of British doctors were either sons of men of the "secondary professional classes," or of tradesmen and (especially in Scotland) of intelligent artisans.[2] It was not so many years earlier that the gap between the university-trained physician and the "apothecary-doctor" had seemed impassable.[3] Gradually, however, improved standards of medical education and qualification had lessened the old distinction.

Whatever his background, there were still in 1870 a number of ways in which a man might enter the medical profession. He might be licensed by the Colleges of Physicians and Surgeons, by the Apothecaries' Societies, or by some of the Universities.[4] The Licence of the Royal College of Physicians of London was recognized by the Local Government Board as the only qualification which enabled its holder to practice medicine, surgery, and midwifery. Other licenses were limited to either medicine or surgery, and it was not infrequent for general practitioners to take only one qualification. Higher qualifications, such as the Membership or Fellowship of the Royal College of Physicians of London, the Fellowship of the Royal College of Surgeons of England, and memberships or fellowships of the Scottish and Irish professional colleges, were obtained by examination or election. Physicians in the nineteenth century still headed the professional hierarchy, although the surgeon, throughout the eighteenth and early nineteenth centuries, had shed much of the trades status of barber-surgeon.

The Medical (Education) Act of 1858 had been a major step towards bringing some centralization and unity in the diverse standards of medical licensing. The Act, which had established the General Medical Council, gave to the Council the function of maintaining a *Medical Register* to admit the qualified and remove from its lists those considered unworthy to practice.[5] As admittance to the *Register* was gained merely by presenting the requisite fee together with the license of one of the authorized medical licensing bodies, the standard of medical education of the private practitioner varied greatly.

Private practitioners were, therefore, physicians and surgeons who differed considerably in their professional qualifications and attainments. In March 1868, the *British Medical Journal* published an analysis of the *Medical Register* which demonstrated that of those 20,014 practitioners who were legally entitled to practice in all branches of medicine and surgery, 3,072 were qualified only in surgery and 1,440 in medicine alone.[6] An attempt to reform this situation was made in 1870, in a Government Medical Reform Bill. This legislation was blocked, however, by the British Medical Association which, at the time, was opposed to any medical bill which did not provide for direct representation by the medical profession in the General Medical Council.[7] The situation was finally remedied by the Medical Act of 1886.

Although registration was not then essential to enable a doctor to practice his profession in the United Kingdom, there was strong reason to comply with the program. Registration was requisite before a medical practitioner could sign death or birth certificates, hold public appointment, or sue for the recovery of his fees in the courts.

The number of registered medical men increased steadily from 20,084 in 1871, to 35,651 in 1900. In proportion to the total population (of the United Kingdom and Ireland), where in 1871 there had been one registered practitioner to every 1,370 inhabitants, by 1900 the ratio had changed to every 1,144 persons.[8] This drop in ratio of patients to practitioners had a deleterious effect on the average income of the general practitioner and was in part responsible for the low fees paid to doctors by sickness and benefit societies at the end of the century.

The Relationship between the Private Practitioner and the State

By 1870, a considerable area of interdependence had developed between the medical profession and the state. Dr. Henry Rumsey described a share of the existing relationship in that year in a speech to the British Medical Association: "The State has for some time recognized the Profession as a whole, by making use of it, through public authorities, for public purposes." And he noted the work of doctors in medical relief of the destitute, in medical care to inmates of asylums and prisons, in medical services to the police, civil service, and laborers in public works, in medical care of soldiers and sailors, and finally, "by medical agency again, the State protects the children and youth of the working classes in factories, workshops and mines, where the keenly-contested race between labour and capital requires constant and vigilant supervision." [9]

Official services rendered to the state by medical men also included the work of public vaccinators, coroners, and medical witnesses. As early as 1870, *The Lancet* commented on the increase in the appointment of medical coroners and the gradual adoption by the public of the idea that the coroner's office should be held by medically qualified men.[10] The reforming *Lancet* was perhaps a little oversanguine, for, at a British Medical Association meeting in 1887, much fault was still found with the coroner system throughout the country and with the absence of medical assessors in courts, where medical evidence was given.[11] Still, by 1879, some coronerships open to medical men were paying substantial salaries ranging from £650 to £2,099.

The remuneration of medical practitioners who served as witnesses at coroner's inquests had been recognized as a necessity by the Act of 1836 (6 & 7, Will. IV. C. 89). In 1864, the submission by an eminent London physician of a handsome bill of £84, for services rendered in identifying a thirteen-year-old skeleton, spurred the Treasury and Home Office to develop a standard allowance for London physicians of ten guineas a day plus expenses.

The private practitioner also acted as an agent of the state in the registration of deaths and in the notification of infectious diseases. Legislation in the last thirty years of the nineteenth century extended his participation in these functions. As Dr. Edward Fox was to observe in his 1894 Presidential Address to the British Medical Association, "the need of medical guidance is permeating more or less every branch of the public service." [12] It was clearly apparent that the state and the doctor were increasingly linked together in the expanding society.

Views of the Individual Private Practitioner
on the State's Role in Health

The British Medical Association, as spokesman for the profession, exerted many and diverse pressures for the extension of government health services. Quite apart from such organized influence, many private practitioners, as individuals, evidenced a serious interest in health reform.

THE EDUCATION OF PUBLIC OPINION

Long before 1870, medical men recognized the need for educating public opinion before government reforms could be instituted. Simon had believed that if England's sanitary reform was to be effected, "the educational onward impulses may be expected to come pretty continuously from members of the Medical Profession and from few others."[13]

It was logical to expect future "educational onward impulses" to come from within the profession. The past work of men like Neil Arnott and John Roberton, friends of the London working classes, and John Ferriar, Thomas Percival, and James Kay-Shuttleworth in Manchester, had sounded some of the first public challenges for state action in sanitary reform. Occasionally, private practitioners, like Southwood Smith, had been absorbed into state medical work, and devoted their lives to the extension of legislation for the protection of the health of the public.

An immeasurable amount of public education in public health was accomplished in the years 1870 to 1900 by private practitioners. The movement for the appointment of the Royal Sanitary Commission had been led by a private physician—Dr. Henry Rumsey. Throughout the country medical men, singly or as representatives of local sanitary groups, were spurring the movement onward.

In 1871, the distinguished Regius Professor of Medicine at Oxford, Dr. Henry W. Acland, delivered a thoughtful and stirring address to the Royal College of Physicians, which was widely reported in the medical and lay press. Its subject was national health, which Dr. Acland defined as "that condition of the individuals of the nation which enables [them] to discharge rightly their respective functions." He noted that the country was rapidly accepting the belief that *prevention* of sickness was a more rational and "sacred" duty than its *cure*.

But Dr. Acland also observed that England still needed to become more familiar with this proposition, and called on the medical profession to show the way.[14]

Acland envisaged a dynamic central health authority which would keep in close touch with the needs of the people. He believed that the state must assist the masses "in what they were unable to do for themselves," and that compulsion of the ignorant in sanitary matters was justifiable, until it was made unnecessary by scientific education.[15]

The speech recognized clearly what Sir George Newman, Chief Medical Officer of the Ministry of Health, was to confirm years later—that an enlightened public opinion was one of the foundations for winning the assent of the community to sanitary government.[16]

Much of the educative influence brought to bear by the private practitioner took place within the doctor-patient relationship. The daily press offered another medium of propaganda, and from time to time, medical men made use of the newspapers to arouse the public against more blatant sanitary evils.

A large degree of medical sanitary education was channeled through such powerful organizations as the National Health Society, the Public Health Section of the National Association for the Promotion of Social Science, and the British Association for the Advancement of Science.[17] Many doctors not engaged in government medical service, as well as some who were, participated actively in the work of these national bodies.

The *Transactions of the National Association for the Promotion of Social Science,* and occasionally the reports of the British Association for the Advancement of Science, contain a variety of papers by private practitioners, as well as by medical officers of health, emphasizing the need for guiding the public toward better standards of health.[18]

Often such education was carried out by simple speeches in the poorest London neighborhoods on such topics as "How to Keep the Home Healthy" and "Cleanliness," as well as by special lectures to more educated, drawing room audiences on "Sick Nursing," "Ambulance," and "Hygiene." [19] The chairmanship of the National Health Society's Public Health Section, which sponsored such activities, was held for many years by a series of distinguished medical sanitary leaders.

Local medical practitioners also served as advisers to the Ladies Sanitary Association, which distributed a variety of sanitary tracts among the lower, middle, and working classes throughout the seventies and eighties. One of the most effective local organizations for educating the public to a wider conception of public health was the Manchester and Salford Sanitary Association. Arthur Ransome, M.D., F.R.S., Lecturer on Public Health at Owens College, was one of the leaders of this Association, which flooded the Manchester area with pamphlets on such basic subjects as "Facts about the Skin," "Causes of Preventable Disease," and "The Teeth and How to Preserve Them."

Still another channel for sanitary educative work were the regional sanitary conferences convened sporadically throughout the last thirty years of the century. The most notable took place in 1875 when Joseph Chamberlain, as Mayor of Birmingham, invited 1,140 persons to the Birmingham Sanitary Conference. Some 700 accepted Chamberlain's summons to the meeting, which aimed to arouse the public to the importance of sanitary questions. The forceful Mayor, who envisaged Birmingham as the Metropolis of the Midlands, had determined that: "In twelve months by God's help the town shall not know itself." The city was to undergo a major sanitary revolution during Chamberlain's term of office.[20]

The private practitioner, by participating as a technical and personal leader in the sanitary educative movement, was steadily helping to formulate new standards of public health. The movement, diffuse and undirected as it was, embraced the education both of the public and its local authorities. But medical practitioners were increasingly realizing, as well, that more than education was needed; central direction had become essential in the complex and evolving industrial society.

PROPOSALS FOR A STATE HEALTH SERVICE

The utilitarian advantages of a central Ministry of Health, spelled out by Bentham as early as 1820,[21] had been reiterated by medical men in succeeding years. During the period 1870 to 1900, plans for a state medical service were advanced from time to time by medical practitioners both within and without the government service. John Simon and medical men testifying before the Royal Sanitary Commission had advocated a more extensive national health organization than eventually evolved in the Local Government Board. Dr. Henry Wyldbore Rumsey, writing just previous to the period of discussion, developed plans for a state medical service on an insurance basis in his *Essays on State Medicine*. In 1874, Dr. Thomas Grimshaw submitted a proposal to the British Association for the Advancement of Science, calling for a reorganization of sanitary administrative areas and a complete executive authority in sanitary government which could exercise constant supervision.[22]

More attention was attracted to the ideas advanced by the distinguished hygienist and friend of Chadwick, Dr. Benjamin Ward Richardson.* Speaking to the Social Science Association's Health Section in the fall of 1875, Richardson outlined a utopian city of health, "Hygeia," with sanitary controls from birth to death. This sanitarian's paradise was to be spotlessly clean, superbly ventilated, and splendidly sunlit. An ardent temperance man, Richardson permitted no alcohol or tobacco in "Hygeia." Disease, in the absence of filth, magically disappeared, and the death rate plummeted to 5 per 1,000. Prevention was the theme and control the means.[23] The speech was published as a pamphlet the following year and was widely quoted in newspapers in England and abroad. In his subsequent address, *Ministry of Health,* Richardson called for a strong central health ministry in England to serve as a model for underdeveloped nations.[24]

Another London physician, Sir Morell Mackenzie (1837–1892), who maintained a lucrative practice as a throat specialist, proposed a State Department of Medicine, with state-paid medical officers available to, but not compulsory for, the public.[25] Mackenzie is far better remembered, however, for his controversial book, *Frederick the Noble,* named for the Emperor of Germany, upon whom he operated for cancer of the larynx.

There were other private medical men who, like Mackenzie, advanced the idea of a state medical service, but who did little to make it a reality in this period. In 1889, J. Brindley James, M.R.C.S., a former President of the West Kent Medico-Chirurgical Society, called for a civil medical service of the Crown, the creation of two medical peers, and a nonpolitical Cabinet Minister of Public Health.[26] In 1895, the Local Government Board took note of an article written one year

* Benjamin Ward Richardson (1828–1896), M.A., M.D. (St. Andrew's), F.R.C.P., F.R.S., qualified as a physician in Scotland and set up practice in London in 1854. He lectured at the Grosvenor Place School of Medicine from 1854 to 1856, and became physician to the Royal Hospital for Diseases of the Chest (then the Royal Infirmary for Asthma) in 1856. Richardson was the founder (1855) of the short-lived *Sanitary Review and Journal of Public Health,* as well as a second journal *Social Science Review and Journal of the Sciences.* He took a leading part in the sanitary movement, writing and lecturing widely on popular health topics. Richardson invented a useful chloroform inhaler, and was knighted in 1893 for his humanitarian and scientific accomplishments.

earlier in *Macmillan's Magazine* by George Mahomed, M.R.C.S., entitled the "State and the Doctor." Mahomed advocated the formation
of a state medical service with uniform standards of entrance.[27]

Proposals like these for state medical services were not numerous,
but they indicated that some private practitioners were thinking in
terms of general state action in curative medicine for a wider section
of the population than was covered by the poor law.

One scheme proposed for state curative medical services which attracted considerable publicity in the eighties and nineties [28] was the
Rentoul Plan, named after its originator, Dr. Robert Rentoul, who
advocated a public medical service for the benefit of a portion of the
wage-earning class. Two departments were to be set up under the Rentoul Plan, one to dispense treatment for the payment of a small cash
fee, and the other, to be managed on a provident basis, with payments
made during health. Dr. Rentoul's primary aim was a reform of the
flagrant abuses in the out-patient services of medical charities. He also
believed such a state system would eliminate "counter-prescribing" by
chemists (druggists) and would reduce abuses in medical clubs for the
working class.[29]

The voluminous correspondence pro and con that developed with
respect to the plan, was so heavy that the *British Medical Journal* in
November of 1889 announced its intention of publishing the letters
in abstract, presenting only the main lines of argument used by the
correspondents. Local branches of the British Medical Association
throughout the country considered the Rentoul Plan at branch meetings. Many labeled the proposals impractical, but felt some investigation of medical charity abuse was necessary. Others feared that such a
government body would only help to reduce the fees paid for medical
service generally.[30] In the autumn of 1889, a British Medical Association Committee investigated the Rentoul Plan, and in the spring of
1890 twenty-two local branches voted on it. A clear majority rejected
the scheme as impracticable, unnecessary, and undesirable.[31]

Although the Rentoul Plan had as its main purpose the elimination
of abuse from the medical charity system (a purpose with which the
British Medical Association's Council was most sympathetic), it nevertheless depended on state intervention in an area of curative medicine
which heretofore had been available only to the destitute. Despite this
rejection, the Rentoul Plan had stirred medical thinking about the
role of the state in curative medicine. The professional organization
of medical men was not willing, however, at this time to accept a "State

Department of Curative Medicine" (for other than the destitute), which might act in competition with their professional interests.

THE MEDICAL JOURNAL AND THE SANITARY MOVEMENT

England's two leading medical journals, *The Lancet* and the *British Medical Journal*, both influenced and reflected the thinking of private practitioners on the state's role in health. Other professional medical journals, like the *Medical Times and Gazette*, the *Medical Press and Circular*, and the monthly *Practitioner*, were less directly concerned, on the whole, with the legislative and political aspects of medicine, and also had more limited circulations.[32]

Both *The Lancet* and the *British Medical Journal* regularly published abstracts of, and editorials on, major parliamentary actions or reports dealing with health matters, and the correspondence columns of the two journals served as a forum for the private practitioner when he wished to air his views. Few general conclusions can be drawn from such correspondence, however sporadic, which cannot be assumed to be necessarily representative of the private practitioner at large.

The most vocal organ of the British Medical Association was, of course, the *British Medical Journal*. For almost the whole of this period (1867–1898) the *Journal* was edited by Dr. Ernest Hart, a courageous medical journalist, sincerely humanitarian in his views. Hart may have been looked upon askance by some medical men—as the historian of the British Medical Association claimed.[33] But, in the dual role of editor of the journal and Chairman of the Association's Parliamentary Bills Committee for many years, he was a highly influential figure. Under Hart, the thoughtful editorials of the *British Medical Journal* were alive to the basic conflict between *laissez faire* and that developing body of thought which urged:

> Let the community recognize that it has a corporate duty towards the most unfortunate—towards the crippled combattants who are helpless . . . in the struggle with the strong. Let it apply the great power of its corporate wealth and corporate organizing power to make life at least tolerably human for those who, if left to their individual energies would go under, to our harm as well as their own.[34]

As the years went by, Hart expanded and improved the *Journal's* coverage, indirectly making history in medical journalism and attracting an ever-widening audience of medical men.

A close second in circulation was *The Lancet,* long the voice of the Wakleys, father and sons. *The Lancet* had a long history of pleading for state action in many areas of public health. The repeated commissions of investigation initiated by *The Lancet* into housing, food adulteration, factory working conditions, and the distress of the poor in London, were designed to publicize conditions in need of reform. The forceful language of the Wakley editorials again and again urged the private practitioner to take note of public health problems ripe for state intervention. At times, *The Lancet* despaired at the apathy of the government and the public, rasping bitterly: "The future historian will record with wonder that the men of the Victorian age would meet, and write, and agitate, and petition in order to save one murderer from the gallows, while at the same time they suffered honest citizens to die like rotten sheep rather than pass a law to prevent the dealers in drinking-water to adulterate it with sewage." [35]

When the central government's health functions were merged in the Local Government Board in 1872, *The Lancet* observed that in the prevention of disease, "the Government must exercise for the people a paternal function." *The Lancet* recommended concentrating all sanitary powers in the hands of a cabinet minister who would supervise the entire health of the nation. "Recognizing the great principle that the people ought to be the best interpreters of their own wants, and not treated like children in the old feudal days, immediate legislation must also ascertain what they cannot do for themselves; secure them the clean dwellings they require, give them fuel, air, water and unadulterated food." [36] In the same vein, when the Disraeli Government failed in 1875 to substantiate their campaign promises for strong health measures, *The Lancet* was sharply critical.[37]

As media for the dissemination of sanitary statistics, as active supporters of sanitary legislation and centrally directed government action in many areas of public health, the leading medical journals were a constant guide to the private practitioner.

Organized Medical Pressure for Central Government Action

LOCAL MEDICAL SOCIETIES AND GROUPS

Local medical societies in the years 1870 to 1900 were surprisingly apolitical and unconcerned with broader issues of state intervention in health. Primarily preoccupied with local medical problems, they also served as media for the exchange of professional information and for promoting professional-social interests of their members. *The Proceedings and Transactions of the London Medical Society,* for example, are chiefly a record of special medical case histories in this period. A few of the Society's annual orations dealt with topics hinging on the practitioner's role in the society in which he lived. Records of the London Medical Society, however, show little concern with political or administrative problems of state medicine.

Medical reformers in the eighteen-forties and fifties had found support within the local medical societies for medico-political questions. Provincial society meetings, as reported in the medical journals, displayed more regard in these earlier years for questions of sanitary reform and improvement of poor law medical care. But even the Manchester Medical Society, which in the late thirties and forties had agitated for the reform of the poor law, in subsequent years was little involved in political aspects of public health.[38]

The correspondence files of the Local Government Board, nevertheless, contain scattered instances of pressure brought to bear by local medical societies upon the central government. Petitions for a systematic inspection of schools were sent to the Board in 1879 by the Sheffield-Medico-Chirurgical Society and the Northumberland and Durham Medical Society and, in 1880, by the York Medical Society.[39] A group of eighteen medical practitioners of Kingston on Thames in May of 1888 petitioned the Local Government Board on a pending Infectious Diseases Notification Bill.[40] From time to time, the medically directed Manchester and Salford Sanitary Association also sent memorandums to the Board on central sanitary legislation.

Toward the close of the nineties, a number of local medical guilds were formed. These new professional medical groups were formed partly because of the difficulties associated with contract or club practice, and partly because some practitioners believed that the British Medical Association paid insufficient attention to medico-political and medico-ethical matters. One of the earliest of the new guilds, the Manchester Medical Guild, founded in 1895, discussed such topics as the abuse of medical charities, club practice, and the promotion of the teaching of ethics in medical schools.[41] In April, 1896, they supported a parliamentary bill on the registration and training of midwives, and in 1899 considered the Vaccination Bill.

The new guilds did not, however, take any major role in national health affairs in the closing years of the century. An attempt was made to organize the guilds in May, 1900, when Dr. Samuel Crawshaw of Ashton under Lyne convened a conference of guild members and general practitioners. Crawshaw, supported by the eminent surgeon Victor Horsley at this meeting, had hoped the prospective organization of guilds might become an alternate (and more effective) group to the British Medical Association. Delegates to the conference, however, passed a series of resolutions which recognized that the general practitioner would be better off aiming for reforms within the British Medical Association to make it more representative of, and politically responsive to, the general practitioner than by setting up a new organization.[42]

For the most part, local medical societies and the guilds seemed content to leave such problems as the state's role in health to the British Medical Association. While records of provincial societies' meetings show occasional discussion of a national aspect of public health, it was with relative infrequency that local groups brought direct pressure upon the government.

THE BRITISH MEDICAL ASSOCIATION

The organization which claimed the right from 1870 to 1900 to speak for the medical profession at large was, of course, the British Medical Association. Undoubtedly, the parliamentary influence the Association was able to command, as the profession's spokesman, was considerable.

In actuality, the Association was not wholly representative of the private practitioner. In 1871, 4,403 medical practitioners in England and Wales were members of the Association, a figure which represented only about 28 per cent of the total registered medical practitioners throughout the country. Within the counties of England and Wales, representation in the British Medical Association varied considerably from as high as 63 per cent in Cumberland to only 13 per cent in Essex.[43]

Membership in the Association had increased fairly steadily from the original 310 who had joined in the founding year (1832), to 1,300 by 1842, and 2,000 by 1865. By 1900, membership totalled 18,000.[44] It is not possible, however, to identify the proportion of members engaged only in private practice, and those employed in government service.

The Association was attacked upon a number of occasions by the independent medical journals for not being broadly representative of medical men. The *Medical Times and Gazette,* which unsuccessfully sought a general practitioners' association, called the British Medical Association "a club of London physicians and surgeons, who once a year visit and patronize their professional friends in the country." [45] Similarly, an editorial in *The Doctor* snarled at the organization "which professes so much and does so little." Claiming it was only repeating complaints of hundreds of members, *The Doctor* protested the monopolizing of the Association's offices by a few: "This open defiance of public opinion is covered by a plausible system of representation, which enables the office-holders to stick to their posts, and to manage the elections, as completely as if they had been carefully trained under French prefects in the worst times of the Empire." [46]

A degree of professional rivalry can be read into the statements of these two journals. It was also inevitable that the Association should be London-controlled, since the busy schedules of provincial doctors precluded frequent travel to London meetings.

Whatever criticisms may be levied at the British Medical Association, the organization was the only national medical group in continuous existence during the period of discussion which could claim to represent the private practitioner, and whose representatives met, treated with, and brought pressure to bear upon government officials and Parliament.

The work of the Association had become so extensive and diversified by the last thirty years of the nineteenth century that its historians, Ernest Little in 1932 and Paul Vaughan in 1959, have only attempted to touch upon it. It is manifestly unfeasible within the limitations of structure and organization of the present study to essay any exhaustive treatment of the political pressures which the Association brought to bear on the numerous public health measures of the period. However, a sampling of its general attitudes towards the state's role in health, together with a glance at some activities of the Association's Parliamentary Bills Committee, may help to capture the flavor of the period.

General Attitudes of the Association to the State's Role in Health. From the time of its founding in 1832 as the Provincial Medical and Surgical Association, the British Medical Association took a lively interest in sanitary reform and the care of the sick poor. As early as 1837, a major committee of the Association had recommended the appointment of a central poor law medical Board to which all poor law medical officers could report. *British Medical Journal* editorials in the early years frequently voiced sharp demands for sanitary reform.

In delivering the Annual Address on Medicine to the Association's

Council in 1872, Dr. Samuel Wilks of Guy's Hospital surveyed the
expanding role of the doctor and called upon medical men to "aim at
a very high standard, nothing less than the improvement and welfare
of the material nature of man." [47] Leaving aside the problem of medicine and the spirit, it is still doubtful if the Council of the British
Medical Association would have adopted this frame of reference *in
totidem verbis* as its political program. Nevertheless, the over-all scope
of its political interests in succeeding years was not too far removed
from this collectivist aim.

As the Association viewed itself, rather fondly, through the eyes of
the editor of the *British Medical Journal* in 1873, it was seen:

> as the greatest and most powerful Association existing in connec-
> tion with any profession in any part of the world; its widely rami-
> fying and yet compact organization, its true and amply representa-
> tive character, its unselfish efforts for great public objects, its zeal
> for the promotion of public health, for the advancement of the
> interests of the public services, for the diffusion and improvement
> of education, for the maintenance of brotherly feeling and of high
> ethical aims; its watchful and intelligent supervision of sanitary
> and medical legislation; its continuous diffusion of scientific
> knowledge, were made apparent in the face of the world.[48]

Certainly, the British Medical Association was zealous in promoting
many measures which invoked further state control in public health,
and certainly, the organization maintained a "watchful and intelligent
supervision" of sanitary and medical legislation.

Ernest Little, in compiling the Association's first history, made a fair
generalization of its program, which is also largely descriptive of its
efforts during the years 1870 to 1900. Little saw the Association as
aiming to advance knowledge on the incidence, cause, prevention, and
cure of disease, providing adequate health services for the whole community "irrespective of individual economic circumstances, by methods
adjusted to the needs of different groups," and promoting progressive
standards of efficiency in medical and ancillary services.[49]

The British Medical Association never formulated a rigid and permanently applicable conception of the central government's role in
public health. In the years immediately prior to 1870, the Association
had fought for the appointment of the Royal Sanitary Commission and
had supported a plan for a strong central health department. To the
eclipse of the Medical Department in the Local Government Board
by the lay management, the Association had responded with steady

censure. Yet it recognized the need for primary local action and never viewed all sanitary reform as the province of a central department.

The Parliamentary Bills Committee. In 1863, with a dawning consciousness of its political role in public health legislation, the British Medical Association set up a Parliamentary Bills Committee. The Committee's function was to review legislation and serve as a liaison with the government on matters affecting the public health and professional interests. The Committee did a sound job and framed many good amendments to bills on public health, which were incorporated in the final acts.

The Parliamentary Bills Committee, which was chaired by Ernest Hart from 1872 to 1897, made known its views within Parliament largely through three men: Sir Lyon Playfair, Sir B. Walter Foster (later Lord Ilkeston) and Sir Robert Farquharson. Foster and Farquharson were qualified medical men. Foster, who had served as Physician to the Birmingham General Hospital, became Liberal M.P. for Chester in 1885 and was quickly recognized in Parliament as an expert on medical matters. Sir Robert Farquharson, who had served in the Army Medical Service and subsequently as a dermatologist at St. Mary's Hospital, London, held office as a Liberal M.P. from 1880 to 1896. Farquharson was also familiar with medical problems of the poor. In writing of his experiences at St. Mary's, he described the six years as a depressing task, "seeing crowds of physical waifs and strays of life, with chronic coughs and dyspepsias, and rheumatisms—half-starved people whose appetites we stimulated with tonics, but whose vacant stomachs we could not hope to fill." [50] Sir Robert subsequently chaired the Parliamentary Bills Committee from 1897 to 1900.

In the readily available pages of the *British Medical Journal* Ernest Hart gave full publicity to the work of the Parliamentary Bills Committee. Hart saw to it that detailed reports of the Committee's discussions were issued immediately after each meeting. The *Journal*'s regular "Medico-Parliamentary" section also provided abstracts of actual discussions in the House of Commons on medical affairs.

The Committee's work spanned the whole program of national sanitary reform in the years from 1870 to 1900. To detail its pressures and manipulations on each piece of legislation is manifestly impossible here, but it is interesting to sample and summarize a report Hart wrote for the year 1871: successful opposition to a Coroner's Bill which threatened to deprive physicians of post-mortem fees; support for a bill for restraint of habitual drunkards and for a measure requiring the registration of baby-farming; prolonged consideration of poor law medical care; support for the consolidating public health Act of 1871; discussions on the Pharmacy Acts Amendment Bill, on the Vaccination Acts Amendment Bills, and Irish poor law medical procedures. In concluding, Hart urged all members of the medical profession to communicate freely with the Committee on measures introduced into the legislature affecting individual or professional interests.[51]

Under Hart, the Parliamentary Bills Committee operated as a thriving political pressure group. But even under the more restrained chairmanship of Farquharson, Hart's successor, the Committee continued to be a powerful spokesman for the Association. A review of the subjects of their activities for 1900 shows the broadening scope both of their interests and of public health itself: the Factory and Workshops Act Amendment Bill; lead poisoning; child labor in mines; vivisection; model milk clauses; poppy cultivation in India; food adulteration; the Lunacy Bill; military hospitals in South Africa; the Army Medical Corps; and many other subjects.

The Committee not only attempted to influence public health legislation which had already been introduced into the House, but collected information and statistical material to persuade members of the government that further legislation was necessary.

This scientific approach to the reform of the public health was characteristic of the Association's efforts even before 1900, and their history was distinguished by a number of special reports compiled by investigating committees. A series of excellent studies on provincial workhouse infirmaries, carried out in 1896 by the British Medical Association, stimulated the Local Government Board's attention to reforms in provincial infirmaries.[52] The new interest in the health of industrial workers, evident in the nineties, was reflected in a Parliamentary Bills Committee investigation into the mortality of women and children employed in factories.

At its 1889 annual meeting, the Association appointed a committee to investigate the state of development and brain power of school children and to bring the results of the investigation to the attention of government education authorities. This committee's reports were widely discussed and were to lead to further investigations, in which the Association was joined by other philanthropic and scientific groups.[53]

The whole area of medical care for the poorer classes was under discussion in the late eighties and nineties, and Medical Attendance

Committees of the Association canvassed the subject. In 1887, one of these Committees recommended that future medical attendance on the poorer classes should be conducted on an insurance basis.

British Medical Association efforts in the reform of medical qualifications had first met success in the passage of the Medical Act of 1858. The Association's continuing struggle to improve and reform the Act of 1858 was finally rewarded in the Medical Act of 1886.

There is obviously no method by which the work of the British Medical Association on behalf of the private practitioner and all medical men throughout the country may be condensed to capsule size and weighed for its significance in the national scale of public health reform. In many areas, the Association was in advance of public opinion, and acted as a leader in community efforts to prevent sickness and alleviate the sufferings of those whom the social machine discarded as physically unfit for immediate use. It is true that the Association acted as a professional group for the welfare of its members. But the wider purposes of serving the community was repeatedly demonstrated in investigating public health abuses, through fostering scientific investigations, and by bringing collective pressure to bear upon the Government to pass necessary health legislation.

At no time did private practitioners, en masse, subscribe to any unified policy on the role of the state in public health. Yet increasingly, in their professional functioning, medical men were being drawn into a closer relationship with government activities and the corporate working of society. It would have been difficult for the private practitioner, who was so often a community source of reference, to stand apart from the sanitary movement of the seventies and eighties. Much of his reforming effort was channeled towards educating public opinion and was expressed in those local and national groups dealing with sanitary reform.

A few far-seeing private practitioners proffered plans for a state health service, the most notable being that proposed by Dr. Robert Rentoul. But medical reaction to such plans did not indicate that the profession at large was ready to concede so great an extension of the central government's role in curative medicine.

The medical journals, acting as media for the dissemination of information on state action, and themselves supporting government intervention in many areas of health, guided the views of the private practitioner. Relatively little pressure for reform came from local professional medical societies. Nor did the new medical guilds of the last decade of the nineteenth century exercise a major role in the public health movement.

In the efforts of the British Medical Association, the only medical group in existence during the period which could claim to represent the private practitioner, medical influence for national health reform was exerted on a systematic and broad scale. The work of the Parliamentary Bills Committee, directed so energetically by Ernest Hart, spanned the whole area of public health in its continuing pressure for central government action. The Association, by its own acknowledgment (and in fact) maintained an intelligent and watchful supervision over all medical and sanitary legislation, and initiated broad-scale investigations into public health evils. Their contribution to the development of collective measures on a national scale for improving the health of the people of England and Wales is a substantial one.

As the century drew to its close, medical men were increasingly aware that fast-moving social and economic changes had brought new definitions of the role of the doctor and of medicine in society. The wise and timely speech of Dr. A. M. Williams, delivered at the Association's annual meeting in 1895, recognized that the great social changes were neither temporary nor casual, and called upon medical men "to ensure that proposed changes and reforms in our professional and public relations shall be steps in advance and not retrograde in respect of the interests either of the profession or the community." For, concluded Dr. Williams, such interests "can in fact never be antagonistic, but must advance or recede together." [54]

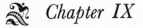 *Chapter IX*

New Patterns of
State Medicine

By 1900 insistent economic, social, and political pressures were moving the English people inexorably towards a more collective and co-operative organization of the state. Those comfortable, protecting watchwords of Victorian solidarity—duty, property rights, and traditional authority—even in their heyday had been underlain by an uneasy prescience of the vast potential of the working classes as a social force. By the turn of the century, this force had pushed its way to the political surface. The changing patterns of state medicine evolving in the personal health services during the first decade of the twentieth century were closely linked to the new concepts of a national society.

The Socio-Economic and Political Background

Economically, during the period 1830–1880, the status of the laboring classes had improved considerably. Individual incomes had expanded, and the prices of primary articles of consumption had declined. Working-class education had been improved, the working-class death rate decreased, and life made physically less hazardous and more comfortable by the steady sanitary improvements. But the gap between rich and poor was still very great, and unemployment caused by fluctuations in the world market had serious effects. The march of urbanization had created many unsolved housing problems of which the lower income groups were most forcibly aware.

The voluntary organization of the laboring classes in the trade unions, however, was gradually to force a redefinition of social policy. The development of the trade union movement had political manifestations in the general elections of the eighties. By 1888 county councils had begun to feel the local influence of trade unions.[1] Towards the end of the eighties, new unions like the Mining Federation, the United Textile Factory Worker's Association, and the General Labourer's Union had already altered the atmosphere of the staid Trade Union Congress. The favorable results of the dock and gas workers strikes in London during 1889 had opened the way to an enrollment of general laborers in the trade union movement, and swelled the political potential of the working class.[2]

By 1895 the trade union movement had become sufficiently powerful to assemble the delegates of a million workers at the annual congresses. Total union membership was now estimated at one-fifth of the entire working population of adult males.[3] The early labor leaders like Thomas Burt and Alexander MacDonald had been elected to Parliament under the auspices of the Liberal Party. Henry Broadhurst, who took his seat in 1880 from the potteries district, also had had Liberal Party support. But in 1892, labor entered the national political arena in its own right when Keir Hardie, John Burns, and J. Havelock Wilson were elected to Parliament as Independent Labor Party candidates. Although none of the Party's twenty-eight candidates who ran for office in 1895 was successful, the new party was to gain strength in succeeding years. Largely as a result of the Taff-Vale decision, which threatened the position of all British trade unions, Labour Party candidates after 1901 began to win by-elections.

The Liberal Party recognized the writing on the wall, only too clearly. If they were to survive, they must make certain of the votes of the laboring classes. There was no alternative but Bismarck's method —social legislation as a bribe and pacifier.[4] The challenge had to be met if the working classes, now rising to political power, were not to extend state intervention still further for their own protection, and at too great a cost to their former masters.

The legislative intervention which followed constituted no startling innovation. It had been building slowly in many areas throughout the nineteenth century. The trend towards centralization had been reinforced toward the close of the century by the creation of larger units of local government and the transfer to county councils of an authority hitherto in the hands of ad hoc bodies. The Education Act of 1902 made public funds available to ensure properly paid teachers and a national standard of public education. Legislation in 1897 brought the Workmen's Compensation Act. The Factory Acts were also consolidated and extended to protect special categories of laborers.

The whole question of land tenure had come anew under scrutiny with the Land Tenure Reform Association in the seventies, and as a result of the wide interest roused by Henry George's *Progress and Poverty* in 1879 and Alfred Russel Wallace's *Land Nationalization* in 1882. In the same year, the Trade Union Congress had passed a resolution in favor of nationalization of the land, while Henry Broadhurst, doggedly appearing in the well accoutered Westminster assemblage in clothes tailored by his wife, had ventilated the grievances of leaseholders before Parliament.[5]

Gradually the old authority of land ownership was being sapped by the demand for greater social justice in the living and working conditions of the British people. At the same time, the problem of urbanization had forced upon the nation the realization that the government's responsibility in directing the use of land could not be ignored. By 1909 the Town Planning Act put further control into the hands of experts.

Eight years previous to the passage of the Town Planning Act, the increasing expenditures on national services for the public welfare had also led to the appointment of a Royal Commission on Local Taxation to consider the distribution of taxation between national and local authorities. No immediate solution to relieve the situation in which local authorities found themselves was arrived at by the Commissioners, however, who, as *The Times* remarked, were "all the more impressed with the extreme difficulty of arriving at any conclusions that can be applied in practice." [6]

The first decade of the twentieth century was clearly a period of considerable flux, in which the government's role was undergoing political revision in many directions to meet the social and economic needs of the larger society of twentieth century England. The immediate cause for this reconsideration of social policy had been the working-class rise to political expression of their needs. Private charity would no longer satisfy the laboring classes, and the cessation of the endeavors of the National Association for the Promotion of Social Science was one of the manifestations of middle-class failure to solve the problems of industrialization.

Scientific Investigation into Conditions of Life

The critical light of scientific investigation, which had been scrutinizing society during the last twenty years of the nineteenth century, greatly facilitated social legislation. Without the necessary analytic and statistical background amassed by the social reformers, public support for further regulatory legislation would have been far more difficult to obtain.

A basic concern with the individual in society underlay the corporate development of state control. But the development of statistical methods, permitting the quantification of masses of social observations, helped to clarify the individual's needs in an industrial society. Sanitary reformers would have been powerless without that background of statistics prepared by William Farr, Florence Nightingale, and their associates.

Statistics and quantitative measurement in England from the eighteen-thirties had led to an awareness of the relation of bad environment to health. Statistics in the last thirty years of the nineteenth century were to lay bare the conditions of work of factory employees, were to vindicate the campaign against disease, to indicate the urgent need for coming to grips with the social problem of longevity and an aging population, and to open the way to further public health legislation.

One of the landmarks of the new investigations into the social scene was that undertaken by Charles Booth (1840–1916) and his associates into laboring conditions in London—an inquiry which occupied seventeen years and seventeen volumes. Booth, the son of a Liverpool corn merchant, had had a successful career as a London shipowner, and after middle life established himself as an authority on social problems. The *Life and Labour of the People in London* was a detailed and vivid description of social and economic conditions in the metropolis in the last part of the nineteenth century. Masses upon masses of statistics added up to a shocking exposure of conditions of life in London districts. Booth's team of investigators included Beatrice Potter (Webb), Sir Graham Balfour, and Ernest Aves.

As Beatrice Webb noted, "In comparison with the preceding generations of social researchers [Booth's] method of analysis constitutes if not the starting point, certainly the first sign post," in the new sociological science.[7] The study revealed through statistical tables that 30 per cent of London's inhabitants lived below a bare subsistence level.

In the early edition of his long study, Booth announced that he had, theoretically, no objections to the socialist approach of "organizing systematically the labour of those who are incapable of finding an undertaking. . . ."[8] He saw this then in the nature of a state charity, socialistic only in the sense of the poor law. The later, and more complete edition of the work, had more guarded conclusions, stressing improvement, first of all, in individual responsibility, and stating that "probably only experience can decide as to what shape collective action, whether monopolistic or not, may easily take." [9]

B. Seebohm Rowntree's 1901 study of poverty in York was also carried out with that "spirit of patient inquiry" which characterized Booth's work. Rowntree, estimating 18s. 10d. weekly as the minimum required to maintain a bare existence for a family of four, found that over 15 per cent of York's wage-earning classes lived in such "primary poverty."

By far the most extensive of the new social scientific inquiries, however, were those undertaken by the Fabian Society, and especially by those "two most remarkable people," [10] Beatrice and Sidney Webb. The Fabians, with their idealistic aim of "reconstructing society . . . in such a manner as to secure the general welfare and happiness," [11] carried out inquiries, organized research teams, and spread before the public the results of their social investigations in readable form.

The flood of Fabian pamphlets which issued from the Society at the turn of the century did not, however, reflect a specific interest in public health reform. Not until 1908 was B. L. Hutchins' "What a Health Committee Can Do" prepared, and in 1911 F. L. Dodd's, "A National Medical Service" appeared.[12] Beatrice and Sidney Webb, however, in 1910 published their *State and the Doctor,* which was based upon their researches in connection with the Poor Law Commission, and which advocated for the country a unified national health service.

Another important inquiry into social conditions was carried out in 1904 by a Privy Council-sponsored Inter-departmental Committee on Physical Deterioration. The Committee had been appointed in response to the publicity aroused over the poor physical condition of many Army recruits, particularly those enlisting for service in the Boer War.

The forceful report of the Inter-departmental Committee indicted overcrowding, atmospheric pollution, and bad conditions of employment as cardinal factors in a physical deterioration primarily confined to the poorest strata. The Committee also pointed to defective milk supplies, decrease in breast feeding, and parental ignorance and neglect. The Committee's only general remedy was a broad-scale scheme of social education to help overcome the paralyzing state of helplessness and despair among the poor. More specifically, they sweepingly proposed the establishment of an advisory council on health, public crèches under Local Government Board supervision, the extension of the service of health visiting, a more complete system of medical inspection in schools, better sanitary conditions in the schools themselves, and the provision of hot meals for school children.

Some medical testimony was taken in the course of the Committee's researches, largely from medical officers of health, school medical inspectors, and certifying factory surgeons. Dr. Eustace Smith also gave evidence on behalf of the Royal College of Physicians, chiefly on nutrition.

While it is doubtful whether much "deterioration" from earlier years of the nineteenth century had actually occurred, the report was, nevertheless, startling to the public. *The Times* characterized it as:

> a very remarkable production and one which indicates a new departure in the manner in which questions of public health are likely in future to be regarded. . . . the whole substance of its recommendations practically turns upon the necessity for improving the health of certain strata of the population by the definite application of medical science to their requirements.[13]

Throughout 1904, as the volumes of the Committee's reports were issued, medical interest ran high. *The Lancet* devoted a number of leading articles to the topic.[14] At the 1905 annual meeting of the British Medical Association, the Section on Industrial Hygiene considered the Committee's report at length. The Society of Medical Officers of Health met in January of 1905, and gave support to the Inter-departmental Committee's suggestions.[15] The *British Medical Journal* pointed out that most of the recommendations of the Inter-departmental Committee had been made in the medical press over the period of a number of years, and that the *British Medical Journal* itself had devoted a series of articles to physical deterioration.[16]

If in many ways naive with respect to the real significance of nutrition, the report of the Inter-departmental Committee on Physical Deterioration, nevertheless, contributed to the public unease about the national health. Together with the Fabian investigations, which publicized unsavory conditions of working-class life at the turn of the century, the report succeeded in highlighting the problems of society's low-income members. Increasingly, such studies showed nineteenth-century humanitarian placebos to be inadequate for the multiplying complexities of a twentieth-century society. Beatrice Webb had said of the Booth investigation that perhaps its most "noteworthy clue . . . was the irrelevance of charitable assistance, whether regarded as a good or evil influence, in determining the social environment of the common people." [17] The time had come when the whole structure of social welfare was under question; and the imminent political power of the laboring classes in their own right made the question more than theoretical.

The State and the Development
of Personal Health Services

In this new climate of social self-scrutiny, the development of personal health services as a state responsibility came at last quite naturally. The year 1907, marking passage of the Education (Administrative Provisions) Act is commonly assigned as the date for the introduction of the personal health services in England. But the shift in emphasis from the sanitary movement to collective provision of personal health services as a form of national security had, in fact, developed gradually during the last years of the nineteenth century. New vistas into conditions of mass ill-health had been opened up in the eighties and nineties by social research in such fields as tuberculosis, the high infant and maternal mortality rates, and the poor health of school children.

The step-by-step growth of the personal health services as a part of state medicine, even in the first decade of the twentieth century, is too detailed for exhaustive treatment within present limits. Topical studies published in some of the areas also make this unnecessary.[18] A survey of some of the highlights is indicated, however, as part of the background to that major step in state intervention which was to be introduced in the 1911 Insurance Act.

In a Presidential Address to the Section of State Medicine of the British Medical Association in 1907, Sir Arthur Newsholme enumerated some of the ways in which community activity had entered the field of public health. A large number of these services were concerned with the control of infectious disease: local authorities provided treatment and hospital care for some of the acute infectious diseases; the medical officer of health in many areas, in addition to inspecting "contacts," gave his services gratuitously in infective disease; many local authorities provided antitoxin in cases of diphtheria treated at home, while others sent out municipal nurses to care in the home treatment of infectious disease; facilities for bacteriological diagnosis of certain infective diseases were made available without charge by many local authorities; and free vaccination was offered to all. Fees of doctors called in by midwives under specifications of the Midwives Act of 1902 were paid by local authorities; education committees were beginning to employ school doctors; and school nurses assisted in applying remedies. Some municipal milk depots, as a part of their service, also offered free medical consultations.[19]

Newsholme, a committed advocate of the extension of public medical services, felt that free medical aid should be given to all who were in need of it.[20] He pointed out that an increasing proportion of total sickness was treated in voluntary and in state- and rate-supported institutions; and that throughout England and Wales, where, in the years 1866–1870, 8.3 per cent of total deaths had taken place in public institutions, by 1901–1903, the percentage had risen to 16.2. In London, the figure was even higher: 16.3 per cent in 1866–1870 and 34.9 per cent in 1901–1904. Newsholme saw the establishment of a complete public medical service as a natural phase in the evolution of the system.

Dr. Newsholme had suggested only some of the developments in public medicine, but even in these, trends towards a growth of personal health services could be detected. Three of the main areas up to 1910 were to be found in efforts to control tuberculosis, more especially phthisis, to check maternal and infant mortality, and to improve the health of the school child. Only after 1910 did the Local Government Board take the initiative in campaigning against venereal disease; and up to 1910 even the medical journals took little interest in the subject as a broad-scale social problem.

The personal health services evolved from the broadening concept of communal needs and functions in twentieth century society. Pressures which had pushed the problems of life of the working-class man to the fore had gradually created a public recognition that sanitation alone was not the answer to communal health. Medical and treatment services were necessary for special classes of the community who required care which they were unable to supply for themselves.

TUBERCULOSIS

More often than not the pale Victorian heroine floating wanly through the literature to sink gracefully into a decline was suffering from pulmonary tuberculosis. Far less dramatic than the epidemic diseases, tuberculosis was continually prevalent in Victorian England, with an average death rate per million of 2,116 in the decade of the seventies. Most physicians considered tuberculosis to be a hereditary, constitutional disease related in some unspecified manner to poor environment. Few hospital facilities for tuberculous patients were available, and those afflicted had little hope of cure.

The publication of Koch's research in 1882 proving the infectivity of tuberculosis, aroused new public interest in the disease. The identification of the tubercle bacillus, unlike other communicable disease, was not immediately followed by the preparation of a prophylactic vaccine. Nevertheless, by the middle eighteen-nineties some community programs of prevention and treatment were underway in England, France, and several other European countries. The United States moved more slowly towards organized community programs against the disease.[21]

In England both voluntary effort and local authority action preceded the central government in fighting tuberculosis. Prominent in rousing community interest for uniform planning of the care of tubercular patients was Dr. Robert Philip.* Philip campaigned unflaggingly for a co-ordinated tuberculosis program to include notification, provision of dispensaries, sanatoria for selected patients who might be cured, hospitals for dying patients, and residential colonies for the guidance of patients in whom the disease was latent.[22]

The National Association for the Prevention of Consumption, founded in London in 1898, also embarked upon an educational program to prevent the spread of tuberculosis. In 1904, a national committee to provide sanitoria for workers suffering from tuberculosis was established. The Charity Organization Society in the same year attempted to have more beds in public hospitals set aside for tuberculosis patients.[23]

Meanwhile, medical officers of health in populated areas throughout England were also beginning to interest themselves and their communities in the problem of tuberculosis. Newsholme in Brighton and Niven in Manchester had fostered local programs of tuberculosis prevention and care. Manchester had adopted voluntary notification of

* Sir Robert William Philip (1857–1939) matriculated at Edinburgh University, taking the M.B., C.M. in 1882 and M.D. in 1887; F.R.C.P. (Edinburgh) 1887; F.R.S. (Edinburgh) 1889; F.R.C.P. (London) 1933. He became interested in tuberculosis during a period of study in Vienna. Philip established the Royal Victoria Hospital for Consumption in 1894. He wrote extensively on the subject of tuberculosis and held the presidency both of the Royal College of Physicians of Edinburgh (1918–1923), and the British Medical Association (1927). Philip was knighted for his work in 1913.

phthisis in public institutions in 1899, and this had been extended to all medical practitioners in 1900. Liverpool instituted a similar voluntary notfication program in 1901.

Local authorities also launched a series of measures aimed at diagnosis and notification and such direct, preventive steps as laws against expectoration in public, promotion of disinfection and cleanliness, and the use of sanatoria.[24]

The organization of a series of national and international conferences on tuberculosis heightened public interest in the disease. A British Congress on Tuberculosis assembled in London in 1901 under the patronage of Edward VII. The royal backing had its traditional uses. "Thousands," commented *The Times,* "who would pass by a meeting of men of science as something too dull for their notice or too mysterious for their comprehension will have their interest and sympathy awakened by the example of His Majesty." [25]

The papers presented to the Congress stressed the person-to-person infectivity of the disease and discussed at length the need for the notification of phthisis and the public provision of sanatoria. England's medical journals carried full accounts of the Congress and supported the call for broader programs to control the disease.[26]

Other large congresses on tuberculosis were to be held in Paris in 1905, in Washington in 1908, and in London in 1909.

In August of 1901, a Royal Commission, consisting largely of distinguished pathologists, was appointed to investigate the relation of tuberculosis in animals and in man. The researches were carried out over a period of thirteen years, but as early as 1904 the Commission, in an interim report, concluded that tubercle of human origin gave rise in the bovine animal to tuberculosis identical with ordinary bovine tuberculosis. In 1907, a further report stressed the relation between the drinking of cow's milk infected with bovine tubercle bacilli and the subsequent infection of man by tuberculosis, and urged the necessity of more stringent measures being taken against the sale of tuberculous milk.[27] This Commission, throughout its long series of investigations carried out by teams of notable specialists, made important contributions to medical science.

Nevertheless, despite the publicity roused both by the work of the Royal Commission and the successive international congresses, public facilities for treating tuberculosis developed slowly. It was not until after the passage of the National (Health) Insurance Act that a Departmental Committee on Tuberculosis was appointed to organize a new tuberculosis service; and not until 1912 did the Local Government Board make all forms of tuberculosis under medical care notifiable.[28]

England's two leading medical journals prior to 1911 gave little encouragement to central government action against tuberculosis. Occasionally, the *British Medical Journal* and *The Lancet* urged the improvement of poor law care for tuberculosis patients and advocated increased charitable provision of beds for phthisis sufferers.[29] But the medical journals were cautious about advocating use of any central government funds to provide sanitoria. British delegates to the 1908 International Tuberculosis Conference in Washington stressed co-ordination between local authorities and charitable organizations, as had the medical journals.

Scotland's Local Government Board in 1906 attempted to rouse local authorities to their responsibilities regarding tuberculosis. In 1908, the Local Government Board for England and Wales issued special tuberculosis regulations for poor law care. More broadly, in the following year, England's Board urged the use of educational measures to prevent the spread of tuberculosis; they advocated bacteriological diagnosis by detection of tubercle bacilli in the sputum, and the use of well-organized tuberculosis dispensaries, particularly in large towns. The Board also pointed out that under the Public Health Act of 1875, sanitary authorities had the power to provide sanitoria treatment for patients, whether or not they received poor relief. "Considerations of finance will need to be borne in mind," continued the Board's prudent administrative memorandum, "and it is to be remembered that thoroughly efficient sanitoria for consumptives need not be built upon expensive lines. Before embarking on any large scheme, each sanitary authority should consider what it can do with arrangements already available." [30]

This significant memorandum of the Board, which *The Lancet* hailed as "the first official document which—perhaps without knowing it—foreshadows a fusion between preventive medicine and sick relief," [31] followed an investigation carried out for the Board in the previous years by Dr. H. Timbrell Bulstrode. Bulstrode had praised the effectiveness of sanitoria treatment at an early stage of tuberculosis, but felt further study was necessary before it was certain that notification of phthisis was a significant factor in reducing its prevalence.[32]

In 1911, Arthur Newsholme, as Medical Officer of the Local Government Board, reviewing the whole national problem of tuberculosis, admitted that the majority of tuberculosis cases were still not treated in

their early stages. The National (Health) Insurance Bill, with its promise of sanitoria, would if passed, Newsholme felt, help to provide for
early recognition and treatment. Every sanitary authority, Newsholme
urged, should arrange for free examination of sputa, and for training
the patient and his family in the necessary hygienic precautions.
"Above all, patients suffering from advanced disease should be treated
under sanitary conditions which are satisfactory in every respect." [33]
Within the old theme of state prevention there was now clearly linked
a responsibility to cure.

In actuality, although pulmonary tuberculosis was still the most
formidable of the endemic diseases, the national statistics for England
and Wales pointed to a steadily declining death rate for the four
decades from 1871 to 1910: 219 per 100,000 of population (1871–
1880); 178 (1881–1890); 139 (1891–1900); and 117 (1901–1910).[34] Newsholme attributed this decrease to a combination of factors favoring
increased resistance to tuberculosis—better sanitation and housing,
improved working conditions, more wholesome and abundant food
and clothing, as well as more efficient medical attendance than in the
past.

By 1910, the *British Medical Journal* was still cautious about advocating sanatoria:

> The question of sanatorium treatment, as at present conducted,
> is still in the crucible of professional opinion, and there are not
> wanting those who entirely distrust it as a final solution of the
> problem. . . . We are in no sense opponents of sanatoriums, but
> their mission is, in our opinion, educative rather than curative.[35]

Only the beginning steps toward national community responsibility
for the care of tuberculosis patients had been taken by the close of the
twentieth century's first decade. Many smaller local sanitary authorities
had done little for the control or treatment of tuberculosis.[36] The issue
of how much should be attempted on a local and how much on a
national level was inextricably bound to the problem of local vs. central funding. Further national action, however, was imminent under
the National Insurance Act.

The medical press had recognized the need for public action to control tuberculosis, but had also sounded reservations on the extent of
such service to be provided by the state. Local action joined to charitable efforts, felt the medical journals, might well be expanded before
national funds were called upon. The initiative for extending state

treatment of tuberculosis came from diversified sources in the first decade of the new century, with no major campaign undertaken by any one medical group. The Local Government Board had prodded local authorities to establish preventive and curative services for tuberculosis, but by 1910 the results of their admonitions were still tentative.

MATERNAL AND INFANT MORTALITY

Like the sanitary advances, the personal health services developed under the banner of prevention. Society's focus, however, had begun to extend beyond the environment to the individual and to social groups of special vulnerability. Infants and parturient women, recognizably more susceptible to health hazards, had stirred new public concern by the turn of the century.

The source of this community solicitude sprang from the continuing high infant mortality rates (see table). Indeed, although the general death rate had declined steadily, infant mortality had increased in the nineties to a record 1899 high of 163 per 1,000 births for children less than one year old. Any appraisal of the five-year figures from 1860 on could only be sobering and alarming—the more so because England's birth rate had fallen continuously since 1870.

TABLE 3. Infant Mortality [37]

| | Average Death Rates per 1,000 | | | | | Relative Mortality Figures (1861–1865 death rate = 100) | | | | |
| | *Age in years* | | | | | *Age in years* | | | | |
	0–1	1–2	2–3	3–4	4–5	0–1	1–2	2–3	3–4	4–5
1861–1865	155	69	37	25	18	100	100	100	100	100
1866–1870	157	63	32	22	16	102	92	88	88	90
1871–1875	154	59	28	19	14	100	86	77	76	81
1876–1880	145	58	27	17	13	94	85	74	68	74
1881–1885	139	53	23	15	12	90	78	64	60	69
1886–1890	144	53	22	14	10	93	78	61	56	58
1891–1895	151	52	21	14	10	98	76	58	56	58
1896–1900	156	49	19	13	9	101	72	53	52	50
1901–1905	138	41	16	11	8	90	60	44	44	46
1906–1908	124	37	15	9	7	80	53	41	36	40

Humanitarian roots of the infant welfare movement were linked to the early nineteenth-century legislation to protect the working child. By the late sixties public interest turned toward the protection of infants, aroused by the evils of baby-farming. Dr. J. B. Curgenven, Honorary Secretary to the Harvein Society and one of the pioneers for infant protection, brought pressure to bear on the Home Office to draw up legislation. Ernest Hart, with his characteristic reforming vigor, in 1868 joined the campaign fostered by Curgenven's new Infant Life Protection Society. Widespread public interest in the whole subject developed in 1870 over the sensational murder trials of two "baby-farmers," Margaret Waters and her sister Sarah Ellis, responsible for the deaths of a number of infants boarded in their care.

The first Infant Life Protection Act, requiring the registration of births and deaths of infants in baby-farming establishments, passed Parliament in 1872. Weaknesses of the law, however, still permitted many abuses. Following the notorious case of Mrs. Dyer, who strangled and tossed into the Thames the infants she was paid to care for, a second Infant Life Protection Act was passed in 1897. This was subsequently replaced by the Children Act of 1908.[38]

The need for providing instruction for infant care was also recognized by the nineties, and Manchester's medical officer of health, Dr. James Niven, organized a team of voluntary "health visitors" to advise mothers in their homes. In St. Pancras, Dr. John F. J. Sykes opened a school for mothers in 1907, and his example was copied in other areas of England. The French scheme of furnishing free milk to mothers also began to be copied in a number of English cities with the support of voluntary societies, as early prototypes of the infant welfare centers. All such measures assisted in lowering infant mortality.

The child welfare movement which evolved in England at the turn of the century paralleled the development in many European and American cities of stations to encourage breast feeding or to provide a safe substitute in clean milk. Such "milk stations" gradually became "well-baby clinics," providing medical care for infants and young children and instruction to mothers. In France Pierre Budin, Professor of Obstetrics at Paris, pioneered in establishing by 1892 a system of infant consultation centers, upon which many other countries modeled similar programs. By 1907 France had 497 child welfare clinics. In New York Nathan Strauss provided funds in 1893 to develop a series of milk stations which he supported until 1919. New York City, in establishing in 1908 a Division of Child Hygiene within its City Health Department, became the first city to assume community responsibility for providing a comprehensive child health program.[39]

Meanwhile, a major effort had been underway for some years in

England to curb the use of untrained, incompetent midwives. From 1876 on, the London Obstetrical Society in co-operation with the British Medical Association repeatedly attempted to persuade the Government to institute legislation requiring state registration of midwives. Several medical members of Parliament introduced a bill for this purpose in 1890. But none of the long series of such attempts was to meet success until 1902, with the passage of the Midwives Act prohibiting (as of 1910) the practice of midwifery by unregistered women.

During the twelve-year period since the introduction of the 1890 Bill, the medical profession was split in its attitude towards midwife registration. The British Medical Association and General Medical Council repeatedly urged the principle of protecting women in labor from untrained midwives.[40] Despite this, considerable professional opposition to the various bills had developed. Underlying medical objections was the fear that registration might set up an inferior but apparently state-approved, body of practitioners.[41]

The controversy simmered on throughout the nineties, despite support for a registration program given by a Select Committee on Midwives Registration of 1892, and again, the British Medical Association opposed registration bills of the nineties, as unlikely really to eliminate unqualified midwifery.

The controversial Midwives Act of 1902, as finally passed, stipulated that no woman might "habitually and for gain attend a woman in childbirth otherwise than under the direction of a qualified medical practitioner unless she be certified under the Midwives Act." [42] As first introduced, the bill contained no penalties for unqualified practice, and the British Medical Association's Council formally dispatched a memorandum to Parliament opposing the whole measure. Even when the bill was amended in Committee to provide a penalty for the *habitual* unqualified practice of midwifery, the Association refused to be placated,[43] and its *Journal* expressed irritation that the measure was able to command parliamentary support from such influential medical personages as Robert Farquharson and Sir Michael Foster, M.P. for the University of London.

The practical Dr. Farquharson, who represented West Aberdeenshire, observed in the debate, however, that he "took his stand upon the ground that it was high time that something should be done." He pointed out to the House of Commons that the General Medical Council in 1899 had resolved that the "absence of public provision of midwives was to be regarded as productive of a large amount of grave and fatal disease among the poorer classes," and noted that the Council urged upon the Government the importance of passing some measure for the education and registration of midwives. Although Dr. Farquharson did not agree with all of the provisions of this bill, he "was not one of those who refused something because they could not get everything." [44]

The Lancet, during discussion on an earlier midwives bill of 1900, conducted an opinion poll of medical men on the subject. Of 7,250 communications received, 1,547 supported the bill, 640 were indifferent and the remaining 5,000 opposed the measure. *The Lancet* felt medical opinion had changed little by 1902 and continued its opposition to the new bill with the words: "To leave the parturient poor to the mercies of the GAMPS is cruel, but to supply them with a semi-educated grade of medical attendants is no kindness. If the first could lead to disasters, the second would seem as inevitably to make for tragedies." [45]

The pragmatists settled for the possible, however, and the 1902 bill was enacted. Many of the medical fears proved to be groundless, even as the number of certified midwives increased (between 1906 and 1909, the number certified jumped from 956 to 5,934). In 1910, a Departmental Committee investigating the working of the Midwives Act of 1902 concluded that the Act was a factor in reducing the death rate from puerperal septic diseases. [46]

In the fifteen-year period which preceded 1903, the highest death rate from the puerperal septic diseases was 202 per million females living, in 1893. This had dropped to 118 in 1902, the lowest figure in this period being 109 in 1898. The Midwives Act came into operation in 1903, and in that year, the puerperal death rate dropped to 97. By 1907, it had fallen to 81. [47] Maternal mortality, nevertheless, was still high at the end of the first decade of the twentieth century.

Following the passage of the Midwives Act, however, public attention turned again to the need for reducing the high infant death rate. Sir Walter Foster, on behalf of the British Medical Association, raised the problem in Parliament in the summer of 1904. Addressing his questions, on the relation of medical out-relief to infant mortality, to the Local Government Board, Foster urged that medical relief and special foods should be made more available to the poor for their infants. Mr. Walter Long, who replied for the Local Government Board, stated (albeit equivocally), that there did not appear to be sufficient grounds for issuing a circular on this matter to Boards of Guardians. For, claimed Mr. Long, the high rate of infant mortality was largely due to improper feeding and "this was by no means confined to the children of the pauper class." [48]

Although the Local Government Board took no immediate action, the problem of infant mortality was increasingly prominent in sanitary circles and in the public eye. *The Times* published a series of articles on the subject in November 1904, commenting:

> It is, after all, as a question of morale that we are compelled, in the last resort, to consider the slaughter of the innocents which we have described, and its probable or possible consequences to the nation. This almost stationary expenditure of infant life owes much of its significance to its association with a falling birth-rate, and with the conditions which such a birth-rate implies.[49]

Almost two years later, the Local Government Board acknowledged the seriousness of the problem with a National Conference on Infantile Mortality, held at Westminster Hall. John Burns, the Board's President, opened the meeting with a call to the medical profession and the medical journals to help form a healthier public opinion. In round numbers, Burns continued, 100,000 infants died annually "from neglect, carelessness, thoughtlessness and ignorance." [50] The conference, as a whole, passed a resolution urging the Education Department to offer to senior class girls instruction in personal hygiene, diet, and on the weaning of infants.

A second National Conference on Infantile Mortality was convened in March of 1908. Again John Burns presided, and hailed the results of the first conference as exceeding "his most sanguine expectations." Local authorities all over the country had been stimulated, Burns noted, and Parliament, in passing the Notification of Births Act of 1907, also had a share in the good work.

The Notification of Births Act, requiring notification to medical officers of health of every birth within thirty-six hours, applied only to areas in which the local authority adopted the Act, with subsequent approval by the Local Government Board. Its significance in reducing infantile mortality stemmed from the fact that early notification enabled health visitors to seek out the mother and child at a time when their guidance could be most effective.[51]

This Act did not carry the blessings of the whole medical profession. Indeed, medical representatives in Parliament had attempted to persuade the House of Commons that the obligation of notifying should not be placed upon the attending physician. The *British Medical*

Journal deplored passage of the Act with the penalty clause for failure to notify within the required time, noting with rich self-pity: "It is a very unsatisfactory ending, and we fear exemplifies only too well the unsympathetic attitude which the House of Commons is ready to assume towards the medical profession." [52]

The Lancet, however, took a broader view, commenting on the utility of the measure and the fact that many physicians had urged the principle of early notification. Even *The Lancet,* however, complained of the penalty clause: "That the State should demand from a medical man what is a public duty without providing any adequate remuneration for such a service is hardly equitable." [53]

Among the major causes of infantile mortality were the diarrheal diseases. Summer diarrhea carried off thousands of infants each year, the weakest children first. Although the mid-twentieth century has bypassed the causes of such diseases, it was clear to those at the beginning years of the century that civic cleanliness campaigns aided in reducing diarrhea death tolls, and studies of the disease made in the first decade of the twentieth century emphasized the significance of domestic cleanliness in the feeding of infants.[54]

By 1909, the problem was sufficiently serious so that the Local Government Board undertook a special nationwide study of the incidence and control of the causes of infant mortality. Their conclusions and recommendations stressed the importance of the detailed investigation of all infant deaths, emphasized the value of health-visiting, and urged adequate training for midwives and community instruction of infant hygiene.[55] The Board's Medical Officer, Arthur Newsholme, in commenting on the report, echoed Simon in his broad social conscience: "Failure to recognize conditions of life favoring disease and difficulty of access to prompt and efficient medical treatment form important causes of excessive child mortality. Action favoring such recognition and treatment," continued the far-seeing Newsholme, "will do much to equalize the possibilities of healthy child life in the different social strata." [56] Newsholme's social strata were still fixed, but he knew disease to be the great leveler. A chance for the children of all strata to grow to a healthful maturity was his professional aim. Once launched upon such a road, society could not turn back. The mothers who knew their children *need* not die, could no longer accept an impersonal fate —disguised, or not, as the will of God.[57]

The infant and maternal welfare movement was diffuse and uncoordinated, with marked variations in different local areas. The medical profession, while upholding the need for protecting infants and mothers in childbirth, nevertheless found themselves in the official position of opposing the two major legislative enactments in aid of the movement: the Midwives Act and the Notification of Births Act. The principle of the Midwives Act, however, was one which the British Medical Association and other medical bodies had accepted; their grievance was the understandable fear that the registration system, as enacted, might create an inferior body of "specialists" who would threaten the profession's interests. Numbers of medical men, however, did support the Midwives Act as the best legislation which could be obtained to eliminate a serious evil.

By 1909, the Local Government Board's survey of the whole problem of infantile mortality marked the central government's serious attention to its responsibilities in this area of the personal health services.

THE HEALTH OF THE SCHOOL CHILD

Once society had recognized its corporate health as a national resource and had begun to scrutinize the personal health of special groups, school children stood revealed as a natural laboratory. Universal primary education had been established in England by the Education Act of 1870. It was not until 1891, however, that Lord Salisbury's Act abolished elementary school fees. Although masses of British children were now daily brought into the schools, public interest in their physical well-being grew slowly in the last twenty years of the nineteenth century.

Countries like France, Germany, and Sweden roused themselves to the need for medical care for school children well before England. School medical services were set up in Brussels in 1874, throughout Sweden in 1878, and in Paris in 1879. In the United States, Boston was the first large city to establish organized medical inspection of schools (1894), followed by Philadelphia and Chicago (1895), and New York (1897). By 1900 most of the large towns of Germany had school doctors.[58]

By the eighties, a few British doctors began to concern themselves with school health. A Birmingham physician, Dr. Priestly Smith, published a speech in 1880 on "Short Sight in Relation to Education." Two years later, Dr. Clement Dukes, physician of the Rugby School, published an article entitled "Health at School," subsequently to be expanded into a manual of school health which went through four editions over the next thirty-three years.[59] By 1884, Dr. (later Sir) James

Crichton-Browne had prepared for the Education Department a report on the mental health of London's elementary school children.

At a meeting in Glasgow of the British Medical Association's Section on Psychology in August, 1888, Dr. Francis Warner, a pioneer in child health, called for action to assist mentally deficient school children. Warner noted that school children formed one sixth of the entire population, and urged "scientific examination" of children in schools as a matter of social importance.[60] Stimulated by Warner's speech and sensitive to the rising public interest in school health, the British Medical Association later that year appointed a committee to study the average development and condition of brain power among elementary school children. This committee's first report, issued in 1889 and based upon an examination of 5,440 children, attracted considerable attention, and gained the co-operation of the Charity Organization Society, the Sanitary Institute, and other groups.[61] Special schools were established for feeble-minded children in London and in five provincial centers, and the *British Medical Journal* urged provision of further special schools as well as regular medical inspection of school children.[62] By 1902, Bradford, Birmingham, Hull, and London had appointed medical officers with special duties in connection with the health of school children. London had formed a Medical Officers of Schools Association, and in Leeds and Sheffield public medical supervision had been made available for physically and mentally defective children.

Further impetus was given to the school hygiene movement by the reports of the Royal Commission on Physical Training (Scotland) of 1903, and the famed Inter-departmental Committee on Physical Deterioration of 1904. Both groups advocated the medical inspection of school children and more attention to school hygiene, and both committees tossed in a further recommendation that provision should be made for feeding school children by voluntary organizations, with safeguards to prevent abuses of the system.[63]

All too many children of the poor in the great cities dutifully attended elementary classes in accordance with the law but had no food at breakfast or lunch. Voluntary schemes to remedy this were worked out in several local areas. But the use of public funds for such purposes still raised questions. Even *The Times* observed callously:

> We do not forget those 122,000 children in London going to school unfed. . . . But, after all, are they any worse off going to school unfed than if they remained at home unfed? They are only brought more into evidence, and the spectacle seems to throw some

of us off our economic balance altogether. But the resources of civilization founded upon economical competition are surely not yet exhausted.[64]

Hungry children were far more publicly apparent in schools, which was unfortunate for the delicate economic balances of some of *The Times'* readers. The whole problem came to a head in the appointment in 1906 of the Inter-departmental Committee on Medical Inspection and Feeding of School Children Attending the Public Elementary Schools. This committee's report praised the work carried on in local medical inspection of schools, feeling it had done "much toward bringing to view defects, the treatment of which secures the child from unnecessary suffering." They noted, however, that conditions were far from perfect and that there was "much opening for improvement." [65]

The Lancet's reaction to the report of the Committee of 1906 was one of full support for their recommendation of medical inspection, but the problem of feeding the school child left this medical journal in a quandary. It was "clearly indefensible," *The Lancet* acknowledged, to force a child to attend school when, because of lack of food, it was not in a state fit to benefit from the instruction. But, on the other hand, worried *The Lancet,* any attempt to set up a public system of free meals for indigent children might encourage lazy or careless parents to shirk their duties further.[66]

Despite such concerns, some central action in the current climate was inevitable, and Parliament passed the Education (Provision of Meals) Act of 1906. Under its authority, local education authorities were empowered to provide meals for school children when private funds were insufficient or not available. The public sums expended, however, were to be pegged to a rate of not more than a halfpenny per meal. Voluntary aid was linked with public aid in this Act, as the local authorities were authorized to assist voluntary committees in the work.[67]

It was not until two years later (1908) that a U.S. city (New York) provided school lunches for children.

Meanwhile, the question of providing for national school medical inspection had gathered increased momentum in England. The preventive values of medical inspection of school children were advocated by the British Medical Association and the medical press. The *British Medical Journal* in 1905 and 1906 continued to urge state-supported medical inspection of schools, but suggested that local private practitioners be employed to carry out the job.[68]

An Education Bill brought in during 1906, which contained a clause to provide medical inspection, was not supported by the British Medical Association and failed in passage. The Bill was permissive only insofar as its application to medical inspection, and the Association urgently demanded that this be made compulsory. Sir Victor Horsley, the eminent brain surgeon, led a delegation of Association members to the Board of Education urging not only compulsory inspection but the setting up of a medical department within the Board of Education.[69]

In 1907, however, compulsory school medical inspection was finally written into the Education (Administrative Provisions) Act. The Second International Congress on School Hygiene had been held just preceding the introduction of the Education Bill, and, as the first Chief Medical Officer for the Board of Education wrote: "The fact that almost every civilized country was represented by medical men of high place, gave the whole question of school hygiene a place of added importance in public opinion." [70] The Congress of School Hygiene of 1907 showed that England had lagged behind other countries in its public interest in school hygiene. The compulsory feature of the pending Education Bill, however, was to place England in the lead in school hygiene. Section 13 1 (b) of the Act provided for the "medical inspection of children immediately, before or at the time of or as soon as possible after their admission to a public elementary school," making inspection a duty of the local education authority.

The Education (Administrative Provisions) Act of 1907 constituted a major piece of social legislation, and is considered the legislative beginning of the personal health services. The law created a medical department within the Board of Education and authorized a full-scale medical inspection service. Treatment, as such, was not encompassed, but the future direction was clear. As first Chief Medical Officer to the Board of Education, Dr. (later Sir) George Newman was, for 28 years, to exercise broad humanity, professional competence, and skill in public persuasion.*

Action in the early months of the newly formed school medical sys-

---

* Sir George Newman (1870–1948), a Quaker, was educated at King's College, London, and Edinburgh University. M.B., C.M. (Edinburgh) 1872; M.D. (Edinburgh) 1895; D.P.H. (Cambridge) 1895. Senior Demonstrator of Bacteriology and Lecturer on Infectious Diseases, King's College, 1896–1900; Medical Officer of Health, Finsbury, 1900; Chief Medical Officer to the Board of Education, 1907; Medical Officer, Local Government Board, 1907; Chief Medical Officer, Ministry of Health, 1919–1935; K.C.B. 1918; C.B.E. 1935.

tem appeared to be slow. Shortly after the establishment of the new medical department, the *British Medical Journal* noted that the Education Department had been forced into medical inspection by the House of Commons, and doubted that the permanent officials would insist upon effective medical inspection systems.[71]

Nevertheless, the Board of Education accepted the Act, and sent forth an official circular to local authorities, even advising them to "keep in view the desirability of ultimately formulating schemes for the amelioration of the evils revealed by medical inspection." [72] This, of course, was the inevitable conclusion. Medical inspection of school children could only reveal the widespread need for medical care. By the end of 1908, medical inspection in London had demonstrated that the bulk of London's elementary school children were in poor health. Existing provisions for their medical care were inadequate. In school after school, hundreds of children suffered from discharging ears, ringworm, tuberculosis, and other illnesses and physical deficiencies. Numbers more were badly in need of dental and ophthalmic care.

A special subcommittee of the London Education Committee, including representatives of all the London hospitals and also Sir Victor Horsley on behalf of the British Medical Association, was formed to explore the medical needs and possibilities for treatment of London's school children. The subcommittee's majority urged the immediate setting up of school clinics under the London County Council. A minority suggested that the Council should merely utilize existing institutions, giving financial help, if necessary.[73]

The *British Medical Journal* recognized fully that the state was now "committed to the policy of providing medical relief, not only for the legal pauper and for the small wage-earning and casual labour classes, but also to giving or procuring proper care for sick or defective children of school age." [74] The problem was how to administer the treatment.

By June, 1909, the British Medical Association's Parliamentary Bills Committee had recommended that the Association oppose referring school children to the public medical charities. While countenancing their treatment in "provident dispensaries" on an insurance basis, or under contract, the Committee suggested that it would be much better to use private practitioners and pay them from public funds. "It is the duty of the State," intoned the *British Medical Journal* in the spirit of the times, "to do its utmost to prevent the physical deterioration of its citizens, on whose efficiency the future of the nation rests." But

not at the expense of medical charities supported by voluntary contributions or by "exorbitant demands on medical staffs!" [75] A deputation from the Metropolitan Counties Branch of the British Medical
Association, led by Sir Victor Horsley, called upon George Newman
in the spring of 1910 to urge the formation of a regular school medical
service, entirely independent of charitable institutions.[76]

Meanwhile, a second report from the Special Subcommittee on
Schools of the London Education Committee revealed that 43,746
London children suffered from bad vision, discharging ears, and ringworm. No further provision for treatment had been agreed to. The
problem was becoming acute. Parents, unable to pay for medical care
for their children, were obligated under the Prevention of Cruelty to
Children Act to apply to Boards of Guardians. But few Guardians had
furnished medical care to school children. Gradually, in view of the
failure of the poor law authorities, local health authorities in many
areas of England had begun to supply medical care to poor children.[77]

The situation was still fluid by 1910. In London, charity hospitals
were being used by the Education Authority to care for school children.
In other parts of the country, the local public health authority made
provision. The Board of Education's new medical department had
ordered that school medical services make use of existing machinery
of medical and sanitary administration, rather than to create new agencies to multiply the already multiple jurisdiction. But the Education
authorities had at least by 1910 begun to provide medical inspection
and supervisory health services.

Surveying the first two years of work of the Board of Education's
medical department, George Newman expressed justifiable satisfaction. "No one," wrote Newman, "can read the record of the work undertaken by the Local Education Authorities today without noticing
the marked progress which has taken place in the attention given to
the care and education of the abnormal and ailing child." It was true,
as Dr. Newman recognized, that "in this comprehensive work of
amelioration only a beginning had been made." [78] But it was a beginning.

The medical journals, too, were impressed with the accomplishment of the school medical service in its short period of existence. The
British Medical Journal praised Newman for full reporting on actual
investigations of illness in school children.[79] *The Lancet* was gratified
that the new medical department had not merely collected statistics,
but had "brought about a new social condition among us, under which

thousands of children are now receiving physical aid, and in a second-ary manner, moral support." [80]

British physicians had a creditable share in the start of the school health movement. The British Medical Association's efforts had stim-ulated the interest of scientific and charitable organizations in the subject. Local programs of school medical inspection had been pre-ceded by national concern, stirred up by the recommendations of the Royal Commission on Physical Training for Scotland and the Inter-departmental Committee on Physical Deterioration. With the passage of the Education (Provision of Meals) Act of 1906 and the Education (Administrative Provisions) Act of 1907, the health of the school child was recognized as a specific duty of the state. By 1910, no over-all solu-tion had been found to the problem of how to treat the ills revealed by school medical inspection services. The British Medical Association, too, was still feeling its way on medical treatment for the school child, caught partly between a desire to retain vested professional property rights and acceptance in principle of the right to medical care for school children unable to purchase it. The suggestion put forth by the *British Medical Journal* was a state subsidy to private practitioners for attendance on the poor school child. The Association opposed state subsidy to charitable organizations which might agree to treat the sick school child at the expense of the doctors. A final solution was still pending in 1910.

With the development of the school medical service in the first decade of the twentieth century, the Chief Medical Officer for Schools could say with reason that "the fact emerges that the centre of gravity of our public health system is passing in some degree from the environ-ment to the individual, and from problems of outward sanitation to problems of personal hygiene." [81]

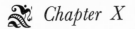 *Chapter X*

Further Paths to State Curative Medicine

THE DEVELOPMENT of the personal health services was rooted in accepted state authority for preventive health measures in communal protection. That the government should go beyond the poor law and assume responsibility for ensuring medical treatment for wide segments of the English public appeared far from certain in the opening years of the new century. Yet, by 1900, signs of growing public dissatisfaction with voluntary medical services and with poor law medical care were clear for those who would read them.

The Medical Advance

A remarkable change in public attitude toward medicine took place from 1850 to 1900. The therapeutic nihilism characteristic of the fifties [1] was now replaced by eager expectation of cure. With this was evolving among large sections of the public a conviction of the individual's right to medical care. This alteration in popular outlook, brought about by revolutionary advances in the medical sciences, underlay the growth of government action for curative medicine in many European nations. Even a brief glance at some of the great medical developments in the second half of the century makes this change in public attitude understandable.

Advances in surgery, perhaps the most dramatic, stemmed from the successful American introduction of ether into surgical practice in 1847 and of chloroform the following year in Edinburgh by Sir James Simpson. Once shown to be effective, anesthetic procedures were rapidly adopted in Europe and America.[2] American surgeons went on to develop additional methods of local anesthesia. Not only was untold suffering thus relieved, but surgeons now had the time to develop new operative techniques.

Abdominal surgery in 1865 was still very limited. Although ovariotomy was then performed more frequently than in early years of the nineteenth century, the mortality was still over 30 per cent. Very rarely were the spine or cranial cavity explored. Until the adoption from 1865 on of the antiseptic techniques of Lord Lister (1827–1912), hospital gangrene, pyemia, septicemia and erysipelas ran wild through every surgical ward. Many surgeons, indeed, wore the same frock coats from year to year in unwitting pride at the encrusted filth which testified to their numerous operations.[3] Lister, who initiated his revolutionary methods after reading the research reports of Louis Pasteur on the role of microorganisms in fermentation, finally saw his techniques (subsequently refined by others) introduced into surgical practice throughout the western world. America, however, took almost twenty years after Lister's innovation before completely accepting antiseptic and aseptic methods in surgery.[4]

Until the last quarter of the nineteenth century, with the emergence of bacteriology as a science, no rational body of facts existed for the prevention and treatment of infectious disease. The rapid bacteriological discoveries and the subsequent development of preventive vaccines could not fail to engender a new and optimistic outlook towards both medicine and the future possibilities of scientific investigation.

Meanwhile, progress in chemical physiology and diseases of metabolism had indicated that the prevention and cure of some disorders lay in the study of interrelating body systems. Research on the ductless glands from the late eighties on revealed the existence of hormones influencing other areas of the body and body metabolism. As early as 1891 thyroid extract was successfully employed in the treatment of myxedema.[5]

The new discoveries accelerated the trend towards medical specialism. Hughlings Jackson (1835–1911), pioneered the newly evolving field of neurology with his work on the localization of brain lesions. Opthamology and pediatrics also emerged as professional disciplines by the close of the century. By 1895 Wilhelm Roentgen (1845–1923) had discovered the mysterious "X ray" or Roentgen ray, and the science of radiology was born. And in 1899 the use of X rays had developed so rapidly that a British physician noted that they formed part of the machinery of every properly equipped hospital.[6]

The utilization of such scientific progress in medical practice, together with the longer training required of medical specialists, ultimately raised the costs of both medical and hospital care. Medical fees in the United States rose markedly even before the close of the nineteenth century. The English middle and upper classes in 1900 could still afford to purchase the new medical care directly from their private physicians. A majority of the working class had no such financial resources. By the turn of the century a variety of alternative paths to medical treatment had developed.

Voluntary Effort in Medical Care at the Beginning of the Twentieth Century

Curative medical services in England, apart from the poor law facilities, followed a strong tradition of voluntary support. From the establishment of the great London hospitals in the eighteenth century,[7] charity donations formed the economic basis for the free medical care given annually to hundreds of thousands of working-class men and women. By the last quarter of the nineteenth century, the whole question of voluntary effort in curative medicine was under continual discussion and investigation. Charitable institutions and doctors alike were dissatisfied with the system as it prevailed, chaotic and unsupervised, in the large urban centers.

Hospital Charities Abuse

The free medical treatment available at the voluntary hospitals of London and other large English cities was supported by private philanthropy and such regular charitable institutions as the "Hospital Saturday" and "Hospital Sunday" Funds.[8] Complaints from medical sources that hospital charity was being abused by working-class people who could afford to pay for outpatient medical care were not new. In the first years of the twentieth century, however, such complaints multiplied and received wider publicity. The Charity Organization Society claimed that the number of outpatients attending the 92 London hospitals increased from 1,082,259 in 1887, to 1,448,026 in 1897 and to 1,584,987 in 1900.[9] A 1905 study by *The Lancet* of general, special, and cottage hospitals in London, as well as of convalescent homes, showed a total of 5,451,675 outpatient visits to all types of hospitals in 1904. The total Hospital Sunday Fund award to these institutions that year was £ 56,398.[10]

Medical practitioners attending patients at the voluntary hospitals received no payment, as such, and there was little direct check on the capability of patients to pay. Not only did physicians see the situation as unfair, but the floods of patients applying for free treatment made outpatient care, of necessity, cursory.

Various attempts had been made to delimit free hospital treatment. The Medical Committee of the Charity Organization Society throughout the seventies had inveighed against the abuse of free medical services, in pamphlets, letters to *The Times,* and occasional speeches.[11] In 1875, an inquiry conducted among outpatients at the Royal Free Hospital concluded that 4 to 6 per cent of the patients were able to afford the services of a private practitioner, 49 per cent could pay "provident dispensary" rates, and 12 per cent, who were destitute, were entitled to poor relief.[12]

The situation deteriorated instead of improving towards the end of the century. The *British Medical Journal* noted irately in 1893 that after a quarter of century of agitation and innumerable acknowledgments of such abuse, no attempt was being made to work out a plan to check the system.[13]

Dr. Samuel Squire Sprigge,* the perceptive Assistant Editor of *The Lancet,* pointed out in 1905 that many workmen who subscribed, for example, to the Birmingham Hospital Saturday Fund through penny-weekly subscriptions, looked upon this not as a small gift to charity, but as a contribution which entitled them to free care. In some northern industrial towns of England workmen, Sprigge noted, were now even claiming a right to have a voice in governing the hospitals.[14]

A British Medical Association Charities Committee had investigated the whole subject in 1896 and reported that the deeper the inquiry went, the more widespread were the evidences of the abuse of hospital charity which turned up.

Medical groups could not agree, however, that a government-directed hospital service was the answer. Even the liberal *Lancet,* in its 1905 "Special Supplement in Support of the Metropolitan Hospital Sunday Fund," took issue with the suggestion that the time had come

* Sir Samuel Squire Sprigge (1860–1937) qualified in medicine at St. George's Hospital in 1887 after attending Cambridge. He joined *The Lancet* as Assistant Editor in 1893 and became its Editor in 1909, serving in the position until 1937. The author of *The Life and Times of Thomas Wakley,* Sprigge wrote his thoughtful study, *Medicine and the Public,* as his Cambridge M.D. thesis. He was knighted in 1921, elected F.R.C.S. in the same year and F.R.C.P. in 1927.

for London hospitals to be supported out of government funds, claiming that this was too great a drain upon the public's purse.[15]

THE PROVIDENT DISPENSARY

As an alternative to hospital charity, many of the upper working class chose to join a "provident dispensary." The introduction of this institution early in the nineteenth century had met some medical opposition. By 1870, provident dispensaries were more favorably received among medical men.[16]

Provident dispensaries were operated as a local insurance scheme, under which, for the payment of from one to tuppence weekly, a working-class man could receive medical care. Proceeds were shared by the attending doctors. Persons eligible to join were usually limited to workingmen and servants.[17] As a rule, provident dispensaries were organized as semipublic institutions with wealthy subscribers who did not derive medical benefits but who shared in the management.

Even the provident system had its abuses, and some medical men felt that provident institutions were patronized by persons who could easily afford a private practitioner. The *British Medical Journal,* however, by 1875 supported an extension of the provident plan, with proper precautions taken by managing committees to prevent abuse, saying: "We would warn those members of the profession who differ from us, that it is a mistaken principle to try to delay the inevitable." [18]

In 1881, under the sponsorship of James Stansfeld, M.P., and Dr. Alfred Carpenter, President of the Council of the British Medical Association, a movement was started to organize provident dispensaries in all districts of London, run on a "friendly society" basis, but including not only the working class male subscriber but his wife and children.[19] Throughout the late eighties and nineties, however, medical men continued to complain that provident dispensaries encroached upon their professional incomes. As with hospital charities, medical men felt that a much more affluent class of workingmen resorted to provident dispensaries than actually needed such services. When in 1889, a group of Birmingham citizens started a Consultative Medical and Surgical Institution to be run on a provident basis, the venture failed because of lack of co-operation of Birmingham medical men.[20]

The number of provident dispensaries continued to grow, nevertheless, and by the nineties the correspondence columns of the *British Medical Journal* bulged with complaints. Even its editorial policy, formerly sympathetic to the cause of provident dispensaries, began to worry about this matter "of grave and growing importance. It may well be asked," continued the *Journal*, "how the yearly increasing numbers of our profession are to gain a living if this multiplication of provident departments of hospitals, provident dispensaries, medical aid societies and clubs, with their miserable rate of remuneration, is to continue." [21]

CONTRACT PRACTICE IN MEDICAL CLUBS AND FRIENDLY SOCIETIES

The low-income worker of the nineteenth century could also secure medical care through a local medical club or a friendly society. Friendly societies had sprung up after the decay of the guilds in the seventeenth century. Very few offered medical aid benefits until the late eighteenth century, but friendly society medical aid plans were to spread rapidly throughout England in the second half of the nineteenth century.

For a small weekly insurance payment, usually not more than four-pence, members of the friendly society could expect a doctor's care in time of illness. Physicians who participated in such programs were employees of the friendly society, serving on a contract basis. Occasionally, large friendly societies united, forming friendly society institutes, which might own buildings and employ one or more full-time doctors to treat subscribing members.[22] Some friendly societies negotiated contracts with nursing homes; others even built their own.[23]

Medical clubs and medical aid societies and works clubs were conducted on a similar system, except that they did not provide the other social and protective services of a friendly society. Private medical clubs were often established directly by local doctors for their poorer patients, in which case there was no intermediary between doctor and patient as when the doctor was employed by a friendly society. Works clubs were based on an employer's contract for medical care for workmen in one type of employment, together with their families.

Once started, contract practice for medical care within friendly society membership spread rapidly. As early as 1837, Dr. Henry Rumsey noted that "the occupation of the medical attendant had hitherto been nearly doubled" by the mutual aid benefits.[24] By May 1884, 42 amalgamated friendly societies in England offered contract medical service to some 164,000 members. From the eighties on, friendly society membership grew rapidly, and the medical journals and contemporary accounts of the societies constantly referred to the increase.

The evaluation of the effectiveness of treatment rendered under this type of contract practice depends upon whose account of the service is read. Those glowing descriptions of benefits as described in friendly society literature contrast markedly with the accounts rendered by physicians in the contemporary medical journals. As early as 1856, beneficiaries of the service were complaining of the careless and insufficient medical attendance and of lack of confidence in their surgeon. Dr. Rumsey offered an oversimplified explanation for this—that members of a friendly society were aware that their medical contractor was underpaid, which "naturally rendered them suspicious as to the proper fulfillment of the contract." [25] Even members of General Medical Council, however, had doubts about the quality of some contract practice. In June, 1893, that organization's Committee on Medical Aid Associations recommended to the Council that any medical practitioner should be cited by the Council for acting in a "reprehensible manner" if he held a medical aid appointment with duties so onerous he could not do justice to his patients; if he gave certificates not justifiable on medical grounds; or if the group for which he worked used canvassing to attract members. A majority of the conservative General Medical Council, however, voted against adopting this report.[26]

A certain unprepossessing, if not shabby, aura continued to cling to contract practice, however. Beatrice and Sidney Webb, writing in 1910, observed that the club doctor was often looked upon publicly as an inferior kind of practitioner.[27] An even more serious limitation to friendly society medical care was that few societies provided treatment to women, children, or persons suffering from venereal disease or alcoholism. "Taken together," the Webbs pointed out, "these excluded classes must amount to more than three-fourths of the population." [28]

The medical profession itself was divided on the subject of contract practice. Large numbers of doctors participated in the system. It could not have operated otherwise. Many doctors, especially in the early part of the century, had initiated contract practice in their own districts, as a form of personal charity to their poorer patients. The complaints which poured into the correspondence columns of the medical journals in the last twenty years of the nineteenth century were directly related to conditions of work under the societies.

One of the cardinal points of dissension was the physician's inability to set his own fee, and his resultant complaint that he was underpaid by the friendly societies who hired him. The contracts were usually set at about four shillings a head, sometimes less if the societies could find a doctor willing to serve at lower rates. In the average private medical club established by doctors for working-class patients, the usual fee by 1905 was five shillings per head or higher.[29]

Other sources of conflict between doctor and friendly society lay in unsatisfactory relations with secretaries of friendly societies and the absence of written contracts specifying exactly what services the doctor would be required to perform. Major surgical operations and care in childbirth were, however, generally excluded by mutual understanding. Lack of tenure and the unprofessional advertising utilized by some friendly societies added to the medical unease. Another most bitter complaint of doctors was the absence of any wage limit for the beneficiaries of contract practice in friendly societies and medical aid associations.

The profession as a whole took the abuse of contract practice so seriously that widespread organized efforts were made by the doctors to remedy the situation. In the last decade of the nineteenth century a number of local medical societies were formed—largely to oppose the evils of contract practice (as perceived by physicians)—at Cork, Eastbourne, Folkstone, Hartlepoole, Kidderminster, and elsewhere.

The most bitter struggle between doctors and friendly societies raged at Cork in 1894. The medical practice of Cork physicians had fallen off steadily with an increase in friendly society medical benefits in that city. Cork doctors claimed that numbers of substantial citizens, with incomes up to £1,000 a year, were joining the clubs at the same low rate as poorer members of the societies. When the societies sought to extend this benefit to the families of all members, a concerted protest went up from the doctors of the area and the medical officers employed by the societies. The clubs, paying no attention to the doctors' cries, suddenly found themselves faced with mass resignations, and the physicians of the town formed an association to support the club doctors. In an effort to crush the medical strike, the friendly societies brought in scab doctors, but public opinion in this instance supported the Cork doctors, and the imported practitioners made little headway, the patients leaving the clubs.[30]

The British Medical Association constituted a forum for the violent complaints which filled the pages of its *Journal* year after year. In 1900, the *Journal* devoted a regular column to the subject headed, "Contract Medical Practice." Letters, news items, and editorials were published in the column, and a standing notice in the advertisements of the *Journal* was directed to "Medical Men Who May be Thinking of Applying For Appointments In Connection With Clubs or Other Forms of Contract Practice," warning against particularly poor contract situations.

By far the most important investigation of contract practice was carried on from 1903 to 1905 by the Medico-Political Committee of the British Medical Association. Pursuant to the instructions of the 1903 annual meeting of the Association, the committee sent out 12,000 questionnaires to individual practitioners who were engaged in various forms of contract practice. In response, 1,548 returns were received, and of these, 692 were from doctors who stated that they were not engaged in any form of contract practice. In all, a total of 856 replies were received from doctors participating in contract practice, and the committee also utilized the reports of local medical societies.[31]

In its final report the Medico-Political Committee recognized that certain classes of the community clearly required some means of insuring the cost of medical attendance through paying small premiums. "The considerations which lead to this conclusion," their report continued, "can hardly be set aside even by the most strenuous opponents of contract practice."[32] The committee, nevertheless, felt a number of reforms in contract practice to be vital to the medical profession: increased payment for doctors' services; the distribution of contract work among all practititioners in a district; abolition of canvassing; and recognition of a doctor's right to refuse to admit to his contract practice persons he deemed "unsuitable as to financial position."[33]

Most significantly, however, the report which was written by the Association's Secretary, Mr. (later Sir) J. Smith Whitaker, recommended that the profession support the adoption of a form of local public medical service, open to every practitioner in any district, that it give the profession control of contract practice, and that it do away with the irritations caused by the friendly societies. The British Medical Association report in full constituted partial recognition of the need for sharing the risks of illness among members of the community—even if doctors demanded the right to judge who were, and who were not, eligible.

While not in itself a form of state intervention, the contract system under friendly society and other auspices did represent an increasing role played by members of the community in sharing the risks of the individual's illness. Friendly society medical care, as it expanded towards the close of the nineteenth century, became more and more an invasion of what had been the private-property sphere of the medical man. The profession was disturbed by the growth of the contract system, not only because it affected its financial interest but because, as the system operated, it was impossible to provide the kind of professional service to the patient which doctors felt was essential. There is evidence of medical discontent and discord, and finally even direct strikes. Opposed to this is the positive evidence that, as the societies spread, more and more doctors were employed in this form of medical practice.

It is not possible to determine the total number of physicians employed full-or part-time in contract practice in the opening years of the century, but it seems significant that out of 12,000 questionnaires sent out by the British Medical Association's Contract Practice Committee, so few replies were received. If the average doctor had actively resisted the spread of this form of socialized medicine, the Association should have had a greater response.

The subject of contract practice was to come under consideration again, when Lloyd George based his 1911 National Insurance Bill upon friendly society participation. The whole problem of contract practice, with its complex pro's and con's, is a study in itself. It forms a part of a discussion of the profession and state intervention only insofar as its rapid development by the turn of the century demonstrated the growth of community sharing of the risks of illness. In its 1905 investigation of contract practice, the British Medical Association recommended the adoption of locally organized public medical services. Further proof of the acute need for publicly supported medical care was to emerge in the work of the newly created Royal Commission on the Poor Laws and the Relief of Distress.

The Royal Commission on the Poor Laws and the Relief of Distress, 1905–1909

As has been discussed earlier,[34] by 1900 stirrings of a new public attitude towards the treatment of the poor were clearly perceptible. Nineteenth-century society had been satisfied with relieving destitution, with little effort to prevent it. By the turn of the century, criticisms on the work of the Charity Organization Society had multiplied.[35] Even more unpopular was the unimaginative, unprogressive Local Government Board, plodding along, wholly unable to adapt to the changed social climate in any of its far-flung responsibilities—poor law, public health, town-planning, and housing.[36]

The numbers of persons applying for poor relief, including medical relief, were rising steadily, as were the costs. From 1890 to 1899, the expenditures from the poor rates for relieving the poor rose from £ 6,418,106 to £ 8,161,532. Although the increase in numbers receiving relief was also accompanied by a growth of estimated population (28,448,239 in 1890 to 31,397,078 in 1899),[37] the Local Government Board's staff was increasingly concerned over the extent of the "drift away from the principles of 1834." [38] By 1909, in a population estimated at 35,756,615, one person in every 40 received poor relief, at a total cost of £14,717,098. Some 30 per cent of these received poor law medical care costing £896,711.[39]

The appointment in 1905 of the Royal Commission on the Poor Laws and the Relief of Distress was not, however, based on any general public demand. The Conservative Government took the step just before leaving office. Sidney and Beatrice Webb attributed the Commission's creation to the energetic new head of the Local Government Board's Poor Law Division, James Stewart Davy, and the Board's President, the philosophical Gerald Balfour, "who recognized the public advantage of a precise dissemination between opposing principles." [40]

The Times welcomed the appointment as a practical one, noting that there had been no such inquiry for about seventy years, during which vast changes in the country's economic and social conditions had taken place. "Few human arrangements are so perfect as not to call for a revision after such a period," observed the editors calmly.[41]

Neither had the medical journals raised any clamor for a general investigation of the administration of poor relief. The *British Medical Journal* observed the Commission's appointment dispassionately, merely regretting that the Prime Minister had not appointed more medical men to the Commission.[42] Similarly, *The Lancet* wished for one or two additional medical men on the Commission.[43]

Despite these passing complaints of the medical journals, the composition of the Royal Commission's membership was to be largely responsible for the thoroughness and scope of its investigations. *The Times* had commented: "What we want is impartial and expert consideration, from which political bias has been banished as completely as possible." [44] As the Commission was appointed, the selection appeared to fulfill this need; it was preponderantly composed of experts drawn from either social investigation or poor law administration. Among some of the better-known appointees were Sir Samuel Provis, Permanent Secretary to the Local Government Board, George Lansbury, Charles Loch, Octavia Hill, and Beatrice Webb. The Commission was headed by Lord George Hamilton, who had had official administrative experience as Chairman of the London School Board and as Secretary of State for India.

The controversy between those who fought the battle for deterrence and the exponents of the new scientific social reform ebbed and flowed during the Commission's hearings, and appeared even in their consideration of the extent of medical assistance to the poor. Beatrice Webb illuminated the situation within the Commission during negotiations when recording in her diary:

> In listening to the evidence brought by the Charity Organization Society members in favour of restricting medical relief to the technically destitute, it suddenly flashed across my mind that what we had to do was to adopt the exactly contrary attitude, and make medical inspection and medical treatment compulsory on all sick persons, to treat illness, in fact, as a public nuisance to be suppressed in the interests of the community.[45]

To obtain evidence on the conditions of poor law medical treatment, the Commission called upon medical superintendents of poor law infirmaries, district medical officers concerned with outdoor relief and medical officers of health.

A variety of medical evidence was presented to the Royal Commission; the information submitted had, naturally, variation in points of view. A central question in the Commission's scrutiny of poor law medical care was whether or not medical care for the destitute should be merged with the functions of sanitary authorities into one, official medical service. The Local Government Board's Medical Officer, Sir Arthur Newsholme, urged such unification on the grounds that it would foster the early recognition and treatment of disease.[46] Newsholme was backed in this view by a majority of the medical officers of health testifying before the Commission. Their liberal position was typified by the statement of the Medical Officer of Health for Sheffield, Dr. Harold Scurfield: "Practically, I am in favour of giving medical attendance to anybody without pauperization, that is free medical service." [47] A number of poor law medical officers, like Dr. Nathan Raw, also called for the establishment of a unified national health service.[48]

The British Medical Association, which not only presented a lengthy memorandum to the Commission, but whose representatives offered additional testimony, was forced to admit that the profession was divided on the advisability of creating a state medical service.[49] The Association faithfully suggested a variety of improvements in conditions of work of the poor law medical officers. The Association also recommended that standards of nursing and medical facilities of poor law infirmaries should be equated with those of the great voluntary hospitals; that special medical and surgical assistance should be obtainable, as necessary, in poor law infirmaries; that county poor law infirmaries could be improved through amalgamation; and that better provision should be made to treat cases of venereal disease. The British Medical Association went on record, however, as opposing the municipal maintenance and control of voluntary charitable hospitals.[50]

As the testimony on medical care of the poor continued, the Royal Commission began to feel that a special investigation on indoor and outdoor medical relief was essential. They assigned the task to Dr. John McVail, County Medical Officer for Stirlingshire and Dumbartonshire. An experienced public health man, McVail had served as President of the Society of Medical Officers of Health, and a member of the Council of the British Medical Association. His report was thorough, and urged a more dynamic role upon the Local Government Board.

McVail felt first that the Board should possess, and exercise, much more extensive powers to compel Boards of Guardians to take proper action. The administrative areas of Boards of Guardians should be enlarged, he recommended. Both indoor and outdoor medical relief should be subject to regular and systematic inspection by medical inspectors of the Local Government Board. More public attention should be paid to the control of phthisis. McVail also suggested separate treatment facilities for imbeciles and epileptics, and the extension of poor law hospitalization to dependents of able-bodied persons whose care would involve either loss of work by their able-bodied relative or the risk of spreading disease.

McVail was guarded, however, upon the thorny topic of a free medical service:

> Trying to think of the subject, not as a medical man, but rather as a member of the general public, I am bound to say that I shrink from the contemplation of any scheme by which the whole community would have a right to medical advice paid for out of Imperial taxes or local rates. . . . it seems to me that preventive medicine could be better applied to a system of medical provident institutions than to a universal rate-provided medical service.[51]

Nevertheless, McVail acknowledged fully that the poor law medical program was neither adequate nor self-sufficient. Both rural and urban medical relief under the poor law, he continued, was "a cripple supported on two crutches—the general hospital on one side and gratuitous medical work on the other." The medical relief provided for paupers was quite inadequate, McVail felt, in dealing with some of the most important medical problems of the time, such as the healthy rearing of children, control of phthisis, and early preventive treatment of disease.[52]

The problem of medical care for the poor was, of course, only a part of the whole poor law investigations. In 1909, after four years of extensive researchers, the Report of the Royal Commission was issued in its now famous two-part form—the Report of the Majority of the Commission, and the dissenting Minority Report, which was signed by the Reverend Prebendary H. Russell Wakefield, Mr. Francis Chandler, Mr. George Lansbury, and Mrs. Sidney Webb.[53]

In its broad administrative lines, the Majority Report recommended that the poor law medical service should continue in England and Wales, separate from the public health service administered by local authorities. The Commissioners, recognizing that sickness was one of the chief causes of pauperism, felt it necessary to "continue a system of therapeutic treatment" without any additional restriction.[54]

The Majority Report vigorously opposed the establishment of a free medical service, however, on the grounds that those inevitably increasing numbers who availed themselves of such service would lead to the state providing for practically the whole population, and that such a service would inevitably tend to "kill all the existing voluntary organizations for medically assisting the sick poor" and would ruin the practice of the majority of private medical practitioners. Finally, they noted darkly, the cost of gratuitous medical assistance would make its adoption prohibitive.

The majority of the Commissioners acknowledged defects in existing poor law medical service in quality and extent. Any remedies for such defects, they emphasized, should be consistent with the premise that medical assistance should not be made "so attractive that it may become a species of honourable and gratuitous self-indulgence instead of a somewhat unpleasant necessity resorted to because restoration to health is otherwise impossible." [55]

Even the Majority Report, however, was far more progressive than anything John Burns and his Local Government Board envisaged. Their Report put on record the majority's belief that medical relief and the poor law deterrence principle should be separated. They suggested the establishment of a Medical Assistance Committee associated with the poor law, which would include representatives of the provident medical societies. Public medical assistance they then saw organized on a provident basis with the assistance committee paying the fees of those who could not provide for themselves.

It was the Minority Report, written largely by the eloquent Beatrice Webb, which called for basic changes in society's attitude toward poverty, and which demanded wide-scale Government intervention to control the labor market and to increase capital expenditures in the downswings of the trade cycle.[56] The Minority Commissioners also urged establishment of a uniform county public medical service to eliminate extensive overlapping and renounced the principle of deterrence in medical relief.

The Minority Report did not, however, look kindly on improvements in the quality or extent of poor law medical care which might tempt more citizens "voluntarily to range themselves among the destitute."[57] The establishment of a unified medical service [58] on public health lines would not, the minority Commissioners felt, involve a *free* provision of medical services to any and all applicants. Parliament, they felt, could legislate a code of charges for services, which would make it possible to recover the costs of medical treatment from those able to afford it.[59]

Despite its reservations with respect to providing treatment for all who might apply, the whole Minority Report recognized a corporate duty for curative treatment to those in need of it. As the Webbs later described the Minority Report, its spirit was an acceptance of the "fundamental principle that social health is not a matter for the individual alone, nor for the Government alone, but depends essentially on the joint responsibility of the individual and the community for the maintenance of a definite minimum of civilized life." [60]

Both the Majority and Minority Reports proposed a revolutionary change in the country's administrative structure through the abolition of Boards of Guardians and poor law areas. Both reports concurred in the surrender of the principle of deterrent poor law and less eligibility. Both reports anticipated a vast extension of public provision for the sick poor, and felt it necessary to separate mental deficients from the general poor law medical treatment.[61]

Reaction from the medical journals to the report of the Poor Law Commission was immediate and extended. Indeed, the *British Medical Journal,* in 1908, on hearing a rumor that the Commission might recommend the adoption of a public medical service observed sharply: "the egg on which the Commission has been sitting so long is already addled . . . that the medical profession would not agree to becoming a branch of the Civil Service," and that "such a plan as a remedy would be almost useless." [62] In January, 1909, the *British Medical Journal* again anticipated the Royal Commission's report with the observation that, although a great deal was expected from the forthcoming report, it could not alter economic conditions. "Short of recommending a scheme of universal compulsory sick assurance on the German plan, it is difficult to see what it can propose except an extension of the non-contributory state system of aid in incapacity and old age which has been developing in this country during the present generation." [63]

When the Commission's Report was finally issued, a lengthy analysis of the two documents was prepared by the *British Medical Journal,* but with a suspicious comment on the Minority Report: "while a free medical service for all is disavowed it is generally felt that the tendency of the recommendations is in that direction." [64]

So strong was medical interest in both documents that a special Poor Law Reform Committee was appointed in June, 1909, to consider the findings of the Royal Commission as they affected the medical profession. Somewhat lamely, this committee in presenting its conclusions to the Council of the British Medical Association stated only that any system of medical assistance which might be adopted must include two principles in order to be satisfactory to the medical profession. First, medical services rendered to the state should be paid for by the state, and, second, payment should be adequate and in direct accordance with the professional services rendered.[65]

In a major editorial on July 3, 1909, however, the *British Medical Journal* granted that the profession accepted the following points:

1. That the present medical service for the poor is in urgent need of reform.

2. That co-ordination of all public and voluntary medical agencies is necessary to prevent the present overlapping and consequent waste of money and energy.

3. That charitable medical institutions are greatly abused by people who are not fit objects for charity, and that every inducement ought to be held forth for the poorer classes to make self-provision against sickness.

4. That preventive as well as curative measures ought to form part of any medical service.

The *Journal* admitted that "it is inevitable that what appear to be

the selfish interests of the profession will loom largely in our debates."
Yet, they felt the success of any public medical service to be contingent
on the just recognition of the physician's rights.[66]

Officially, the British Medical Association took no position during
the 1909 poor law discussions on the idea of a nationally operated
medical service. Dr. James Smith Whitaker, speaking on behalf of the
Association at a meeting of the Poor Law Medical Officers Association,
stated that "at present" the Association had no opinion on the matter.[67]
The *British Medical Journal* in October disavowed holding a brief for
either the Majority or Minority Report, and suggested taking points
from each.[68] At the beginning of 1910, however, the *British Medical
Journal* attacked state-supported free medical care in an editorial as
not only outside the range of practical politics, but as "altogether
subversive of the principle that there is a responsibility of the individual toward the State as well as of the State towards the individual." [69]

When the Prevention of Destitution Bill (inspired by the Minority
Report and later to be shelved) was discussed in the House of Commons, the *Journal* commented impartially on the debate and upon the
government's position that any attempt to reform the existing poor law
system was a long, difficult task which could not be successfully undertaken in one session, or even in one Parliament, except with the good
will of all parties concerned.[70]

The Lancet's reaction to the reports of the Royal Commission indicated a greater awareness of the great social changes responsible for
the whole scrutiny of social policy at the opening of the twentieth
century. *The Lancet* recognized the Commission's work as "one of the
most important documents dealing with the social life of this country
that we have ever read." Noting that preventive medicine was the crucial consideration in all efforts to relieve poverty, *The Lancet* deplored
the old poor law's inelastic regulations which had been "dragged,
resisting and protesting, hither and thither in vain attempts to make
them meet situations undreamt of by those who designed them." [71]

As a journal, *The Lancet* took no stand upon either the Majority or
Minority Report. Its editors, however, opened their pages to a group
of medical men and social investigators, led by Dr. H. Beckett-Overy,
M.D. (Edinburgh), F.R.C.S. (England), Somerville Hastings, M.S.
(London), F.R.C.S. (England), and Arnold Freeman, the nonmedical
social investigator, who appealed to *The Lancet's* medical readers to
support the minority proposals for a well organized and unified public
health service.[72]

Despite the wide public interest in the work of the Royal Commission on the Poor Laws, the Government declined to undertake any thorough overhaul of the poor law system. Indeed, the controversy over the Lloyd George Budget, which followed shortly after, distracted attention from the Commission's proposals.

If the Government could have summoned full parliamentary backing for legislation to effect the sweeping reorganization of the nation's local government required by the Royal Commission's recommendation, it would still have had to choose between the proposals of the Majority and Minority Reports. Twenty years were to elapse before legislation combining features of the two reports was to be incorporated in the Local Government Act of 1929.[73]

In 1909, Local Government Board officials desired no such revolutionary changes. John Burns, its President, made no mention of the Commission's work in his annual report, although one of his inspectors, Philip Bagenal, admitted the Majority and Minority Reports had aroused "fresh public interest" in poor law reform.[74] Burns did, in the immediately succeeding years through a series of circulars, initiate certain reforms aimed at improving the conditions of outdoor medical treatment and indoor and outdoor nursing care.[75]

As far as medical participation in the work of the Royal Commission may be surveyed, a majority of the medical officers of health, and the medical heads of the departments most concerned with public health and poor law medical relief, supported a unification of the two services. Throughout the body of testimony collected from government-employed medical men, a large degree of sympathy was expressed for an extension of a state medical service to classes other than the destitute. In actuality, such extension had already occurred in the broadening of treatment given in the new poor law infirmaries.

The McVail investigations also concluded that extensive reforms were necessary in the administration of poor law medical relief, but Dr. McVail was reluctant to agree to a public medical service, open to all comers.

The medical profession, as represented by the British Medical Association, failed to commit itself conclusively on the proposal for replacing poor law care with a central state medical service. Its opposition to the municipalization of voluntary hospitals intimated its resistance to broadening the government's administrative role in the curative medical services. Nevertheless, the Association recognized the need for considerable improvement and extension of existing poor law medical care, despite its reluctance to endorse either the Majority or Minority Report.

The Royal Commission's recommendations failed immediate implementation, but they had an important educational influence and served as a reservoir for future reformers. With the Commission's investigations, the whole area of state responsibility in curative and preventive medical service was thrown wide open. Both the Majority and Minority Reports signified, unquestionably, that a new approach to poor law treatment and the public health services was essential.

As the new century's first decade closed, political necessity and political circumstances were to push aside any comprehensive approach to community health in favor of the more limited state health insurance.

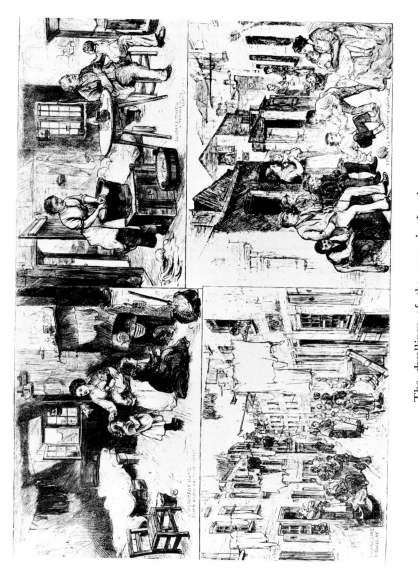

The dwellings of the poor in London

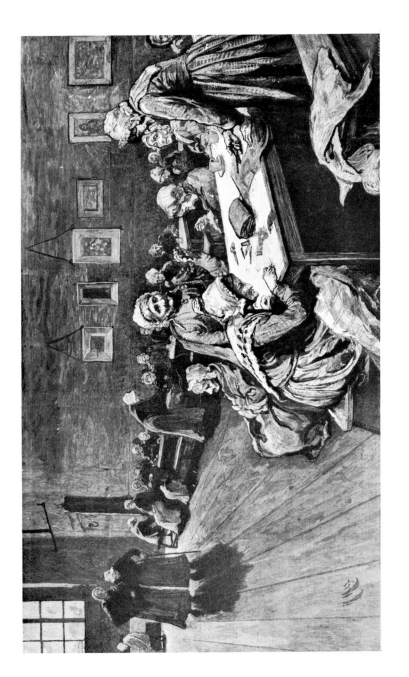

Old Age—a Study at the Westminster Union

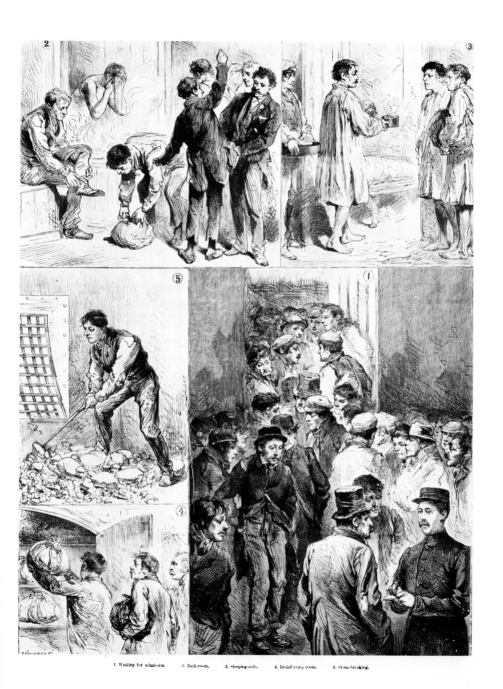

1. Waiting for admission. 2. Bath-room. 3. Sleeping-cells. 4. Disinfecting room. 5. Stone-breaking.

Sketches at a "Casual Ward"

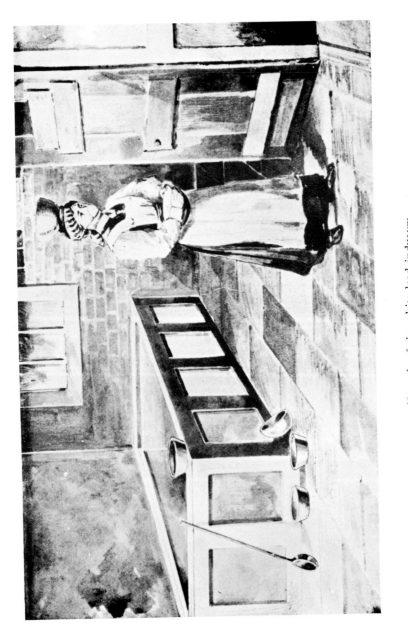

Hazards of the white lead industry

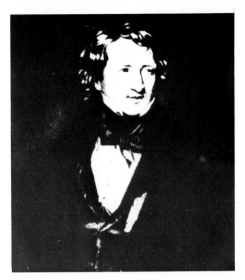

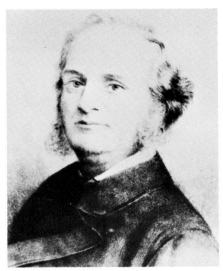

Thomas Wakley, Sr. (1795-1862), editor of *The Lancet*. Courtesy of the National Library of Medicine

Ernest Hart (1835-98), editor of the *British Medical Journal*

REPRESENTATIVES OF THE MEDICAL PROFESSION IN PARLIAMENT

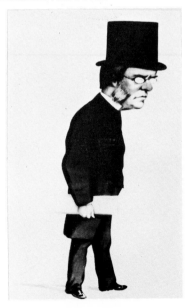

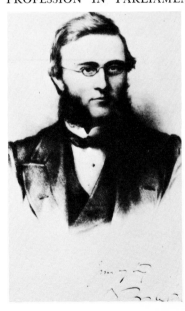

Sir Lyon Playfair (1818-98). Cartoon from *Vanity Fair*, Feb. 20, 1875

Sir (Balthazar) Walter Foster (1840-1913)

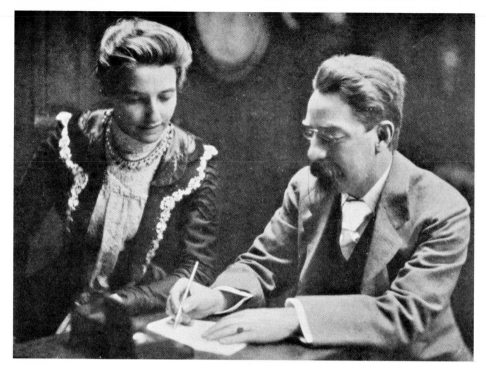

Beatrice Potter Webb (1858-1943), and Sidney Webb, Lord Passfield (1859-1947). From Beatrice Webb, *Our Partnership* (by permission of Longmans Green Co.)

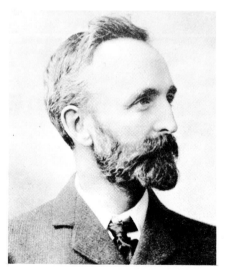

Sir Arthur Newsholme (1857-1943). From Arthur Newsholme, *Fifty Years in Public Health* (by permission of Mr. Keith A. B. Wilson)

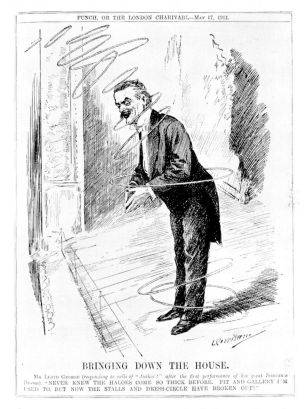

"Bringing Down the House"—Lloyd George Introduces
the National Insurance Bill. Cartoon by L. Ravenhill
from *Punch,* May 17, 1911, reproduced by permission

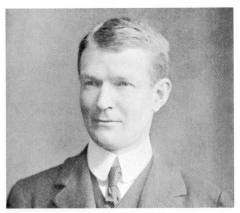

William John Braithwaite (1875-1938). From
W. J. Braithwaite, *Lloyd George's Ambulance
Wagon* (by permission of R. M. Braithwaite)

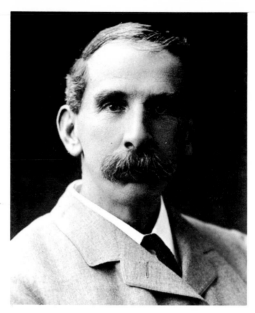

Sir Victor Horsley (1857-1916). Photograph by G. C. Beresford, from Stephen Paget, *Sir Victor Horsley, A Study of His Life and Work* (by permission Constable and Company, Ltd.)

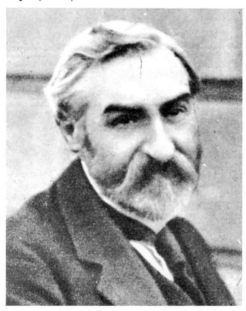

Sir James Smith Whitaker (1866-1936), medical secretary of the British Medical Association, 1902-12. From Ernest Little, *A History of the British Medical Association, 1832-1932* (reproduced by permission of the Secretary of the British Medical Association)

Chapter XI

The Medical Profession and the National Insurance Act

> If I had to sum up the immediate future of democratic politics in a single word, I should say "Insurance." That is the future—Insurance against dangers from abroad, insurance against dangers scarcely less grave and much more near and constant which threaten us here at home in our own island.
>
> Winston Churchill, Speech at the Free Trade Hall, Manchester, May 23, 1909.[1]

THE National Insurance Bill of 1911 was floated out upon a public opinion primed for a new approach in social medicine. The Act was to be a political masterpiece of Lloyd George; but the background to its popular reception had been building for years—in the disturbing facts unearthed by the new breed of social investigators, in the growth of the personal health services, in the spread of club insurance schemes, and in the steady push to political power by organized labor.

The forthright reports of the 1909 Poor Law Commission, although politically fallow for years to come, kindled fresh public interest in the plight of the poor. Tireless efforts of the Fabian publicizers stirred the new social conscience still more deeply. Every working-class home feared the sudden loss of work, and actual unemployment throughout England and Wales remained chronic and severe, little relieved by the Distress Committees of the Unemployed Workmen Act (1905). Strikes and lockouts already marked labor's unrest and its surge toward "direct action." The Liberals, party of that "gigantic straddle" between middle class and radical working class,[2] returned from the revolutionary "People's Budget" elections in 1910 without a clear majority, politically dependent on the support of the Labor Party and Irish Nationalists. But the Parliament Act of 1911 was only months away from limiting the power of the House of Lords to block social reform.

The years between 1909 and 1914 were to be profoundly significant for the English people. At the summit, the brilliant Edwardian society played out its Indian summer of privilege in blind, if graceful, confidence born of the past.[3] On the Continent, the Kaiser and his general staff grew bolder. At home, strikes increased and palliatives kept pace. After long agitation, the Old Age Pensions Act was passed and came into force on January 1, 1909. A noncontributory scheme—paying pensions of only five shillings a week to workers over seventy with weekly incomes below ten shillings—the Act brought half a million persons into a new form of financial dependency on the state. The country, groping its way to community answers, was ready for new ideas, and the government possessed the men to implement reforms. Neither the Majority nor the Minority Reports of the Poor Law Commission had recommended national insurance as the primary solution. Insurance solved none of the basic economic problems of society, yet it could appeal alike to the man of property and to the worker. In the months to come, insurance was to become a magic word, lighting a new social future.

Background to the Bill

The political architect of the National Insurance Bill was David Lloyd George, then Chancellor of the Exchequer in Asquith's Government. Entering Parliament in 1890 from Caernarvon at the age of 27, this adopted son of Wales had moved swiftly to political power in the Liberal Party. In the service of his genuine humanitarianism and hatred of privilege, Lloyd George could exercise courage, personal magnetism, political resourcefulness, and an earthy shrewdness.[4] All were to be called upon in the ensuing battle for health insurance.

Touring Germany in 1908, Lloyd George had been greatly attracted by what he was shown of German social insurance. Beset by a hacking and worrisome throat ailment, he warmed to German sanatoria and the German government's campaign against tuberculosis. The Chancellor's experience with the public cost of free grants under the Old Age Pensions Act had also shifted his interest towards a contributory insurance program. By early 1910, he had already tentatively begun to explore the possibility of an English national insurance scheme with associates and some representatives of the friendly societies.[5]

The concept of government-sponsored sickness insurance was not new. The House of Commons in both 1773 and 1789 passed old age and sickness plans for the laboring poor, which failed to obtain support in the House of Lords.[6] The U.S. Congress established the first compulsory, prepaid medical care program in the U.S. for merchant seamen in 1798, imposing a charge of twenty cents a month to be withheld from the wages of each seaman on U.S. vessels. This Act in behalf of sick and disabled seamen had a long history of precedent, not only in the collection of "hospital money" from salaries of seamen in the various American colonies, but in sixpenny wage deductions for seamen of the Royal Navy to support a seamen's hospital at Greenwich.[7] Meanwhile, voluntary sickness insurance plans in friendly societies and other mutual aid groups developed steadily in England and on the Continent during the nineteenth century.

By 1911, many European nations had passed legislation providing various forms of compulsory social insurance for sickness, accidents, and old age. The German system, with its Sickness Insurance Act of 1883, was the model on which most of the subsequent legislation was based—Austria (1888), Hungary (1891), Luxemburg (1901), Norway (1909), and Switzerland (1911).

Although the German insurance plan was largely Bismarck's brainchild, it was no accident that Germany was the first Western European nation to adopt such legislation. Prussia experienced a strong medical reform movement during the 1848 revolutions. Rudolph Virchow (1821–1902), the brilliant German pathologist, together with liberal medical colleagues, advocated a state health program under a Ministry of Health, which would have made it the state's duty to care for the physical welfare of all its members. Virchow's plans were checkmated with the failure of the 1848 revolt. But in the years which followed, the German states developed many local sickness funds, membership in which was compulsory for certain groups of wage earners. German physicians, therefore, were thoroughly familiar with the concept of sickness insurance and did not oppose the introduction of Bismarck's measure in 1883. In fact, unlike English and French physicians, German doctors of the eighties seem to have given little thought to the introduction of compulsory health insurance. Bismarck's Act, of course, was passed at a time when German medicine was in the midst of the most dramatic of the bacteriological discoveries, when physicians were preoccupied with the rapid scientific advances, and when medical men from America and throughout Western Europe flocked to German laboratories and hospitals for postgraduate training.[8]

Russia, a vast country of over one seventh of the earth's total land area, and with heterogeneous peasant populations, had taken a different path to public responsibility for medical care in the nineteenth century. Three years after the abolition of serfdom in 1861, Alexander II established the Zemstvo system to decentralize administration—in which district and provincial assemblies in the European provinces were responsible for the health and welfare of their communities. The Zemstvos built small hospitals and appointed government physicians financed by local taxation. The quality of such medical care was not high during this period. Even by 1914 Russia had no central government medical authority and health conditions were very bad. From 1901 to 1911 infant mortality in Russia averaged 244 per 1,000 births.[9]

In 1910 the Russian medical program had little to offer to an urbanized England which had moved far ahead of Russia in public health. But the German insurance system had already proven its worth in industrialized countries, and the Chancellor of the Exchequer was determined that it should do the same in England.

Although Lloyd George conceived the plan of national insurance for England and carried it through Parliament, the development of the Bill was left to an altruistic young civil servant, William John Braithwaite (1875–1938), then Assistant Secretary to the Board of Inland Revenue. In his memoirs of that hectic year with Lloyd George, Braithwaite records how he was sent for by his superiors in December, 1910, and told that Lloyd George wanted someone to go to Germany for his insurance scheme. A tentative plan had already been drawn up by Treasury staff.[10] After a whirlwind visit to Berlin, and nights of poring over German insurance statistics and reports, Braithwaite went back to England to put a Bill together. By mid-February, a memorandum was ready, together with supporting papers on methods for the collection of contributions.

Although at least one of the Fabians, Sir Leo Chiozza Money (1870–1944), had advocated health insurance for England, the Webbs and the Fabian Society as a whole opposed Lloyd George's plan violently. Beatrice Webb noted in her diary that during the years 1909 to 1911 she and her husband had lost touch with the Liberal cabinet ministers.[11] But Lloyd George invited the Webbs to one of his famous breakfasts at the end of February, 1911, to unfold his new scheme. Braithwaite, who was also present, described their immediate opposition. "Sickness should be prevented, not cured," cried the Webbs, as they "singly and in pairs" leaped down Lloyd George's throat![12] The Fabian Society was thereafter to remain firmly opposed to the Bill, seeing it as a stopgap which would brush aside the comprehensive recommendations of the Minority Report.

Yet, a strong case could be made in 1911 for national health insurance. Voluntary insurance plans, carried out by friendly societies, primarily covered workers who were employed on a regular basis in the stronger trades. The woman wage earner was rarely protected, and persons in irregular employment who worked for low wages were unable to provide such insurance for themselves. Lucy Masterman, wife of the Liberal Member of Parliament, C. F. G. Masterman, described her experiences as a voluntary worker in the Charity Organization Society during the winter of 1906, and the plight of those with no voluntary health protection: "[There was a] sense of utter helplessness when a railway porter or a builder's labourer got ill or lost his job. The family were swept into destitution before they could take breath, and the uncertain and capricious stream of private charity was hopelessly inadequate even to defer disaster."[13]

Introduction of the Bill

Lloyd George, in introducing his Bill into the House of Commons on May 4, 1911, emphasized the fact that not half the workingmen of the country carried any insurance for sickness, and not a tenth for unemployment. Few could afford the premiums, he cried. Stressing that the Bill was a noncontroversial measure, the persuasive Chancellor then suggested that there was agreement on the evil to be remedied, agreement as to its urgency, and a "general agreement as to the main proposals upon which the remedy ought to be based."[14]

As the bill was introduced into Parliament, it aimed at bringing within a scheme of compulsory contributory health and unemployment insurance the country's whole wage-earning population, estimated at about 15,000,000 persons. Modeled in part on the German legislation of 1883–1889, the Bill provided for the compulsory collection of contributions from employers and employees. Male employees were to contribute fourpence a week, female employees threepence, the employer threepence for each employee, and the state was to contribute tuppence.

The payments guaranteed medical attendance, drugs, sanatoria treatment for tuberculosis, and maternity benefit for the insured woman worker or the wife of an insured male worker to the extent of a thirty-shilling payment. In addition, a sickness benefit (10s. for the first 13 weeks for men, 7s. 6d. for women, and 5s. for the second 13 weeks for men and women alike) was to be paid to the insured worker during his absence from work owing to illness or mental or bodily disablement. Benefit payments were to commence at the age of sixteen and cease at the age of seventy. Medical attendance was to continue throughout life. Unlike the German system, the Bill did not include a burial payment provision, thus making it more acceptable to the friendly societies.

The money benefits were to be administered by existing friendly societies and trade unions already operating health insurance plans. In order to qualify for participation in the government program, friendly societies first had to be recognized as "approved societies" by the Insurance Commissioners. Such approval was based on the fulfillment of certain conditions, including the cardinal requirements that the society could not be run for profit except by distributing its benefit to members, and that each society must be subject to the absolute control of its members.[15] The imposition of qualification as an approved society was recognition of the need for government control over the administration of voluntary insurance carriers.[16]

Trade unions might participate in the Act by forming approved societies and, if smaller than a membership of 10,000, by pooling the risks in association with other societies. From an actuarial point of view, friendly societies stood the most to gain, as their own financial reserves would be freed by the new insurance reserve.

In the original Bill, local Health Committees were to be constituted for every county and county borough, one third of the members to be appointed by the county or county borough, one third by the approved societies, and the final third by representatives of deposit contributors, resident in the area, or by the Insurance Commissioners in default of this. In addition to administering the Insurance Act, the local Health Committees were to make general reports and recommendations with relation to the needs of the county or county borough, and to provide for lectures and the publication of information on questions relating to health, as they felt necessary or desirable.[17]

It was an ambitious and far-reaching scheme. Although the insurance principle was a familiar one, central government compulsion was another matter. Fundamental to the Liberal Party's defense of such compulsion was the view that insurance was concerned with the individual not as an individual, but as a member of the social community, endangered by his inability to provide for medical treatment.[18] The government believed that the great majority of the British people would welcome this form of compulsion. Leo Chiozza Money in his *Insurance Versus Poverty* claimed that the average audience anywhere in England accepted compulsion for insurance as a social obligation. Yet he recognized that many persons in the "leisured classes" still had no realization that "the great masses of our people labour under a degree of economic compulsion so intense, so effective, and so inexorable that it would be incredible if it were not an accomplished fact." [19] At the other end of the scale, some members of the Labor Party were either opposed to the contributory principle or, though friendly, were still suspicious of Lloyd George.[20]

Whatever the reservations, they failed to mar the immediate, cordial reaction to the Bill. In the House of Commons the welcome was immediate. Ramsay MacDonald rose to say: "so far as the Labour Party is concerned, we shall certainly co-operate with the Chancellor of the Exchequer in every way we can to make his scheme effective." [21] Austen Chamberlain spoke on behalf of the Conservatives: "Speaking for my honourable Friends, as well as for myself, we shall respond to the appeal made by the Chancellor of the Exchequer in the spirit in which it was made. We are delighted to see the attention of Parliament turned to this matter." [22] John Redmond, after contenting himself as leader of the Irish Nationalists with reminders of social evils extant in Ireland, also announced approval of the Bill.[23]

The Times praised the measure but also sounded one of the first notes of caution:

> The purpose is to avert the consequences of misfortune among the poorer classes of the community by the application of the principle of insurance on a gigantic scale . . . No one will question its desirability; but of its feasibility many doubts will be entertained. It can be done, of course. It is only a question of paying . . . We do not take a pessimistic view, and we do believe that the benefits are worth paying for, but we think the scheme will need a great

deal of readjustment before it is satisfactory, and that plenty of time will be required for the task.[24]

Beatrice Webb attributed the Bill's splendid reception to Lloyd George's "heroic demagogy." The Chancellor, she felt, had taken every item which could be popular with anyone and stirred them into a Bill representing a gigantic transfer of property from the haves, to the have-nots—"enough to make the moderate and constitutional Socialist aghast." [25]

Clouds began to gather after the first acclaim, and by the second reading of the Bill all parties concerned were ready for a pitched battle of divergent interests. From those who were to be most concerned in the operation of a National (Health) Insurance Act, the medical profession, uneasy murmurings had arisen even before the Bill had been introduced.

Early Medical Reaction to the Bill

Lloyd George's plan for national insurance was drawn up with little or no consultation with the medical profession—a source of great irritation to the doctors. Throughout 1910 and early 1911, however, the British Medical Association had been canvassing its members' sentiments on national health insurance.

In its 1905 Report on Contract Practice, the Association had recommended the establishment of locally operated public medical services to meet the overwhelming medical needs of the class just above those aided by the poor law.[26] In testifying before the Royal Commission on the Poor Laws, its representatives had recognized the need for considerable extension of poor law medical care. The Association had been reluctant to commit itself to either the Majority or Minority Report. Doctors were well aware, however, that the government might initiate an insurance scheme. Lloyd George had given warning of his health insurance plans during the discussions on the Old Age Pensions Bill.

In February 1910, the *British Medical Journal* began to grumble that the effect of any form of medical insurance on private practice and medical charities would be far-reaching, and suggested that a departmental committee should inquire into the whole subject.[27] Five weeks later, the *Journal* acknowledged in an editorial that the country would not tolerate the present state of affairs. "The parlous condition of general hospital funds will . . . sooner rather than later, compel boards of management to accept State control in return for State assistance, on any terms that the State chooses to impose." [28] Once again, the *Journal* suggested that a centrally directed medical service might be organized under British Medical Association auspices.

Later in April, 1910, the *Journal* took note of political statements of Asquith and Balfour indicating that sickness insurance was to be put forward by the government, with the words, "This is, undoubtedly, a very serious outlook for the profession, but we cannot stand still and lament the fact, we must endeavour to discover how the intellectual and financial independence of the profession may be secured under the new order of things which seem to be at hand." [29] The same issue of the *Journal* sounded the rising alarm over the possibility of a continuation of the evils of club practice under an insurance plan: "We believe that we express the definite and settled opinion of general practitioners when we assert that the profession will resist to the uttermost any continuance, much more any extension of the club system for medical attendance under the friendly societies, or of the haphazard and pernicious club system that has grown up under the German insurance." [30]

Throughout the second half of 1910, local branches of the Association met to discuss the problem of state sickness insurance. The Medical Secretary of the British Medical Association, Dr. James Smith Whitaker, spoke to the South Wales and Monmouthshire Branch in November of 1910, and stressed the growing national consciousness of the individual as a national asset, which was now combined with the acceptance of a new degree of state intervention in "matters which were formerly left to individual or to voluntary action." [31] Smith Whitaker urged the need for a careful study of the whole subject by the profession and the necessity for united action in response to whatever proposals the Government might put forth.

Letters on the subject of a state medical service and state health insurance began to enter the correspondence columns of the *Journal* even before the Bill was introduced into Parliament. From the University of Liverpool, Dr. Benjamin Moore, Johnston Professor of Bio-Chemistry, wrote to advocate the adoption of a plan of nationalized state medical service as financially beneficial to the young medical practitioner, and of obvious advantage to the community as a whole.[32] His opponents, however, were not many issues of the same magazine behind in denouncing any such plan as Dr. Moore contemplated.

Four days after Lloyd George introduced his measure into the House of Commons, the *British Medical Journal* brought forth a special issue devoted to the Bill, giving an outline of its principal features. The *Journal* pointed out that a Special Committee within the British Medical Association had been working on the problem for the last year, as it might affect the interests of the medical profession. A Special Representative Meeting was announced for Wednesday, the 31st of May to consider the official position of the Association in relation to the Bill.[33] Even before the meeting, the Association had started to canvass members of Parliament and committees of the Liberal and Unionist parties. Letters poured into the *Journal's* editorial offices from doctors throughout the country, reflecting an intensity of feeling which the editors had never before seen.[34]

The first official editorial reaction of the *British Medical Journal*, nevertheless, was restrained:

> The National Health Insurance Bill is in its conception one of the greatest attempts at social legislation which the present generation has known, and seems destined to have a profound influence on social welfare and the health of the community. . . . The members of the medical profession, as good citizens, will approve the objects of the scheme as they would any other well-considered scheme for the benefit of the community, but as its provisions must affect their pecuniary interests, as well as the future development and status of their calling, more seriously than those of any other profession, they are bound to examine it with care and even in a critical spirit.[35]

The first response of *The Lancet* was even more guarded. After describing the features of the Bill, the editorial came to the point at once —the basic fear that the income of medical men would be adversely affected by the measure. While accepting the principle of the Bill as good, *The Lancet* emphasized that "the benefits to the country of national insurance against invalidity shall not be obtained at the undue cost of the medical profession." [36]

Other medical groups at first demonstrated the same ambivalence. The Royal College of Physicians of London sympathized with the objectives of the Bill, but expressed earnest hopes that sufficient time would be permitted for the medical profession to study the provisions of the measure as they might affect medical interests. The Royal College of Surgeons of England, meeting on June first, resolved directly that the Bill should be amended to remove the administration of the medical service from the hands of the friendly societies, that the medical profession should be represented on all committees administering the service, and that the insured be permitted a free choice of medical practitioner.[37] The Royal College of Surgeons of Edinburgh also approved the aims of the Bill, but emphasized the great need of more time for the profession to study the provisions.[38] The General Medical Council appointed a special committee to consider the Bill, which recommended that the government be urged to amend the measure in a number of features involving medical treatment.[39]

Local branches of the British Medical Association, meeting throughout the country in the last part of May and the early days of June, 1911, passed numberless resolutions objecting to various features of the measure. At the Manchester meeting, when the Chairman commented that the Bill would place doctors under the control of friendly societies, loud cries of "No! Never!" filled the hall. So crowded was the meeting that physicians were standing on window ledges, and hundreds jammed the stairs, unable to get in to the hall.[40]

At a special representative meeting held on June 1, 1911, in the Royal College of Surgeons, which was attended by Lloyd George and Braithwaite, the Association proclaimed its famous "six cardinal demands." The Bill, cried the doctors, must be amended to provide the following features:

1. An income limit of £2 a week to be applied to those receiving the medical benefit.
2. A free choice of doctor by the patient, subject to the consent of the doctor to act.
3. Medical and maternity benefits to be administered by the proposed health committees instead of by the friendly societies.
4. The method of remuneration of medical practitioners adopted by each health committee to be fixed according to the preference of the majority of the medical profession of the committee's district.
5. Medical remuneration to be fixed at an amount which the profession considered adequate. (The Representative Body later determined to demand 8s. 6d. as the minimum capitation fee, exclusive of medicine and extras).
6. The medical profession should be adequately represented on the central and local administrative bodies which might be set up to administer the scheme.[41]

The delegates attending this representative meeting, however, also indicated in the resolution carrying their six cardinal demands that they approved the objects of the bill and wished to co-operate in their attainment.

Lloyd George was at his politic best as he met these "representatives of scores of furious meetings of doctors breathing blood and fury." [42] The Chancellor assured his audience in flowing language of his good will towards physicians:

> You may take it from the very start that the axiom which you have laid down is also the axiom which I would accept—that what is best for the profession is in the long run best for the patient, and that any kind of feeling of wrong, of injustice, or of irritation—I mean of just irritation which may rankle in your breasts in respect of the arrangements in this Bill, must be detrimental to the healing value of the measure itself. [43]

Braithwaite rejoiced as Lloyd George calmed the doctors, noting later that he did not believe such a triumph of personality possible in England. [44] But the surface peace soon faded. The profession was already suspicious of Lloyd George's charm and of a difference between his words and his intentions. *The Lancet* warned that when Lloyd George's response was examined more closely, setting aside the charm of his manner, it was clear that the Chancellor had promised "little more than his own personal support, if an easy opportunity for giving it should arise." [45]

The June first meeting had, in fact, only opened the fight between Lloyd George and the doctors. Despite the Chancellor's charm, it rapidly became clear that much of the ensuing bitterness was due to the personality of the Bill's sponsor. Dr. Alfred Cox, who became Medical Secretary of the Association during the course of the battle, remarked that if any other Minister but Lloyd George had introduced the Bill there might have been less violent opposition. But, especially to Conservatives within the profession "Lloyd George was like a red rag to a bull." [46] Cox related the attitude of the Chairman of the Council of the British Medical Association, Dr. J. A. MacDonald, towards the Chancellor, by describing MacDonald's confession that he "had to keep almost superhuman control over himself in these deputations. I remember him saying on one occasion when we left Whitehall, 'If you fellows only knew how hard I find it sometimes to keep my hands off him.' " [47]

Lloyd George, however, was well able to repay the attacks on him launched in the medical journals. At Birmingham, his "Wrangle in the Sick-Room" speech sent medical temperatures soaring:

I had two hours discussion with the medical men themselves the other day. I do not think there has been anything like it since the days when Daniel went into the lion's den. I was on the dissecting table for two hours, but I can assure you they treated me with the same courtesy as the lions treated my illustrious predecessor. You must remember, this discussion about what they ought to be paid is an old one. I cannot say that I care very much for this wrangle in the sick room; it is unpleasant, and may well become unseemly; all the same it has got to be settled. For the moment I am the buffer state. The doctors say to me that 6s. is not enough, and they cuff me on one side of the head. The Friendly Societies say "How dare you give so much," and I get another cuff this side of the head, and between them I can only receive it with that Christian meekness which characterizes politicians.[48]

The Bill in Passage

As the summer wore on the campaign grew more intense. The man who was to become president of the British Medical Association the following year, Sir James Barr, denounced the measure as a step towards socialism. Dr. Alfred Cox noted shrewdly, however, that some of the most vigorous opponents of the measure were consultants who would not be directly affected by the Bill.[49] There were others, however, like Dr. Lauriston Shaw of Guy's Hospital, and Sir Victor Horsley, the brain surgeon, who held more liberal views.

Within Parliament, Dr. Christopher Addison was the main spokesman for the Association in attempting to push through the six cardinal points. Addison recorded how, in an effort to change the controlling role given the friendly societies in the Bill, he canvassed almost every member of the House of Commons.[50] In debate on the Bill's second reading medical objections to many features affecting medical interests were raised by Dr. Addison, Mr. H. W. Foster, and Sir Robert Finlay. In the committee stage, medical pressures were exerted to their fullest.

Meanwhile in July, 1911, the Association, aiming for a united front, circulated a pledge for the signature of all its members:

I, the undersigned, hereby undertake that, in the event of the National Insurance Bill becoming law, I will not enter into any agreement for giving medical attendance and treatment to persons insured under the Bill, excepting as shall be satisfactory to the

medical profession and in accordance with the declared policy of
the British Medical Association; and that I will enter into such
agreement only through a Local Medical Committee representative of the medical profession in the district in which I practise,
and will not enter into any individual or separate agreement with
any approved society or other body, for the treatment of such
persons.[51]

The pledge was signed by 26,000 practitioners in the summer of 1911,
and the Association started a "Central Insurance Defense Fund." In
all, the British Medical Association was to spend £53,000 on the campaign. More than £134,000 was pledged.[52]

By the time the Bill reached committee stage, the Association's protests began to get results through amendments based on some of the
six cardinal points. Dr. Christopher Addison introduced one of the
most significant amendments and carried it with a large majority in
committee—namely that the administration of medical benefit be
transferred from the approved societies to the health committees,
which, by amendment, had become insurance committees. Four of the
six points had been written into the Bill by the third reading, but the
Government arbitrarily refused to consider any £2-income limit, and
the House of Commons voted against this amendment. The *British
Medical Journal* on August 5, 1911, noted that the profession had
made itself felt and had achieved a very large measure of success.[53]
The medical profession was not pleased either by the "Harmsworth
Amendment," which protected vested interests of medical institutes
(affiliates of the friendly societies), or by the fact that they did not obtain as large a representation as they had hoped for on the local insurance committees. The real time of stress, however, was yet to come
—when the Bill became law.

Lloyd George allowed only five days for the report stage of the
Bill, and the Conservatives attempted to push through a resolution
during the third reading which called for a longer period, in which the
measure should be considered by the House and the country. The
resolution was rejected and the Bill went to the House of Lords on
the sixth of December.

Dr. Addison spoke in the House of Commons in the final hours of
passage:

I think not one of us in this House would be willing to wait until
we had a perfect measure. As one who has supported this Bill, I
have not been sparing in criticism of it, but from the very begin-

ning I felt that to lose the measure would be a catastrophe to the
health of the country. What does it do? It provides, for the first
time, something which will combine fifteen millions of the working class in one common bond to promote one another's good
health.[54]

Asquith led the measure to its final acceptance with the words:
"the House, in reading this Bill a Third Time, are conferring upon
millions of our fellow-countrymen by the joint operation of self-help
and of State help, the greatest alleviation of the risks and sufferings of
life that Parliament has ever conferred upon any people." [55]

The Continuing Storm

The passage of the National (Health) Insurance Act brought no calm
to the profession. Instead, a last ditch fight to defeat implementation
of the Act opened. When the measure was sent to the House of Lords,
the *British Medical Journal* prefaced a lead editorial with the (mis-
quoted) phrase: "Gentlemen, said Washington to his counsellors, let
us all hang together, for if we do not we shall all hang separately." [56]
But already a separation of feeling stirred through medical ranks.

The Bill was not to come into operation, excepting provisions dealing with the establishment of administrative bodies, until July 15, 1912,
while insured persons were not to receive benefits until the expiration
of a six-month period following on the Act's coming into force. Medical
benefit, therefore at the earliest would not come into effect until the
middle of January 1913. The interval was to be rife with friction.

On the thirtieth of November, 1911, the Prime Minister's Private
Secretary had written to Dr. James Smith Whitaker, Medical Secretary
of the British Medical Association, and offered him the post of Deputy
Chairman of the Insurance Commissioners. It was a difficult decision,
and Dr. Smith Whitaker referred it to the Association's Council. The
Council, by a vote of 38 to 3, resolved that Dr. Smith Whitaker was
free to accept the post, on the assumption that the Bill would be passed
regardless of any action of the medical profession.[57]

The Council's action, however, did not find universal support. *The
Lancet* remarked with surprise: "The acceptance by Mr. J. Smith
Whitaker, with the approval of the Council of the British Medical
Association, of the post of Deputy Chairman of the Board of Commis-
sioners to be constituted under the Act, must be regarded as a policy

of compromise on the part of the Association, whose position will be puzzling to all of its ordinary members, and is mortifying in the extreme to some of them." [58]

The mortification which *The Lancet* suggested must be felt was given free reign at a disastrous mass meeting at Queen's Hall on December 19th. Victor Horsley, who rose to defend Dr. Smith Whitaker's step, was howled down with hisses and angry cries of "Traitor." The scene did little to raise the dignity of the profession in the eyes of the public, and the controversy and bitterness went on within the Association's staff. Dr. Cox, who had succeeded Smith Whitaker noted that the internal situation could hardly have been worse. "The die-hards became more embittered and even some of the moderates were shaken by the Whitaker episode. I had a difficult time at meetings, for if I defended Whitaker's action, I was under suspicion as having been promoted through his defection." [59]

Yet all that the group led by Addison, Smith Whitaker, and Horsley, had sought to do was to find a solution to an impossible situation. Horsley regarded the medical profession's mass hostility to the Act as shortsighted and opposed to the country's best interests.[60] Horsley's distinguished colleague in surgery, C. J. Bond, was subsequently to comment of Horsley's view in this:

> He clearly realized that what the world sorely needs is a deeper and wider recognition of the fact that selfishness and the aggressive spirit, although they no doubt had some survival value among primitive peoples and savage tribes, under modern conditions of so-called civilization, they act as brakes on the wheels of human progress.[61]

Nevertheless, the "brakes on the wheels of human progress" continued to grind noisily in the ensuing months. The Council of the British Medical Association had officially recommended, just prior to the passage of the Act, that an attempt be made to work out a further agreement with the Act's new administrative appointees to gain the profession's demands with respect to terms of appointment and remuneration. On December 23, the *British Medical Journal* editorialized that until this was done the doctors should not strike.[62]

The Act already incorporated four of the six cardinal points: free choice of doctor, administration of medical and sanatoria benefits by the local insurance committees instead of by the approved societies, representation on all the administrative bodies established under the

Bill, and a committee of the medical profession in each district to represent all registered practitioners in the area on general questions of the administration of medical benefit.

At a Manchester meeting on December 14, however, a strong protest had been raised against the Council's action. A group of medical men of that city angrily constituted themselves the National Medical Union, whose aim was to persuade all medical practitioners to refuse to work under the Act unless it were amended in accordance with the original demands of the British Medical Association. The National Medical Union censored the officials of the Association for their weak policy towards the government, and in London a Reform Group was started to change the composition of the Association's Council.[63]

Two letters sent to the Editor of *The Times* in early January, 1912, typified the split in the profession. The august Dr. Clifford Albutt, Regius Professor of Physics at Cambridge, could only attack the Act as stifling the growth of medicine, sweeping the country back upon old methods. Instead of the contract system, Albutt suggested payment to doctors for work carried out.[64] Sir Lauriston Shaw, one of the leaders of the Addison-Horsley group, replied on January ninth, pointing out that the one great merit of the Act was the elasticity of its provisions, and the fact that it left the method of remuneration and the amount statistically undetermined. So many features of the Act were still fluid, that Shaw felt the medical profession could mold its future, and he urged their co-operation in the measure.[65]

Meanwhile, the Insurance Commissioners had already been appointed as the central administrative authority under the Act. Sir Robert Morant * who had been serving as permanent secretary of the Board of Education, had accepted the post of Chairman.[66] William Braithwaite, despite his major role in the conception of the act, was thus pushed to the background. To the eyes of the sick and disheartened Braithwaite, Morant's charm vanished "when he spoke to the waiters in a way I should be ashamed to speak to a dog." [67] But Morant was the strong man of the hour, and, with Braithwaite's help

* Robert Morant (1863–1920) was educated at Winchester and New College, taking a theological degree in 1885. After ten years of teaching, he entered the Government's Education Department. An important figure in the passage of the Education Act of 1902, Morant became Permanent Secretary of the Board of Education in 1903. He was awarded the K.C.B. in 1907. Morant served as Chairman of the National Health Insurance Commission from 1911 to 1919.

for a few more months, he plunged into a morass of setting up administrative machinery, hiring staff, placating irate doctors, and interpreting the hastily drawn-up legislation. Among those who were to join the insurance staff were Dr. James Smith Whitaker, as Deputy Chairman of the Insurance Commissioners, Mr. David J. Shackleton, former President of the Trade Union Congress, Miss Mona Wilson, Secretary of the Women's Trade Union League, and John S. Bradbury of the Treasury Department (later Lord Bradbury).

The Commissioners quickly commenced overtures to the profession. A first invitation to discuss the situation had to be postponed, all of the medical bodies invited having declined on grounds of being given too little time to consider the request. Meanwhile, a Special Meeting of British Medical Association Representatives in February of 1912 decided that the Association's Council's report placed too favorable a construction on the Act. A new statement was sent out, which called upon the profession not to work under the Act "unless the minimum demands of the profession are effectually and permanently embodied by the Commissioners in the Regulations, with a view to their subsequent incorporation in an amending Act." [68]

A State Sickness Committee was formed next by the Association, and to it was assigned the drawing up of specific proposals to be submitted to the Insurance Commissioners. A Special Representative Meeting approved the State Sickness Committee's recommendations on remuneration. The Government had offered a fee of 6s. per head, including drugs; the Association now demanded a fee of 8s. 6d. (exclusive of drugs) and forwarded the proposal to the Insurance Commissioners on February 29, 1912.[69]

When his skeleton staff and offices were being organized, Morant decided to institute an investigation into the basis for the doctors' claims to a capitation fee of 8s. 6d. Sir William (later Lord) Plender * was asked to visit six sample towns to determine the average charges for medical treatment; three towns were to be selected by the Commissioners and three by the State Sickness Committee of the British Medical Association.

Sir William's investigation took him through the 1910 and 1911

* William Plender (1861–1946), who was serving as President of the Institute of Chartered Accountants at the time of his work for Morant, had earlier helped to establish the Port of London Authority. He was knighted in 1911. Subsequently, he was to serve as High Sheriff of Kent and of the county of London, and Lieutenant of the City of London. He was created a baron in 1931.

books kept by medical practitioners in Cardiff, Darlington, Darwen, Dundee, Norwich, and St. Albans. He also obtained information from the superintendents in charge of hospitals, infirmaries, and dispensaries in the same towns. A total of 265 medical practitioners were approached in Plender's sample study, and of these, 51 (40 in Cardiff) refused access to their records.[70] Plender found the average annual gross income from visits to patients' houses and attendance at surgeries, less a proportion for bad debts, to be 4s. 2d. per head. Income derived from patients attended under contract was 4s. 1¾d. per head of the total population. These figures, which were rushed into press without consultation with the British Medical Association were considerably below the demands put forth by the State Sickness Committee. The *British Medical Journal* felt the investigation was carried out too hastily, and furiously denounced the deductions as incorrect and one-sided.[71]

Technically, the Act came into effect on July 15, but negotiations between the government and the doctors were then still very fluid. The government offered to raise the fee to physicians to 7s. 6d., but met with no success. Finally, on October 23rd, Lloyd George made an offer of 9s., but the figure was to include the supply of drugs, and it was unavailing. The British Medical Association then demanded that all medical men resign from the Advisory Committee of the Insurance Commissioners. A Representative Meeting of the Association rejected Lloyd George's proposal and urged all members of the profession to unite in refusing to take service under the Act. The vote rejecting service under the Act was 11,219 for refusal, 2,408 for acceptance.[72] Of the votes rejecting service, 9,331 were cast by members of the association, and 1,888 by nonmembers; 1,963 of the votes for acceptance were cast by members, 445 by nonmembers. A total of 13,773 doctors, however, did not vote.[73]

Local medical committees were left free, and the Representative Meeting suggested that they negotiate with the insured persons, offering them a panel of doctors who would attend them on terms approved by the Association, the terms to include the application of an income limit.[74]

Before the final decision taken by the representative meeting, however, fourteen prominent medical men refused to resign from the Insurance Commissioners Advisory Committee. This group included Christopher Addison, Sir Victor Horsley, Arthur Latham, F.R.C.P., Sir Shirley Murphy, and Sir C. J. Bond, F.R.C.S.[75] Dr. Lauriston Shaw of Guy's Hospital and Dr. H. H. Mills of Kensington joined in the secession. On December 13, 1912, at a meeting held in the Holborn Restaurant, London, medical practitioners who were willing to serve under the Act formed the National Insurance Practitioner's Association.

Lauriston Shaw (1859–1923), Horsley's distinguished friend and colleague, chaired the dramatic Holborn meeting. Dr. Alfred Salter, later Labor Member of Parliament from Bermondsey, who had proposed the setting up of the new body, stated that the British Medical Association vote was misleading because only half the practitioners attended divisional meetings, and many of those who did attend were intimidated into voting for refusal.[76]

On the eighteenth of December, Lloyd George replied to a letter from the National Insurance Practitioner's Association, which had asked, among other things, whether doctors who took service under the Act would receive the government's support against boycott or intimidation. He could scarcely believe, wrote the Chancellor warmly, "that any such methods could be employed against doctors on the ground that they were engaged in carrying out an Act of Parliament!" If any attempt were made to intimidate doctors anywhere in the country, he concluded, the Government would support them "by every means in their power." [77]

In Birmingham, a group led by Dr. J. B. Brash, invited Addison to present the views of the new Association. A resolution supporting the National Insurance Practitioner's Association was carried, and a panel in Birmingham was assured.

Despite the opposition of the British Medical Association, the Insurance Commissioners were able to build up a skeleton staff against the medical benefit's coming into force on January fifteenth. By January third, they had published a list of 10,000 doctors willing to serve on the panels. To doctors who were already employed under panel service, the 9s. capitation fee meant a large improvement in their incomes. Despite lurid warnings in the Northcliffe Press,[78] it was clearly apparent that the Insurance Act would be manned for operation by the scheduled date.

Doctors throughout the country then clamored to be admitted to the panels and called upon the Association to release them from their pledges. Recognizing that the strike which had never started was ended, a Special Representative Meeting of the Association, on January 18, 1913, resolved to release all practitioners from their pledge. National

Health Insurance Medical Benefit was in force, and the public rushed to sign. In Stepney, the popular Dr. Harry Roberts was besieged by East End patients queueing on stairs, in bedrooms, and bathrooms to sign the pink cards and join his panel. It was still unbelievable to great masses of people that one could see the doctor and be given a bottle of medicine "for nothing," and so they came by the scores to test it out.[79]

The Act and the Association

At first glance the British Medical Association appeared to have lost the Insurance struggle. Furious doctors' letters to the *British Medical Journal* criticized the way the Association conducted the final battle. But the dramatic climax in January, 1913, obscured the very real gains which the Association had obtained, primarily to further the professions' interests.

The manner in which the Act had been framed, with almost no consultation with representatives of the medical profession, had been responsible for much of the uproar. Lloyd George in March, 1911, had explained his plan to some medical officers of health,[80] and subsequently claimed he consulted with two other bodies of medical men before introducing his Bill.[81] In the haste with which the Bill was put together, Lloyd George, in fact, had never seriously consulted representatives of the doctors. In actuality, he and Braithwaite had done far more in early talks to appease the friendly societies.

Despite such understandable provocation, the British Medical Association never attempted to introduce any fundamental changes in the Bill which might improve its public health implications. True, one provision of the Act (Section 63) dealt with action to be taken in areas where excessive illness among insured persons was revealed. The Association did not, however, attempt to improve the Bill in regard to larger questions of co-ordination with the public health authorities.[82]

The Act covered only a segment of the population—almost entirely the adult male wage earner—and then only for short-term risks.[83] Even Lloyd George viewed the legislation as a temporary expedient. The medical benefit did not include major operations, specialist services, nurses, diagnostic X-ray, or general hospital services. The *British Medical Journal* took note of such weaknesses,[84] but the Association had not seen fit to incorporate them in its "cardinal points."

As a body, the British Medical Association was primarily concerned with its own administrative and pecuniary status under the Bill; and the last-ditch fight in the closing days of 1912 revealed a vocal majority still determined to secure a service which would be available only to those employed at very low wage scales.

Within the Association's ranks, however, was a group of far-sighted men who recognized the important community benefits of national health insurance. Names like Addison, Shaw, and Horsley led the small roster of both eminent consultants and private practitioners, who believed it the physician's social responsibility to accept service under the Act. Their influence, in conjunction with the Association's failure to maintain effective controls over medical men throughout the country, threw the victory to the Government.

To what extent those private practitioners who enrolled immediately in the panels were inspired by economic interest rather than a belief in the Insurance Act as a national necessity is, of course, not ascertainable. Immediately after the Act's coming into force with respect to medical benefit, British Medical Association membership declined sharply,[85] presumably because the Association had been unable to maintain an effective control over the whole profession in a question of vital economic interest to all.

From the outset the British Medical Association had accepted the need for some form of public medical service and had recognized in the Bill a measure for community good. The long years of strained relations with friendly societies, however, intensified the doctors' fears of an approved society control under the new measure. Subjectively, their resistance to the Bill can also be linked to prevailing professional dislike of any form of lay control over interests of the medical brotherhood.

But by the start of 1913, they had capitulated, and only sporadic outcries could be heard thereafter. A measure of the physicians' acceptance of the Act as a working reality by 1917 is reflected in a statement of the Association's Insurance Act's Committee. They found the degree of current unanimity, over a subject formerly so controversial, to be remarkable. Not only, observed the committee, did physicians now approve the system in the main, but substantial numbers favored an extension of health insurance, both to provide additional treatment facilities and to make the service available to a broader segment of the community.[86]

With the passage of the Act, England entered a new era in state intervention for public health. To the earlier Government obligations in preventive medicine there were now added widespread responsibilities in the provision of curative medicine and personal health services. If individualism was threatened by the growing corporate society of the twentieth century, the individual, unquestionably, had now become of greater personal concern to the state. For the maintenance of personal health had become the specific responsibility of society.

Chapter XII

The Medical Profession and Government Action in Public Health by 1912—A Perspective

THE PASSAGE of Lloyd George's Insurance Act demonstrated, as never before, the radical change in public outlook which had taken place in England between 1870 and 1912. Central government compulsion for health and welfare had become acceptable to a degree considered intolerable in the eighteen-seventies. Simultaneously, the scope and direction of public health expanded from sanitary reform to the provision of curative medicine and personal health services. During the same years the physician's relationship to government evolved from the independent professional, loosely linked to community authority, to a status close to that of a state agent.

Many forces contributed to this great shift in public attitude and practice. Scientific developments in the prevention and treatment of disease created new horizons of health. Medical research emerged as a valuable public function, and the Insurance Act of 1911, in annually setting aside one penny per insured person for medical research, confirmed the state's investment in scientific progress. Advances in the use of health statistics substantiated the need for governmental action for corporate health. The value of the preventive campaign was reflected in the increase in average life expectancy of ten years for men and nearly eleven years for women between the years 1871–1880 and 1910–1912. Over the same period some 235,000 lives were saved annually, 64 per cent of which could be attributed to reduced mortality from acute and chronic infectious diseases.[1]

As an outgrowth both of the scientific advance and the new statistical approach, the word of the expert now carried greater weight in the government. Simon's struggle with lay administrators ended in defeat, although his expert tradition survived within the Local Government Board's Medical Department. While the expert serving in a bureaucratic milieu of any age can face problems similar to Simon's, the twentieth century was to place greater reliance on technical advice. Sir Arthur Newsholme, as Chief Medical Officer of the Local Government Board, was able to extract the promise from the Board's President that before any recommendation of the Medical Department was vetoed on the advice of the lay secretariat, Newsholme would first be given the opportunity of presenting his case in person.[2]

A further and major factor in the changed public attitude towards government intervention was the political rise of the working class and the publicizing of their economic and health needs by the late nineteenth-century social reformers. No longer did working-class men and women passively accept the gross inequalities in distribution of wealth which left them in the bleak poverty accompanying industrialization. Even to middle-class humanitarian reformers it was finally evident that voluntary charity was irrelevant in the massive social and economic degradation of the cities. The problems of the working class were now a community responsibility in the larger social structure of the twentieth century.

The development of the personal health services marked the start of a new public value of individual health, in a society whose national health might only be as strong as that of its weakest members. As the surgeon and humanitarian C. J. Bond wrote in 1912, "We now realize that the possibility of a healthy and happy life must be within the reach of every citizen, rich and poor, in every community, if that community is to escape the stagnation and decay which eventually overtook . . . ancient civilizations." [3]

National health insurance was the political substitute for a thorough overhaul of the public health services, preventive and curative, indicated by the reports of the Poor Law Commission of 1909. One of the great weaknesses of Lloyd George's insurance scheme was that it was pieced onto existing services, rather than being welded into a co-ordinated program of prevention and cure. The medical assistance available under the Act was limited. Only wage earners making less than £160 a year were covered by the Act, and no provision was made for their dependents. While services of a general practitioner were available without charge to those insured, there was no provision for medical consultant services or hospital treatment. Nevertheless, the National Insurance Act of 1911 constituted an unprecedented advance in government action to provide medical care to a large segment of English society.

Clearly, the British medical profession had an important share in extending the government's role in preventive and curative medicine from 1870 to 1912. It was largely through his own actions that the physician became a key figure in the state's health programs. Medical officers in government service were among the first to recognize the need for extending state action. The natural sequel to Simon's interventionist outlook in preventive medicine was Sir Arthur Newsholme's simple but "socialist" statement: "In the interest of the public health medical services should be readily available for all needing them, and not confined, as at present, to insured persons, to persons under the poor law, to mothers and children under the limited conditions of maternity and child welfare schemes, and of the school medical service." [4]

The British Medical Association and other representatives of the profession were influential in bringing about the creation of the Royal Sanitary Commission. During passage of the public health acts of the early seventies, medical men demanded reforms and attempted to secure revisions of legislation which did not extend far enough to meet sanitary needs.

Between 1871 and 1900, the Local Government Board's medical officers never advocated central government responsibility for the whole of preventive and curative health functions. Their weak administrative position, combined with the existing separation of government health activities, made strong central medical action an improbability. Nevertheless, the Board's medical men did forward sanitary and preventive health programs and must be credited for much of the reduction in incidence of infectious disease by the end of the century.

Poor law medical officers, while devoting much effort to improving their own status, nevertheless urged improvement of medical care to the poor repeatedly. Individual parish doctors worked under difficult conditions, and by 1909 defects in poor law medical treatment were still grave. Local deviations from the centrally established formula of a more liberal administration of sick relief negated the efforts of the Poor Law Medical Officers Association to obtain uniform improvements in medical care. The Association did achieve a measure of success in attempting to persuade the central government to remedy abuses in medical treatment under the poor law.

Similarly, the Society of Medical Officers of Health extended the state's interest in many areas of public health. Never supporting an indiscriminate widening of government health functions, the Society made its decisions upon individual problems as they arose. In expanding its interest during the eighteen-nineties to the personal health services, the Society kept step with contemporary social developments.

Private practitioners, over the years from 1870 to 1900, were drawn into closer linkage with the state, and their responsibilities to the state increased. The notification acts, registration of birth and death requirements, and extended participation in judicial processes—all brought the private practitioner within a larger framework of government health action. Private practitioners helped significantly to educate public opinion for better sanitary standards. A handful, recognizing the urgent need for low-cost medical care, developed plans for a state health service before 1900. By 1905, a large body of opinion within the British Medical Association had acknowledged the necessity of some form of public medical service. The British Medical Association preferred such service to be established locally and operated under the direction of the medical profession rather than the government.

While opposing some public health measures on grounds of professional interest, the Association supported many national collective measures to improve the health of the people of England and Wales. Medical men as a group had increasingly recognized the change in concept of "public medicine" in the new society of the twentieth century. The Association supported in principle the development of state intervention for the personal health services. Yet, on several occasions, it opposed, as contravening their professional interests, central legislation extending government control in this area.

Vested professional interests were largely responsible for the dramatic medical clashes with the Government in 1911 and 1912, when the British Medical Association made a determined attempt to limit insurance to those earning two pounds weekly or less. But in the months before the introduction of the Bill, the Association took a realistic view of the situation, recognizing that some form of state health insurance was a political and economic necessity. Yet, although well aware that the Insurance Bill provided little or no co-ordination with existing public health services, the Association, during the passage of the Act, made no effort to alter the Bill on these grounds. As a body, the Association acted primarily in its own administrative and pecuniary interest in its demands for changing the Bill.

However, there were within the ranks of the British Medical Association a number of medical men (some of them leading consultants) with a vision broader than their own pockets, who succeeded in revolting from the official policy. It was due to the efforts of these practical humanitarians within the Association, as well as to numbers of practitioners outside its orbit, that the government succeeded in establishing the initial panels. Less than five years after activation of national health insurance, the Association's Insurance Act's Committee found that a majority of doctors serving under the Act wished it broadened to cover a larger section of the population and to improve and extend available services.

From an international perspective, England led the nineteenth-century world in the sanitary advance, just as she had pioneered in industrializing her economy. Industrialization had carried with it alternations to living and working conditions which threatened the health of the nation if not met by community action. But England lagged behind several Western European nations from ten to thirty years in assuming government responsibility for some of the personal health services and in adopting national health insurance for workingmen. This delay may partially be explained by the slower political development of an articulate labor movement in England than took place in countries like Germany and Austria.

The over-all British advances in the assumption of national responsibility for public health from 1870 to 1912 come into clearer perspective by even a brief contemporary contrast with the United States. England, during the last thirty years of the nineteenth century and the first decade of the twentieth century had a 60 per cent population increase, emerging in 1912 as a nation of 36,539,636. The United States, which numbered 39,818,449 persons in 1870, counted 91,972,266 persons by 1910—a phenomenal growth in which immigration played a large part.[5] Almost one seventh of the U.S. population in 1910 was foreign born.

The same years were a period of unprecedented industrial expansion and an extraordinary growth of urban centers in the United States. Although the western frontier still offered great acres of rich, uncleared territory to the hardy, the industrial cities of the East and Middle West teemed with poverty, slums, malnutrition, and disease.

Prior to 1872 only three states—Massachusetts, California, and Virginia, together with the District of Columbia—had established boards of health. Only two states maintained registers of births, deaths, and marriages which had any claim to accuracy.[6] As in England, fear of contagious disease forced national action. In 1879, after one of the most severe yellow fever epidemics ever to invade the country, Congress created a temporary National Board of Health responsible directly to the President of the United States. Like England's early General Board of Health, this agency was unpopular and short-lived. Its authority was ill defined. The medical members of the National Board of Health seemed overzealous, and Congressmen, imbued with strong states' rights concepts, resented the new federal whiplash. A re-enactment bill in June, 1883, failed to pass.[7]

The basic American political framework, with its problem of federal-state relationships, delayed national action for public health until it became clear that state and local governments were unable to handle many health and welfare problems.[8]

Throughout the nineteenth century, most of such health functions as were exercised by the federal government were carried out by the Marine Hospital Service, founded in 1798 to care for sick and disabled seamen. The Constitution of the United States delegated no express powers for the public health to the federal government. In consequence, such federal health functions as were undertaken related to constitutional provisions dealing with the regulation of commerce, taxing to promote the general welfare, making of treaties, and supervision of federal territory and reservations. The power to regulate commerce provided the federal government with the exercise of police powers over interstate and national affairs and was an important basis for the initiation of federal health action. Thus federal jurisdiction in 1912 covered such matters as international health relations (quarantine, medical examinations of immigrants, negotiating and implementing international health agreements, reporting the occurrence of epidemic disease, and control of interstate spread of disease); scientific research and investigations; collection and dissemination of information relating to public health and sanitation; and the medical care of beneficiaries specified by federal law.[9] Acts of Congress, authorizing specific federal health functions and appropriating funds to carry out such responsibilities, were necessary to develop a federal health program.

In 1902, the Marine Hospital Service was renamed by Congress the Public Health and Marine Hospital Service, and in the same year the Service was authorized to regulate use of such biologic products (in interstate or foreign traffic) as viruses, serums, vaccines, and antitoxins. In 1912, Congress, in passing a bill authorizing field investigations and research, renamed the federal authority the United States Public

Health Service. But the Public Health Service remained within the U.S. Treasury Department. It was not until 1953, seventy years after the demise of the National Board of Health, that Congress established a Department of Health, Education, and Welfare, and once more a national health agency existed in the United States.

During its lifetime the Marine Hospital Service, limited though its powers were, gradually extended its activities in control of epidemic disease. A young officer of the Marine Hospital Service, Dr. Joseph J. Kinyoun, after touring European scientific research centers in the eighteen-eighties, established one of the first bacteriological laboratories in the United States. From this early "Hygienic Laboratory" on Staten Island, New York there ultimately developed by the mid-twentieth century the largest medical research organization in the world—the National Institutes of Health at Bethesda, Maryland.

But the early basis for sanitary reform came not from the federal government but from local and state authorities. By the close of the nineteenth century local community action had at least laid a basis for the development of public health programs.

Many American physicians aided the growth of local sanitary programs, as individuals and through their state medical societies. While the American Medical Association during the seventies supported the establishment of a National Board of Health and agitated for legislation on vital statistics and on the sale of food and drugs, the Association had relatively little influence on nineteenth-century legislation.[10]

Although a few American communities initiated maternal and child welfare programs and school health services before the close of the first decade of the twentieth century, no parallel to England's National Insurance Act developed in the United States. Public responsibility for curative medicine was limited to the destitute in the U.S., and the adequacy of such care varied widely from state to state. The American colonists brought with them the English poor law under the basic English common law. Unlike England, no national supervision in the U.S. guided the quality of medical assistance to the destitute. America during this period never had large segments of her society on poor relief, as did England. Most sick paupers in the United States, if not cared for by charitable organizations, were treated in local almshouses during the nineteenth century and early years of the twentieth century.[11]

The only provision for medical care by the federal government was that gradually authorized by law for special classes of federal beneficiaries—merchant seamen, Indian tribes, personnel of the Army,

Navy, and Coast Guard, persons suffering from leprosy, federal government employees injured on duty, and other small miscellaneous groups.[12]

It was not until the decade after the passage of Lloyd George's Insurance Act that any real start was made in formulating social policy in America. Although by 1910 every leading European country had adopted workmen's compensation legislation, only four of the United States—Maryland, Massachusetts, Montana, and New York—had passed laws providing for some form of compensation. Several of these laws were shortly thereafter declared unconstitutional.[13] Sickness insurance, available from U.S. mutual societies, fraternal organizations, and similar private groups, covered only a small proportion of those in need of it—the aristocracy of the working class.

The American Association for Labor Legislation, organized in 1906 with a small intellectual membership composed primarily of economists, social workers, and political and social scientists, led a brief struggle in the U.S. in 1912 for national health insurance.[14] During 1912 compulsory health insurance was adopted by the third-party Progressives, headed in this election by Theodore Roosevelt. But with the election that year of Woodrow Wilson, the Progressive Party and its broad social platform went down to defeat.

Social insurance continued to interest a number of American reformers, including some medical men, in the decade from 1910 to 1920. The American Association for Labor Legislation established a Committee on Social Insurance in 1912. Three members of this Committee were liberal physicians, who also served on the American Medical Association's Committee on Social Insurance after its creation in 1915: Drs. Alexander Lambert, I. M. Rubinow, and S. S. Goldwater.

The American Medical Association, established in 1847, took no stand against health insurance until 1920, when its House of Delegates formally resolved that the Association "declares its opposition to the institution of any plan embodying the system of compulsory, contributory insurance against illness, or any other plan of compulsory insurance which provides for medical service to be rendered to contributors or their dependents, provided, controlled or regulated by any State or the Federal Government." [15]

During the years 1911 to 1912, when the Lloyd George Insurance Act was evolving in England, the *Journal of the American Medical Association* published regular letters from its "London Correspondent" which were unfriendly to the Act. But the *Journal* also carried a series of articles in support of England's new program of government-sponsored medical care. The Association's Committee on Social Insurance, a few years later, praised the British system and indicated considerable sympathy for compulsory health insurance legislation in the U.S.

In November, 1912, a lead editorial of the *Journal of the American Medical Association* gave lengthy and thoughtful consideration to the implications of the Lloyd George Act. The editor noted that although the law was "probably the most revolutionary, so far as medical practice is concerned, of any measure yet introduced in an English speaking country, the controversy between the government and the physicians has been almost entirely over the question of compensation and not over the principles on which the act is based." [16] The *Journal* pointed out that the English law marked the beginning of a new era for society and physicians. The modern physician had become a "health officer for the State, working for the general good rather than as a private, professional or business man." Some similar arrangements, the *Journal's* editor felt, "will, sooner or later, be considered on this side of the Atlantic." [17]

More than half a century was to pass before the United States—in 1965—reached a period when even limited national health insurance stood a serious chance of passing the United States Congress. In the period 1910 to 1920, before American Medical Association opposition had coalesced, the American Association for Labor Legislation and the liberal physicians who favored compulsory health insurance did not have the support of organized labor. They failed to develop an effective national organization to back their program and underestimated the strength of vested interests of commercial insurance companies and of many members of the American medical profession.[18] Although several states, led by California, established commissions to study compulsory health insurance, neither major political party, for many years to come, seriously thought of adopting platforms in favor of national compulsory health insurance.

American society with its deeply rooted tradition of individual freedom, its dislike of governmental regulatory powers, and its many economic and educational opportunities for those who would work to improve their lot, was not ready to agree that the workingman was unable to provide independently for his medical care.

Neither had the United States in the first decade of the twentieth century come to a realization of the national value of a healthy population. In a country richly endowed with material resources and with an unlimited supply of cheap labor through immigration, there had been little need to think in terms of conservation. Theodore Roosevelt had organized a National Conservation Commission in 1909, and aroused some public interest in the preservation of natural resources. A Committee of One Hundred on National Health in the same year prepared for the National Conservation Commission a *Report on National Vitality: Its Waste and Conservation.* The report demanded that "The National Government should at least exercise public health functions: investigations, dissemination of information, and administration . . . and . . . remove the reproach that more pains are now taken to protect the health of farm cattle than of human beings." [19] The Committee's report did not suggest national health insurance, however, and its general reproaches fell on deaf ears.

But across the Atlantic Lloyd George's Act was in operation by 1912. With the support of the British medical profession, some 15,000,000 wage earners were now partially covered against the risks of illness. Over the succeeding years the benefits and the number of employed persons covered expanded steadily. And finally in 1946, England, with all levels of her society united as never before through the agonizing struggle for survival in World War II, took the step of providing comprehensive medical care to all persons in the country. Postwar America enthusiastically accepted the concept of large-scale federal support for medical research, but no bill to establish any form of national health insurance passed the Congress.

The English system proved costly, and no government could guarantee to its citizens that all medical care performed under its support would be uniformly excellent. Private medical care offers no such guarantee. But both under the Lloyd George Insurance Act of 1911 and the National Health Service Act of 1946, the individual was assured a free choice of physician, while local committees and a national administration worked together to improve standards of care.

America and England, while united by deep ties of tradition and language, have not followed identical social paths. National planning in a country of over 190,000,000 persons living in fifty federated states, can never parallel legislation in a nation of some fifty million people, governed by a single Parliament, directly responsible to the electorate. But in 1965 Americans, too, entered into a new age of social responsibility, with an awareness that if the nation is to realize its full potential, all members of American society must participate in its growth. To do so, sound health, and the means of curing illness, must be more widely accessible. The cruel cycle of poverty and disease can only be broken by a major national undertaking. Yet health is purchasable—in large part. And the United States at this stage of her development cannot renounce her new maturity, or the communal obligations of such maturity.

The question of what paths towards national health this country will now take is profoundly significant for all Americans.

Notes and References

Introduction

1. The population statistics and national sickness and mortality returns cited, unless otherwise stated, are those for England and Wales and not the United Kingdom (including Scotland and Northern Ireland) as it exists today. During the years of this study, of course, no Irish Free State existed. The Registrar-General of Births, Deaths and Marriages recorded the statistics for England and Wales.

2. Stephen Smith, *The City that Was* (New York: F. Allaben, 1911), *passim.*

3. Howard Kramer, "Agitation for Public Health Reform in the 1870's," *J. Hist. Med. and Allied Sciences*, Vol. 3 (1948), p. 477.

4. See on this point: C.-E. A. Winslow, *The Evolution and Significance of the Modern Public Health Campaign* (New Haven: Yale University Press, 1923), p. 25; Huntington Williams, "The Influence of Edwin Chadwick on American Public Health," *Medical Officer*, Vol. 95 (1956), p. 273; W. G. Smillie, *Public Health, Its Promise for the Future; a chronicle of the development of public health in the U.S., 1607–1914* (New York: Macmillan & Co. 1955), pp. 244–245.

Chapter I. The Profession, Parliament, and Public Health in the Seventies: Three Legislative Landmarks

1. Brian D. White, *A History of the Corporation of Liverpool, 1835–1914* (Liverpool: University Press, 1951), pp. 48ff.

2. *The Times*, Oct. 5, 1869, p. 7.

3. *Ibid.*

4. Simon's lifework is written in the pages of his *English Sanitary Institutions* (London: Cassell & Co., 1890), 2nd ed. (London: Smith, Elder & Co., 1897); and his collected *Public Health Reports*, 2 vols. edited in 1887 by Dr. Edward Seaton and published by the Sanitary Institute. A slim volume of the *Personal Recollections of Sir John Simon, K.C.B.* was privately printed (London: The Wilton's Ltd. Printers, rev. 1894). Some biographical information on Simon is available in various obituaries (see listings in bibliography), and in the *Dictionary of National Biography*, Supplement II, Vol. 3, pp. 316–318. A comprehensive and authoritative biography of Simon was published at the end of September, 1963: Royston Lambert, *Sir John Simon 1816–1904 and English Social Administration* (London: Macgibbon & Kee, 1963).

5. *Annual Report of the Medical Officer of the Privy Council, for 1868–1869*, p. 20ff. (These reports will hereafter be cited as *Ann. Rep. M.O.P.C.*)

6. *Ibid.*, p. 29.

7. Memorandum signed Buckingham and Chandes, Privy Council Office, January, 1867, on file in the Public Record Office under Miscellaneous Memoranda of the Privy Council, 1862–1873, on Public Health and Quarantine.

8. Simon, *English Sanitary Institutions*, 2nd ed., p. 325. The whole memorial appears in the *First Report of the Royal Sanitary Commission*, Appendix, p. xvii. (Hereafter cited as *First Report R.S.C.*)

9. *British Medical Journal*, Jan. 2, 1869, p. 15. (Hereafter cited as *Brit. M.J.*)

10. *Ibid.*, July 24, 1869, p. 91.

11. *First Report R.S.C.*, p. 387.

12. *Ibid.*, p. 408.

13. See the testimony in the *Second Report R.S.C.*, III, of John Liddell, Medical Officer of Health for Whitechapel; Robert Druitt, M.R.C.P., F.R.C.S.; Thomas Heslop, Physician to the Queen's Hospital; A. Bott, Medical Officer of the Witney Union; Dr. William Budd, etc. Dr. Robert Christison, a member of the Royal Sanitary Commission, testified on the need for greater compulsion in relation to pollution of streams by manufacturers in Scotland. See *First Report R.S.C.*, p. 297. Also *The Life of Sir Robert Christison*, edited by his sons (London: William Blackwood & Sons, 1887), Vol. II, p. 236.

14. *Second Report R.S.C.*, III, p. 112.

15. *First Report R.S.C.*, p. 52.

16. *Second Report R.S.C.*, II, p. 196; III, pp. 34 and 53.

17. *First Report R.S.C.*, pp. 99–101, and p. 235; *Second Report R.S.C.*, III, p. 43.

18. *Second Report R.S.C.*, III, pp. 33, 35 and 43; also *First Report R.S.C.*, pp. 231ff.

19. Simon, *English Sanitary Institutions*, 2nd ed., p. 327.

20. *Second Report R.S.C.*, I, p. 36. The functions of the central authority were visualized as keeping the local authorities in the "active exercise of their own functions, remedy defaults, direct inquiries, give advice on local planning, issue provisional orders, receive complaints, issue medical regulations in emergencies, collect reports."

21. A good presentation of the Commission's recommendations appears in Simon's classic, *English Sanitary Institutions*, 1st ed., pp. 322ff.

22. *Second Report R.S.C.*, I, 35ff.

23. *Medical Times and Gazette*, May 7, 1870, p. 497; Mar. 18, 1871, pp. 317ff.; Mar. 25, 1871, p. 353. (Hereafter cited as *Med. Times and Gaz.*) Also *The Lancet*, Nov. 25, 1871, p. 754; *Brit. M.J.* Aug. 19, 1871, pp. 203–207. The Joint Committee had some reservations about the Commission's Report, although they conceded the general excellence of the Royal Commission's work.

24. Simon, *English Sanitary Institutions*, 1st ed., p. 344.

25. This point is considered by William A. Robson in his *Development of Local Government* (London: Allen & Unwin Ltd., 1931), p. 287.

26. Some duties of the Privy Council Medical Office remained with the Council, but all those relating to local government were transferred to the new Board (powers of medical inquiry, supervision of public vaccination, the Disease Prevention Act, and the functions of the Privy Council Medical Office).

27. *Parliamentary Debates*, House of Commons, 3rd series, CCVIII, July 25, 1871, p. 234; July 27, 1871, p. 356.

28. *Brit. M.J.*, Mar. 9, 1872, p. 269.

29. *The Lancet*, Apr. 6, 1872, pp. 476–477.

30. *Brit. M.J.*, Feb. 24, 1872, p. 215.

31. *Ibid.*, Mar. 23, 1872, p. 322.
32. *Ibid.*, Mar. 16, 1872, p. 299.
33. *Ibid.*, Sept. 7, 1872, p. 281.
34. *The Lancet*, Mar. 16, 1872, p. 370.
35. Simon, *English Sanitary Institutions*, 1st ed., p. 373.
36. *The Lancet*, July 27, 1872, p. 125.
37. *Brit. M.J.*, Sept. 28, 1872, p. 347.
38. *Ibid.*, Jan. 23, 1875, p. 119.
39. *Medical Press and Circular*, Jan. 20, 1875, p. 53. (Hereafter cited as *Med. Press and Cir.*)
40. *Ibid.*, p. 52.
41. Lambert, *Sir John Simon*, p. 560; William M. Frazer, *A History of English Public Health, 1834–1939* (London: Bailliere, Tindall and Cox, 1950), p. 120.
42. *The Lancet*, Mar. 13, 1875, p. 376.
43. *Brit. M.J.*, Mar. 20, 1875, p. 386.
44. *Ibid.*, May 15, 1875, p. 701.
45. *Parliamentary Debates*, House of Commons, 3rd series, Vol. 223 (Apr. 19, 1875), p. 1246. Dr. John Lush, M.P. from Salisbury also criticized the Bill for not giving the central authority the right to approve local medical officers of health. *Ibid.*, Vol. 224, May 25, 1875, p. 879.
46. *Ibid.*, Vol. 223, pp. 1256–1257.
47. *The Lancet*, Aug. 28, 1875, p. 318. In a subsequent, more considered, editorial the same journal criticized many of the inadequacies in the law, but recognized that all of the hopes of reformers could not be expected to be fulfilled at one time. *Ibid.*, Sept. 18, 1875, p. 424.
48. *Annual Report of the Local Government Board, 1875–1876*, p. xli. (These reports will hereafter be cited as *Ann. Rep. L.G.B.*)
49. Albert J. Palmberg, *A Treatise on Public Health and Its Application in Different Countries*, translated from the French edition and the section on England edited by Arthur Newsholme, 2nd ed., (London: Sonnenschein, 1895), pp. 3–37. This point is also made in Lambert, *Sir John Simon*, p. 562.
50. *Med. Press and Cir.*, Nov. 24, 1875, p. 432.

Chapter II. The Medical Department of the Local Government Board: Formulation of Policy, 1871–1900

Portions of this chapter were previously published in the author's "John Simon and the Local Government Board Bureaucrats: 1871–1876," *Bull. Hist. Med.*, XXXVII (Mar.–Apr., 1963), 184–194.

1. Simon, *English Sanitary Institutions*, 1st ed., p. 320.
2. Simon credited Farr's reports with having given the Medical Office of the Council "a basis which had not before existed for regular and comparatively prompt inquiry as to sufficiency of local administration." *Ibid.*, p. 318.
3. Joseph Rogers, *Reminiscences of a Workhouse Medical Officer*, edited by Thorald Rogers (London: T. Fisher Unwin, 1889), p. 101.
4. There are numerous complaints regarding the inefficiency of poor law operations in the medical journals in the sixties and seventies. See also Sir Malcolm Morris, *Story of English Public Health* (London: Cassell & Co., 1919) p. 56.
5. *Brit. M.J.*, May 1, 1875, p. 579.
6. Herbert Preston-Thomas, *The Work and Play of a Government Inspector* (London: William Blackwood & Sons, 1909), p. 50.

7. Local Government Board Miscellaneous Correspondence, 1876, No. 58096/76. (These files will hereafter be cited as L.G.B. Misc. Corres.) At the time the correspondence files of the Local Government Board were used for this research and for the study of other medical activities of the Board, the files were under the administrative jurisdiction of the Ministry of Housing and Local Government. The volume of records preserved by the Ministry is considerable. Over 9,000 bound volumes of manuscript and typescript materials of the Poor Law Unions are in existence, in battered but legible condition. The most valuable material for locating central policy of the Local Government Board during the years 1871–1900 is contained in two categories of papers: (1) Local Government Board "Government Office Correspondence" (75 volumes, 1872–1896), and (2) Local Government Board "Miscellaneous Correspondence" (160 volumes, 1872–1900). The "Government Office Correspondence" is particularly valuable, containing detailed material on the Board's adminstrative procedures, drafting of Government Bills, correspondence with other Government offices, internal administrative memoranda and draft orders of the Local Government Board. The Board, at its inception, adopted the useful system of mounting correspondence and memoranda on larger paper and circulating these papers within the Board for official comment. This material, as preserved in the bound files, enables the observer to trace much of the development of the Board's policy. The large file of "Miscellaneous Correspondence" is also useful for interpretations of policy to the public, for origins of policy within the Board, for reports of inspectors, and correspondence with local authorities. All of these unpublished materials are an invaluable supplement to the published annual reports of the Local Government Board, which appear in the *Parliamentary Papers* (hereafter cited as *Parl. Papers*).

8. L.G.B. Misc. Corres., Jan. 20, 1874, No. 3284/74. See also No. 57224/73.

9. Local Government Board, Government Office Correspondence, 1873, No. 78178/73ff. (These files will hereafter be cited as L.G.B. Gov't. Office Corres.)

10. Lambert, *Sir John Simon*, p. 519.

11. *Ibid.*, pp. 521–523 and Zachary Cope, *Florence Nightingale and the Doctors* (London: Museum Press, 1958), pp. 115–119.

12. L.G.B. Gov't. Office Corres., Nov. 25, 1873, No. 73885/73.

13. *Ibid.*

14. Radcliffe (1826–1884), who trained at Leeds School of Medicine, took the M.R.C.S. in 1853. As a surgeon in British parlance he was (like Simon) referred to as "Mr." not "Dr." At varying times, a number of the medical men discussed in this study held different qualifications. It has not been possible to ensure that each was properly referred to as "Mr." or "Dr." at the time he enters the story.

15. Letter of Dr. Edward Smith, Nov. 20, 1873, L.G.B. Gov't. Office Corres., No. 3885/73; see also C. Frazer Brockington, "Public Health at the Privy Council, 1858–1871," *The Medical Officer*, May 1, 1959, p. 244. According to his obituary, Dr. Smith suffered from "personality difficulties." *Brit. M.J.* II, (1874), 653.

16. Lambert, *Sir John Simon*, p. 302.

17. *Ibid.*, pp. 553–554.

18. "Obituary" of Sir John Simon, *Transactions of the Epidemiological Society of London*, New Series, XXIII (1903–04), 253–258. Although anonymous, this obituary from its content is recognizably the product of one of Simon's colleagues at the Local Government Board.

19. Sir John Burdon Sanderson [obituary of] "Sir John Simon, 1816–1904," *Proceedings of the Royal Society of London*, LXXV (1905), 338.

20. Royston Lambert, in his recent biography of Simon, states (p. 555) that the bulk of the Medical Department's documents have disappeared from the Board's files, and asserts that Simon "did write and send many memoranda of protest and

suggestion to his chief." The evidence for such a statement is inconclusive. Many documents relating to work of the Medical Department have been preserved in the carefully bound volumes. It is not possible to say for how long a period Simon continued to express his feelings in formal memoranda to Stansfeld, John Lambert, or Sclater-Booth. The main outlines of their controversy, however, are clear.

21. F.S.B. François de Chaumont, M.D., *Lectures on State Medicine Delivered Before the Society of Apothecaries* (London: Smith, Elder & Co., 1875), p. 152. De Chaumont was later editor of the *Journal of the Royal Sanitary Institute*.

22. Sir Arthur Newsholme, *Fifty Years in Public Health* (London: Allen & Unwin Ltd., 1935), p. 119.

23. *Med. Press and Cir.*, Aug. 18, 1875, p. 123.

24. *Supplementary Report of the Local Government Board by the Medical Officer of the Board, 1874*, New Series II, p. 5.

25. Simon, *Personal Recollections*, p. 23.

26. Simon, *English Sanitary Institutions*, 1st ed., p. 391.

27. *Ibid.*, p. 392.

28. *Annual Report of the Medical Officer of the Local Government Board for 1876*, p. 5. (These reports will hereafter be cited as *Ann. Rep. M.O.L.G.B.*)

29. Alice Smith, *Memoirs of the Buchanan Family, And in Particular of George Buchanan* (Aberdeen: privately printed at Aberdeen University Press, 1941).

30. Personal letter cited in Sir Arthur Newsholme, *The Last Thirty Years in Public Health* (London: Allen & Unwin Ltd., 1936), p. 34.

31. Memorandum from John Lambert to George Buchanan, June 1880, Unnumbered, L.G.B. Gov't. Office Corres.; Memorandum No. B 341K(2), 1882, L.G.B. Gov't. Office Corres.

32. L.G.B. Misc. Corres., No. 98819, 1881. Colonial Office Memorandum.

33. L.G.B. Misc. Corres., No. 48423, 1883, Memorial of the Manchester and Salford Sanitary Association.

34. L.G.B. Misc. Corres., Unnumbered letter of H. March Webb, dated Nov. 30, 1887.

35. S. Gwynn and G. M. Tuckwell, *The Life of the Right Honourable Sir Charles W. Dilke, Bart. M. P.* (London: John Murray, 1917), Vol. 1, p. 504.

36. *Ibid.*, Vol. I, p. 506.

37. Simon, *English Sanitary Institutions*, 1st ed., p. 405.

38. *Ann. Rep. M.O.L.G.B. for 1888*, p. 1.

39. *Ann. Rep. M.O.L.G.B. for 1892-93*, p xl.

40. Simon, *English Sanitary Institutions*, 1st ed., p. 406.

41. C. F. Brockington, "Public Health at the Privy Council, 1858-71," *The Medical Officer*, May 22, 1959, p. 287.

42. L.G.B. Gov't. Office Corres., July 1890, unnumbered draft of the Housing of the Working Classes Act Amendment Bill.

43. L.G.B. Gov't. Office Corres., No. 386781/94, 1894, Sale of Food and Drugs Act (1875) Amendment Bill, 1894.

44. L.G.B. Gov't. Office Corres., March 1895, No. 2754/95, Sanitary Registration Bill.

Chapter III. The Medical Department of the Local Government Board: Disease Control, 1871–1900

1. *Transactions of the National Association for the Promotion of Social Science*

for 1881 (London: Longmans, Green & Co., 1881), p. 69. (Hereafter cited as *Trans. N.A.P.S.S.*)

2. A Glasgow preacher, in 1831, attributed the cholera outbreak to the Lord's wrath at a current attempt to foster a Deceased Wife's Sister marriage bill in Parliament. Cited by Thomas Ferguson, *The Dawn of Scottish Social Welfare, A Survey from Medieval Times to 1863* (London: Thomas Nelson & Sons, 1948), p. 123.

3. William Bulloch, *The History of Bacteriology* (London: Oxford University Press, 1938), *passim.*; Richard Shryock, *The Development of Modern Medicine,* new ed. (New York: Alfred Knopf, 1947), pp. 281ff.; Henry E. Sigerist, *The Great Doctors, A Biographical History of Medicine* (London: Allen & Unwin Ltd., 1933), pp. 368–370; George Rosen, *A History of Public Health* (New York: M. D. Publications, 1958), pp. 294–336.

4. John B. Blake, "Scientific Institutions Since the Renaissance, Their Role in Medical Research," *Proceedings of the American Philosophical Society,* Vol. 101 (1957), p. 47.

5. Frederic P. Gorham, "The History of Bacteriology and Its Contribution to Public Health Work," in *A Half Century of Public Health,* edited by M. P. Ravenel (New York: American Public Health Association, 1921), pp. 72ff.; Howard D. Kramer, "The Germ Theory and the Early Public Health Program in the United States," *Bull. Hist. Med.,* XXII (May–June, 1948) 240–241.

6. See Chapter IV in reference to the auxiliary scientific investigations of the Local Government Board.

7. *Eighth Ann. Rep. L.G.B. for 1878–1879,* p. lxxii. The Board's Medical Department, however, took no part in the granting of these loans.

8. John Snow, *On the Mode of Communication of Cholera,* 2nd ed., much enlarged (London: John Churchill, 1855). The first edition of this work was a slender pamphlet issued in 1849. Snow, a Yorkshireman who believed firmly in temperance and a vegetarian diet, did not publish any further papers on cholera.

9. Edward W. Goodall, *William Budd* (Bristol: Arrowsmith, 1936), p. 97.

10. *Med. Press and Cir.,* Aug. 28, 1868, pp. 188–189.

11. *Trans., N.A.P.S.S. for 1874,* p. 73.

12. Dorsey Jones, *Chadwick and the Early Public Health Movement* (Iowa City: Iowa University Press, 1929), p. 118.

13. Preston-Thomas, *Work and Play of a Government Inspector,* p. 218.

14. *First Report, L.G.B., 1871–72,* p. lv.

15. Miscellaneous Memoranda of the Privy Council, 1863–1873, on Public Health and Quarantine; Minutes of the Privy Council, July 29, 1871.

16. L.G.B. Misc. Corres., Apr. 17, 1874 (unnumbered file).

17. Alice Smith, *Memoirs of the Buchanan Family,* p. 18.

18. W. M. Frazer, *A History of English Public Health, 1834–1949* p. 213; *Ann. Rep. M.O.L.G.B. for 1887–1888,* p. xii.

19. *Ann. Rep. M.O.L.G.B. for 1893,* p xxvi.

20. *Ann. Rep. L.G.B. for 1884–1885,* p. cxix.

21. L.G.B. Misc. Corres., No. 75927/84, July 31, 1884.

22. *Ibid.,* No. 78449ff./84.

23. Simon, *English Sanitary Institutions,* 1st ed., p. 401.

24. Preston-Thomas, *Work and Play of a Government Inspector,* p. 148.

25. *Brit. M.J.,* Aug. 2, 1884, p. 233.

26. L.G.B. Gov't. Office Corres., Vol. 127, No. 658193/93, May 31, 1893; also *Reports and Papers on Cholera in England in 1893,* Supplement to the *Ann. Rep. M.O.L.G.B. 1893–1894,* p. v.

27. *Report on the Inland Sanitary Survey, 1893–1894,* p. vii (Supplement to the *Ann. Rep. M.O.L.G.B. for 1894–1895*).

28. *Ann. Rep. M.O.L.G.B. for 1895–1896*, pp. xx–xxii.

29. *Report on the Inland Sanitary Survey*, Introduction by the Medical Officer, Local Government Board, p. v.

30. *Ann. Rep. M.O.L.G.B. for 1895–1896*, p. xx.

31. Richard Thorne Thorne, *On the Progress of Preventive Medicine During the Victorian Era, Being the Inaugural Address Delivered Before the Epidemiological Society of London, Session, 1887–1888* (London: Shaw & Sons, 1888), p. 60.

32. *Brit. M.J.*, Aug. 17, 1895, p. 442.

33. Gwynn and Tuckwell, *Life of Dilke*, II, 23.

34. *Ann. Rep. M.O.L.G.B. for 1874*, p. 51. See also *The Doctor*, Apr. 1, 1871, p. 72.

35. *Ann. Rep. M.O.L.G.B. for 1874*, p. 54.

36. The method of inoculation, by injecting healthy individuals with lymph from the vesicles of an infected calf, was aimed at producing a mild attack of smallpox in the healthy individual which would render him immune to later infection. See J. R. Hutchinson, "Historical Note on the Prevention of Smallpox in England," in *Report to the Ministry of Health* for the year ending 31 Mar. 1947, Appendix A, pp. 119ff.

37. The *British Medical Journal* of May 23, 1896, pp. 1261–1307, carries a useful résumé of vaccination in England. See also Thorne Thorne, *On the Progress of Preventive Medicine During the Victorian Era*, pp. 5ff.

38. Simon, *English Sanitary Institutions*, 1st ed., p. 311.

39. *Report from the Select Committee on the Vaccination Act (1867)*, *Parl. Papers*, 1871, Vol. XIII, p. iii. A leading article in *The Times* congratulated the Select Committee for dealing severely with the "wild theory" of the anti-vaccinationists. *The Times*, May 31, 1871, p. 9.

40. *Ann. Rep. M.O.L.G.B. for 1874*, pp. 5–6.

41. *Second Report of the Royal Commission Appointed to Inquire into the Subject of Vaccination, 1889–1896*, *Parl. Papers*, 1890, Vol. 39, p. 126. (Hereafter cited as *Royal Comm. on Vaccin.*)

42. *Ann. Rep. M.O.L.G.B. for 1883*, p. iii.

43. *Ann. Rep. M.O.L.G.B. for 1893–1894*, p v.

44. P. A. Taylor, *Vaccination* (London: London Society for the Abolition of Compulsory Vaccination, 1881), Foreword.

45. *Ann. Rep. M.O.L.G.B. for 1886*, pp. ii–iv.

46. *Final Report, Royal Comm. on Vaccin. (1896)*, *Parl. Papers*, 1896, Vol. 47, p. 136.

47. *Brit. M.J.*, May 23, 1896, p. 1300.

48. *Ann. Rep. M.O.L.G.B. for 1898–1899*, p. xii.

49. *Ann. Rep. M.O.L.G.B. for 1899–1900*, p. x.

50. J. R. Hutchinson, *Prevention of Smallpox in England*, p. 120.

51. Simon, *English Sanitary Institutions*, 1st ed., p. 312; *First Report L.G.B. for 1871–1872*, p. lii.

52. *Ann. Rep. L.G.B., 1872–1873*, p. xxx.

53. *Reports and Papers on the Use and Influence of Hospitals for Infectious Diseases* (1882), *Parl. Papers*, 1882, Vol. XXX, pp. 29–30.

54. *Final Report, Royal Comm. on Vaccin.*, 1896, p. 119.

55. L.G.B. Gov't. Office Corres., Vol. 130, unnumbered memorandum on the Bill for enabling County Councils to promote the establishment of hospitals for infectious diseases.

56. *Annual Report of the Registrar-General for 1871*, p. 219; *Annual Report of the Registrar-General for 1897*, p. xviii. The sharp reduction in smallpox deaths is reflected even in contrast with the number of deaths in the two nonepidemic years immediately preceding 1871, i.e., 1,565 and 2,620 respectively.

57. Frazer, *History of English Public Health,* p. 370.

58. Rickett's major work, *The Diagnosis of Smallpox,* was not published until 1908, but as Dr. W. M. Frazer has pointed out, this method of diagnosis had been used by Dr. Ricketts and other for many years before the work was published. Frazer, *History of English Public Health,* p. 371.

59. Dr. R. Bruce Low, "The Epidemiology of Typhus Exanthematicus in Recent Years," Appendix 5 to *Ann. Rep. M.O.L.G.B. for 1914–1915,* p. 33.

60. Thorne Thorne, *On the Progress of Preventive Medicine During the Victorian Era,* p. 19.

61. Thomas H. Bickerton, *A Medical History of Liverpool, From the Earliest Days to the Year 1920* (London: John Murray, 1936), p. 180.

62. *Ann. Rep. M.O.L.G.B. for 1886,* p. xi.

63. William Budd, *Typhoid Fever, Its Nature, Mode of Spreading and Infection* (London, 1873; republished New York, 1931), p. 175.

64. Thorne Thorne, *On the Progress of Preventive Medicine During the Victorian Era,* p. 24.

65. Supplemental Report on Inspections, *Ann. Rep. M.O.L.G.B. for 1873,* p. 13.

66. *Special Supplement to the Ann. Rep. M.O.L.G.B. for 1891 on Enteric Fever in the Tees Valley,* p. viii.

67. *Ann. Rep. M.O.L.G.B. for 1898–1899,* p. xxvi.

68. *Supplement to the 65th Ann. Rep. Registrar-General, Covering 1891–1900,* Part I. p. lxxviii.

69. L.G.B. Misc. Corres. of January and February 1882, Nos. 7374K2/82 and 17522/82. In 1884 infected children were excluded from schools, and closure rules were issued by the Education Department. See Sir Arthur S. MacNalty, *History of State Medicine in England, Being the Fitzpatrick Lectures of the Royal College of Physicians of London for the Years 1946 and 1947* (London: Royal Institute of Public Health and Hygiene, 1948), p. 67.

70. *Ann. Rep. M.O.L.G.B. for 1890,* p. xvii.

71. Richard Thorne Thorne, *Diphtheria* (London: MacMillan & Co., 1891), pp. 217ff.

72. *Supplement to the Sixty-Fifth Ann. Rep. of the Registrar-General,* Part I, p. lxxiv.

73. *Final Report of the Royal Comm. on Vaccin.,* 1896, p. 45.

74. Thorne Thorne, *On the Progress of Preventive Medicine During the Victorian Era,* p. 30.

75. *Ann. Rep. M.O.L.G.B. for 1885,* p. vii.

76. *Supplement to the Sixty-Fifth Ann. Rep. of the Registrar-General,* Part I, p. lxxv.

77. *Report on the Influenza Epidemic of 1889–1890 by Dr. Parsons, with an introduction by the Medical Officer of the Local Government Board,* 1891, p. x.

78. "Memoranda on Epidemic Influenza, March 1895," Appendix to the *Ann. Rep. M.O.L.G.B. for 1894–1895,* p. 199.

79. *Med. Times and Gazette,* Dec. 10, 1870, p. 685; *Brit. M.J.,* June 14, 1873; L.G.B. Misc. Corres., No. 31.759/73 (Petition of the British Medical Association), and L.G.B. Misc. Corres., No. 50.176/74, July 22, 1874 (Memorial of the British Medical Association).

80. *First Report, R.S.C., Minutes of Evidence,* p. 102; *Second Report, R.S.C., Parl. Papers,* Vol. 35, (1871), pp. 57–61.

81. Preston-Thomas, *Work and Play of a Government Inspector,* p. 150.

82. *Transactions, Society of Medical Officers of Health,* 1878–1879 (Annual Report), p. 13. (Hereafter cited as *Trans. Soc. M.O.H.*) *Brit. M.J.,* July 28, 1883, p. 191.

83. Ernest Hart, *The Registration of Infectious Disease* (London: British Medical Association, 1879), p. 3.

84. See L.G.B. Misc. Corres., No. 21370/1876, No. 21370A, 1876 (Petitions of the Northwestern Association of Medical Officers of Health); No. 19586/77, No. 75092/77 (Resolution of the Birmingham Midland Association of Medical Officers of Health); 3978 enc/77, Jan. 2, 1877.

85. *Ann. Rep. L.G.B. for 1883–1884*, pp. cxixff.

86. *Ann. Rep. L.G.B. for 1879–1880*, pp. cxxxii–cxxxiii.

87. L.G.B. Misc. Corres., unnumbered memoranda filed in volumes for October 1887, but dated respectively Feb. 10, 1885; Feb. 13, 1885; and Mar. 1886.

88. *Ann. Rep. L.G.B. for 1887–1888*, p. cl. See also support in *The Times*, Oct. 4, 1887, p. 7.

89. L.G.B. Gov't. Office Corres., No. 108267/87, Jan. 20, 1887.

90. Preston-Thomas, *Work and Play of a Government Inspector*, p. 151; L.G.B. Gov't. Office Corres., unnumbered, Aug. 30, 1889 (Draft Board Order).

91. L.G.B. Gov't. Office Corres., unnumbered memorandum, Sept. 19, 1889.

92. Sir Arthur MacNalty, "The Control of Pulmonary Tuberculosis in England," *Brit. Journal of Tuberculosis and Diseases of the Chest*, XLV (July, 1951), 90–96.

Chapter IV. The Local Government Board: Medical Inspection and the Auxiliary Scientific Investigations

1. Sir John Charles, *Research and Public Health* (London: Oxford University Press, 1961), p. 89.

2. Simon, *English Sanitary Institutions*, 1st ed., pp. 386–387.

3. L.G.B. Misc. Corres., No. 11699613/1895.

4. Simon, *English Sanitary Institutions*, 1st ed., p. 316.

5. L.G.B. Misc. Corres., unnumbered memoranda file, memorandum of Mr. Henley, Feb. 20, 1880.

6. *Idem.*

7. *Ann. Rep. M.O.L.G.B. for 1874*, pp. 133ff.

8. *Ann. Rep. M.O.L.G.B. for 1873*, p. 17.

9. *Reports of Local Government Board Inspectors on the Working of the Public Health Act of 1872, Parl. Papers*, 1875 Vol. 40, p. 9.

10. *Ann. Rep. M.O.L.G.B. for 1898–1899*, p. xix.

11. *Ann. Rep. M.O.L.G.B. for 1887*, p. x.

12. J. H. Bridges and T. Holmes, *Report to the Local Government Board on Proposed Changes in Hours and Ages of Employment in Textile Factories, Parl. Papers*, 1873, Vol. LV, pp. 60–62.

13. *Ann. Rep. M.O.L.G.B. for 1888*, p. v.

14. Morris, *Story of English Public Health*, p. 57.

15. *Reports of Local Government Board Inspectors on the Working of the Public Health Act of 1872, Parl. Papers*, 1875, Vol. XL, p. 9.

16. See especially the "Return Showing Particulars of Local Visitations, Medical Officers of the Local Government Board, from the Date of the Establishment of the Board to 1st January 1880, with Regard to prevalence of Disease in Particular Places, and to Questions therewith connected of Defects of Sanitary Administration," *Parl. Papers*, 1880, Vol. LXI, *passim.;* also evidence of Dr. Edward Ballard before the Select Committee on the Public Health Act (1875) Amendment Bill, Appendix, pp. 157–163, *Parl. Papers*, 1878, Vol. 18, p. 2466.

17. Preston-Thomas, *Work and Play of a Government Inspector*, pp. 143–144.

18. Simon, *English Sanitary Institutions*, 1st ed., p. 405.

19. "Return Showing Particulars of Local Visitations," in *Parl. Papers*, 1880, Vol. LXI, pp. 2–117.

20. L.G.B. Misc. Corres., No. 240b/79, Memorandum dated Jan. 9, 1879. The editor of *The Lancet* had written an irate letter to the Board, asking why his journal had not received recent copies.

21. *Ann. Rep. M.O.L.G.B. for 1882–1883*, p. vi.

22. *Reports of the British Association for the Advancement of Science*, 1874, p. 208.

23. *Ann. Rep. M.O.L.G.B. for 1873*, p. 4.

24. Simon, *English Sanitary Institutions*, 1st ed., p. 316; *Eighth Report, M.O.P.C.*, 1865, p. 20.

25. Brockington, "Public Health at the Privy Council, 1858–1871," *The Medical Officer*, Apr. 3, 1959, p. 185.

26. Simon, *English Sanitary Institutions*, 1st ed., p. 413.

27. *Parl. Debates*, House of Commons, 3rd series, Vol. 224 (June 11, 1875), pp. 1766–1767.

28. Simon, *English Sanitary Institutions*, 1st ed., p. 293; Brockington, "Public Health at the Privy Council, 1858–1871," *The Medical Officer*, May 8, 1959, p. 260.

29. David L. Drabkin, *Thudichum, Chemist of the Brain* (Philadelphia: University of Pennsylvania Press, 1958), pp. 116–117; "Obituary, J. L. W. Thudichum, M.D., F.R.C.P.," *Brit. M.J.*, Sept. 14, 1901, p. 726.

30. Letter of Thudichum to Simon, written during 1869, as quoted in Drabkin, *Thudichum*, pp. 95–96.

31. L.G.B. Gov't. Office Corres., 1879, Vol. 90, No. 8.7.750K(2).

32. L.G.B. Gov't. Office Corres., Aug. 7, 1880, No 69821.

33. L.G.B. Gov't. Office Corres., Letter of Dr. J. L. W. Thudichum, Sept. 19, 1881, unnumbered. By No. 31065K2 of 1882, a further letter from Buchanan advised Thudichum that funds would only be supplied up to Mar., 1883.

34. Thudichum, *A Treatise on the Chemical Composition of the Brain, based throughout upon original researches* (London: Bailliere, Tindall and Cox, 1884).

35. *Brit. M.J.*, Sept. 14, 1901, p. 726.

36. *Ann. Rep. M.O.L.G.B. for 1878*, p. xiv.

37. Simon, *English Sanitary Institutions*, 1st ed., p. 409.

38. Morris, *Story of English Public Health*, p. 64. Sir Arthur MacNalty, "Sir John Burdon Sanderson," *Proceedings of the Royal Society of Medicine*, Vol. 47 (Sept., 1954), p. 756.

39. *Brit. M.J.*, Dec. 10, 1887, p. 1296.

40. *Ann. Rep. M.O.L.G.B. for 1885*, pp. 121 ff.; *Ann. Rep. M.O.L.G.B. for 1894–1895*, p. xxx.

41. Sir Arthur MacNalty, *The History of State Medicine in England*, p. 551.

42. *Ann. Rep. M.O.L.G.B. for 1883*, p. xi.

43. *The Lancet*, Apr. 24, 1875, p. 583.

44. *Brit. M.J.*, Aug. 27, 1887, p. 478. See also *ibid.*, Apr. 13, 1889, p. 853.

45. Letter of Dr. Richard Thorne Thorne to Sir Walter Foster, Apr. 5, 1895, L.G.B. Misc. Corres., No. 47603/95.

46. *Trans. N.A.P.S.S.*, 1872, p. 79.

47. *Ibid.*

48. Beatrice and Sidney Webb, *The State and the Doctor* (London: Longmans, Green and Co., 1910), pp. 223–224.

49. *Trans. N.A.P.S.S.*, 1878, p. 546.

50. *Ann. Rep. M.O.L.G.B. for 1918–1919*, p. vi.

51. Thorne Thorne, *On the Progress of Preventive Medicine During the Victorian Era*, p. 62.

Chapter V. The Poor Law Medical Officers, 1871–1900

Portions of this chapter have previously been published in the author's article, "The Parish Doctor: England's Poor Law Medical Officers and Medical Reform, 1870–1900," *Bull. Hist. Med.* XXXV (Mar.–Apr., 1961), 97–122.

1. Beatrice Webb, *My Apprenticeship* (London: Longmans, Green and Co., 1926), p. 138.

2. Joseph Rogers, *Reminiscences of a Workhouse Medical Officer* (London: T. Fisher Unwin, 1889), p. 239.

3. J. H. Clapham, *The Economic History of Modern Britain: Free Trade and Steel, 1850–1868* (Cambridge: Cambridge University Press, 1952), p. 432.

4. *Ann. Rep. L.G.B. for 1876–1877*, p. xv. The total population at this time was recorded as between 21,000,00 and 22,000,000.

5. The Annual Reports of the Local Government Board during the period 1871 to 1900 irregularly cite numbers of poor law medical officers. For example, the 1874–75 report lists 4,212; the 1876–77 report, 4,233; the 1886–87 report, 4,293 medical officers.

6. B. L. Hutchins, *The Public Health Agitation, 1833–1848* (London: A. C. Fifield, 1909), p. 127.

7. Ruth G. Hodgkinson, "The Medical Services of the New Poor Law, 1834–1871," Ph.D. dissertation, University of London, 2 vols., 1950, Vol. 2, p. 588. A summary of this dissertation was published under the title "Poor Law Medical Officers of England, 1834–1871," *J. Hist. Med. and Allied Sciences*, Vol. 11 (1956), pp. 299–338. As early as 1842 the Poor Law Commissioners in their General Medical Order Number 5 had set up four alternative licensing requirements for poor law medical officers, not all of which, however, required a double qualification in medicine and surgery. See *Ann. Rep. Poor Law Commissioners, 1842*, p. 130.

8. Hodgkinson, "Poor Law Medical Officers," pp. 332–333.

9. Samuel S. Sprigge, *Medicine and the Public* (London: William Heinemann, 1905), p. 146.

10. *Ann. Rep., Poor Law Board for 1868–69*, p. 32.

11. Hodgkinson, "Medical Services of the New Poor Law," II, 712.

12. K. B. Smellie, *A History of Local Government*, rev. ed. (London: Allen & Unwin Ltd., 1949), p. 59. The "Board" had as its ex officio members the Lord President of the Council, the Lord Privy Seal, the Home Secretary, and the Chancellor of the Exchequer, together with the President and two Secretaries.

13. Newsholme, *The Last Thirty Years in Public Health*, pp. 94–95. The correspondence substantiating this statement was not located by the present writer in the files of the Local Government Board. See also Lambert, *Sir John Simon*, p. 557.

14. Henry Rumsey, *Essays on State Medicine* (London: John Churchill, 1856), p. 274.

15. L.G.B. Gov't. Office Corres., Nos. 17557/72 and 17558/72, Mar. 25, 1872. Dr. John Simon commented on Dr. Smith's duties as follows: "according to all I have heard in after years from Dr. Smith on the subject of his work in the office, the old secretarial belief as to the best way of dealing with matters of medical administration, had vigorously survived the fact of his appointment as Medical Officer of the Board; and I understand that he, in relation to such matters, was not expected to advise in any general, or any initiative sense, but only to answer in particular cases on such particular points as might be referred to him." Simon, *English Sanitary Institutions*, 2nd ed., p. 352.

16. Newsholme, *The Last Thirty Years in Public Health*, pp. 92–93.

17. MacNalty, *State Medicine in England*, p. 65.

18. Paul Felix Aschrott, *The English Poor Law System, Past and Present*, 2nd ed. (London: Knight, 1902), p. 207. Dr. Aschrott, a Berlin judge, was a thorough, highly skilled analyst, whose study was recognized by contemporary officials of the English poor law system as an excellent survey. The book was translated from the German by Herbert Preston-Thomas, and issued in two editions (1888 and 1902).

19. *Ibid.*, p. 208.

20. *The Lancet* reported several interesting instances where the Brentford Guardians informed the Local Government Board that they would do nothing to remedy the sanitary situation in their workhouse. *The Lancet* commented on a similar case of open defiance by the local authority, and noted that the Board seemed to be "utterly impotent to enforce commands given out with an air of apparent authority." (*The Lancet*, Jan. 16, 1875, p. 100). Open defiance was probably the exception, but by an easygoing observance of the central orders, local Guardians managed to pursue policies very different than were actually laid down by the Local Government Board.

21. *Ann. Rep. L.G.B. for 1871–1872*, Appendix A, p. 9.

22. Unnumbered circular, L.G.B. Gov't. Office Corres., for 1898, "Extracts from the General Orders of the Poor Law Commissioners, the Poor Law Board and the Local Government Board relating to the Duties of Workhouse Medical Officers."

23. Beatrice Webb, *The Poor Law Medical Officer and His Future* [Papers Used at the Conference of the Association of Poor Law Medical Officers, July 6, 1909] (London: National Committee for the Break-up of the Poor Law, 1909), p. 4.

24. *Brit. M.J.*, Feb. 4, 1871, p. 135.

25. Aschrott, *The English Poor Law System*, p. 187.

26. *Ibid.*, pp. 237–238.

27. Bethnel Green, Fulham, Lewisham, Paddington, Hampstead, and Mile End Old Town. See *Ann. Rep. L.G.B. for 1876–1877*, p. xxvi.

28. Beatrice and Sidney Webb, *English Poor Law Policy* (London: Longmans, Green and Co., 1910), pp. 211–212.

29. Temporary legalization had been granted under the Diseases Prevention Act of 1883, which was renewed annually. This temporary Act ensured that admission under such conditions did not carry with it the stigma of disqualification. An earlier attempt in Section 15 of the Poor Law Act of 1879 had given managers of hospitals optional power to make contracts with vestries for the admission of nonpaupers, but this had not been much applied. By 1900, the Annual Report of the Metropolitan Asylums Board stated they "possessed today hospital accommodation to the extent of upward of 6,000 beds, open to any person of whatever social position who may suffer from certain classes of infectious disease."

30. *Ann. Rep. L.G.B. for 1878–1879*, pp. xxxiiff.

31. *Ann. Rep. L.G.B. for 1883–1884*, p. xxxiv. Most persons admitted to poor law infirmaries suffered from such chronic diseases as bronchitis, cancer, renal disease, "senile decay," and paralysis. *Ibid.*, p. xxxv.

32. Questions 1154 and 1247, *Minutes of Evidence, Report of the Royal Commission on the Aged Poor*, Feb. 15, 1893. See also comments on improved care in the *Ann. Rep. L.G.B. for 1898–1899*, p. 85.

33. The Manchester Guardians, for example, in an effort to exclude all but the destitute poor, forced all who applied to the poor law hospital facilities to enter through the workhouse gate. *Report of the Select Committee of the House of Lords on Poor Relief*, p. viii.

34. *The Failure of the Poor Law*, pamphlet issued by the National Committee to Promote the Break-up of the Poor Laws (no place, 1909), p. 7. There were, however, very few questions raised in Parliament on the subject of poor law medical treat-

ment in the eighties and nineties. Only very occasionally, as in the instance of the management of the Eastern Hospital at Homerton (see *Hansard*, Jan. 23, 1891), was the Local Government Board asked for any public accounting of poor law medical policy.

35. *Ann. Rep. L.G.B. for 1894–1895*, Appendix B, p. 63. See also the statement of Inspector Preston-Thomas in the *Ann. Rep. L.G.B. for 1898–1899*, Appendix B, p. 133.

36. L.G.B. Misc. Corres., No. 42722/89, Paper of the Workhouse Nurses' Association sent to the Local Government Board, Apr. 1889.

37. L.G.B. Gov't. Office Corres., unnumbered memorandum dated Apr. 1, 1892 (in Vol. 150 of 1895).

38. *Ann. Rep. L.G.B. for 1895–1896*, Appendix A, p. 112; *Ann. Rep. L.G.B. for 1897–1898*, Appendix A, p. 27; "Workhouse Infirmaries," *Macmillan's Magazine*, July, 1881, p. 225; *Ann. Rep. L.G.B. for 1893–1894*, Appendix B, p. 133.

39. *Minutes of Evidence, Report of the Royal Commission on the Aged Poor*, 13 February 1894, Questions 13852 and 13856. Lansbury at that time was a Guardian of the Poplar Union. A return to the House of Commons from the Local Government Board, dated Aug. 12, 1896, showed as of June 1, 1896 there were 13,428 sick and bedridden in London infirmaries, with a total of 1,514 nurses for their care.

40. *Ann. Rep. L.G.B. for 1894–1895*, Appendix B, p. 20. See also the report of Mr. J. S. Davy in the same annual report.

41. *Ann. Rep. P.L.B. for 1868–1869*, p. 18.

42. Beatrice and Sidney Webb, *English Poor Law Policy*, pp. 208–209.

43. The annual reports of the Board show the following numbers of paupers attended in outdoor relief (including those both on the permanent medical list, and those for whom orders for attendance were issued):

      1887 (116,267);   1888 (116,218);   1889 (113,072);   1890 (119,041);
      1891 (115,961);   1892 (118,610);   1893 (131,440);   1894 (118,527);
      1895 (132,645);   1896 (116,893);   1897 (112,956);   1898 (110,419).

44. *Minutes of Evidence, Report of the Royal Commission on the Aged Poor*, 1895, Questions 2633, 2638, 17456ff.

45. *Med. Press and Cir.*, Aug. 5, 1868, p. 125.

46. Rogers, *Reminiscences of a Workhouse Medical Officer*, p. xxi.

47. Thomas Hawksley, *Charities of London and Some Errors of Their Administration* (London: John Churchill & Sons, 1869), p. 19.

48. See, in part, *Med. Press and Cir.*, Feb. 5, 1868, pp. 123–124; Apr. 27, 1868, p. 378; May 20, 1868, p. 444; Mar. 18, 1868, p. 249. Also *The Lancet*, Jan. 14, 1871, p. 60; and the *Brit. M.J.*, Apr. 24, 1869, p. 380; Nov. 13, 1869, pp. 539–540.

49. See especially the *Ann. Rep. P.L.B. for 1870–1871*, Appendix, p. 188.

50. (1) Permanency of poor law medical officer appointments and the entire payment of salaries out of the consolidated fund. (2) Adequate and uniform remuneration. (3) Increased salaries for length of service, and promotion to higher inspectorial appointments. (4) Consolidation of the various offices of registrar, vaccinator, medical officer, and medical officer of health, with fitting remuneration. (5) Drugs and surgical instruments to be provided by the Guardians, and dispensers and dispensaries to be established wherever practicable. (6) To obtain for the medical officers the responsible control of all midwifery cases. (7) The provision of a basis for consultation and united action in cases of difficulty. (8) Payment for surgery and midwifery in the workhouses as provided for in district work, and an extension of the list of operations for which extra fees were paid. (9) To raise the status of poor law medical officers, to increase their influence and usefulness, and consequently their remuneration, and to provide a channel through which all the defects of the poor law medical service may be brought to light and "discussed with a view to their

removal or amelioration." See the *Brit. M.J.*, Feb. 4, 1871, p. 134, and *The Lancet*, Feb. 4, 1871, p. 175.

51. *Brit. M.J.*, May 13, 1871, p. 509.

52. *Ibid.*, Feb. 17, 1872, pp. 187–188.

53. *The Lancet*, Apr. 11, 1874, p. 528.

54. L.G.B. Misc. Corres., No. 15574/78 of 1878, "*The Lancet* Memorial."

55. L.G.B. Misc. Corres., No. 52410/78, Aug. 20, 1878. See also *Ann. Rep. L.G.B. for 1878–1879*, p. xliv.

56. L.G.B. Misc. Corres., No. 77841/78, Nov. 13, 1878.

57. The fight for superannuation was bitter. Permissive legislation in 1864 and 1867 had given Boards of Guardians the right to provide for superannuation of union officers. This discretional right had been rarely exercised by local Guardians and, after a lifetime of public service in the community, the parish doctor was usually retired without remuneration.

58. Aschrott, *The English Poor Law System*, p. 87.

59. *Report of the Select Committee of the House of Lords on Poor Relief, 1888,* Minutes of Evidence, pp. 7 and 604.

60. *Ibid.*, p. viii. The report also suggested increased reliance on provident dispensaries and medical benefit funds to reduce the use of poor law medical facilities.

61. The deputation told Sir Walter that paupers were entirely dependent upon "the goodwill and charity of their medical attendants for the administration of anaesthetics. It they had not anaesthetics in any case it was because it was out of the power of the medical man to provide them." *The Lancet*, Mar. 4, 1893, p. 489.

62. L.G.B. Gov't. Office Corres., 1893 (Vol. 127), No. 40904/93.

63. *The Lancet*, Mar. 4, 1893, p. 490.

64. Newsholme, *The Last Thirty Years in Public Health*, p. 78.

65. *The Lancet*, Mar. 28, 1896, p. 860.

66. *Ibid.*, Mar. 6. 1897, p. 661.

67. Rumsey, *Essays on State Medicine*. p. 255.

68. The city of Liverpool, for example, at the end of the century had commenced the erection of a tuberculosis sanitorium for the poor.

69. *Minutes of Evidence, Royal Commission on the Aged Poor,* Questions 14022, 14023.

70. Thomas Mackay, *Public Relief of the Poor* (London: John Murray, 1901), p. 171.

Chapter VI. Local Medical Officers of Health and State Intervention

1. "Our Medical Officers of Health, a Study of the Medical Officers of Health of the Larger Towns in the Seventies," by students of the History Seminar, London School of Hygiene and Tropical Medicine, 1947–1948, *Public Health*, LXI (Aug., 1948), 210.

2. de Chaumont, *Lectures on State Medicine*, p. 35. Sidney Herbert was later created Lord Herbert of Lea. Dr. de Chaumont was overoptimistic in stating that all of these posts were held by full-time medical officers of health.

3. Compiled from annual reports of the Local Government Board, 1875 to 1900. There are no statistics available in the reports to indicate what proportion of these were full-time or part-time appointments.

4. *The Lancet*, Feb. 3, 1872, p. 166.

5. Newsholme, *Fifty Years of Public Health*, p. 142. There were still loopholes after 1892 in the metropolis. The provision read: "after the 1st January 1892 no person can be appointed Medical Officer of Health of any district in the Metropolis

which contained according to the last published census . . . 50,000 or more inhabitants unless he is qualified as a medical practitioner, and also is either registered in the *Medical Register* as the holder of a diploma in sanitary science, public health, or state medicine, under Section 21 of the Medical Act 1886, or has been during three consecutive years preceding the year 1892 a Medical Officer of a district or combination of districts, with a population of not less than 20,000 inhabitants, or has before the passing of the Local Government Act been for not less than three years one of our Medical Officers or Inspectors." *Ann. Rep. L.G.B. for 1888–1889,* p. lv. See also William A. Robson, *From Patronage to Proficiency in the Public Service* (London: Fabian Society, 1922), p. 33.

6. Dr. Alison was very aware of community living conditions as a health factor. Dr. R. P. B. Taafe, Medical Officer of Health for Brighton, advised the National Association for the Promotion of Social Science that Edinburgh was far ahead in instituting instruction in sanitary science. *Trans. N.A.P.S.S.,* 1875, p. 550.

7. C. Frazer Brockington, *Medical Officers of Health, 1848 to 1855* (London: Hodgetts Ltd., 1957), pp. 17–19.

8. "Our Medical Officers of Health," p. 211.

9. *Transactions of the Society of Medical Officers of Health, Annual Report for 1878–1879,* p. 11. (Hereafter cited as *Trans. Soc. M.O.H., Ann. Rep.*)

10. Edward Smith, *Manual for Medical Officers of Health* (London: Knight & Co., 1st ed., 1873; 2nd ed., 1874).

11. See the *Minutes of the General Council of Medical Education and Registration of the United Kingdom, of the Executive Committee* for June 6, 1895, p. 96; Nov. 29, 1895, pp. 470–471; 1900, Appendix XVIII, pp. 627ff. (Hereafter cited as *Minutes Gen. Med. Council.*)

12. *Brit. M.J.,* Jan. 3, 1885, pp. 40–41. See also C. Frazer Brockington, *Short History of Public Health* (London: J. & A. Churchill Ltd., 1956), pp. 34–35.

13. *Ann. Rep. L.G.B. for 1872–1873,* App., pp. 51–52. For a general outline of the duties of local medical officers of health earlier in the century, see the list accompanying the Feb. 12, 1851 letter of Henry Austin, Secretary to the General Board of Health, reprinted as Appendix 1 to Brockington, *Medical Officers of Health, 1848 to 1855,* pp. 39–46.

14. Frazer, *Duncan of Liverpool,* p. 40.

15. *Brit. M.J.,* Nov. 16, 1872, p. 543.

16. L.G.B. Gov't. Office Corres., No. 28758/91, for March 13, 1891; also *Ann. Rep. L.G.B. for 1891,* Appendix A, pp. 1–2.

17. L.G.B. Misc. Corres., 1872, No. 65639/72.

18. Rogers, *Reminiscences of a Workhouse Medical Officer,* pp. 102–103. The *Medical Times and Gazette* advanced the sound argument that the poor law medical officer was already well occupied without further duties, Jan. 28, 1871, p. 99.

19. *Ann. Rep. M.O.L.G.B. for 1874,* p. 14.

20. *Ann. Rep. L.G.B. for 1880–1881,* p. lxi.

21. *Trans. N.A.P.S.S., 1874,* p. 98.

22. L.G.B. Misc. Corres., No. 32822/77 of 1877.

23. *Ann. Rep. L.G.B. for 1880,* p. cvi.

24. Dr. Reginald Dudfield, Medical Officer of Health, Borough of Paddington, prepared a chronicle of the Society's activities from 1856 to 1906, which was published for the group's fiftieth anniversary in a special issue of *Public Health,* the Society's journal. (Dudfield, "History of the Society of Medical Officers of Health," *Jubilee Number of Public Health,* 1906, 198 pp.)

25. In 1869 the name was changed to the Association of Medical Officers of Health; in 1873 to the Society of Medical Officers of Health, and in 1891 to the Incorporated Society of Medical Officers of Health.

26. Dudfield, "History of the Society of Medical Officers of Health," p. 74.

27. An additional "Northern Counties Association" had been in existence from 1875–1882, when it was dissolved.

28. See the reports of the Council of the Society of Medical Officers of Health for years specified. The figures include fellows, members, and associates.

29. Dudfield, "History of the Society of Medical Officers of Health," p. 51.

30. Edwin Chadwick, *Essay on the Means Against the Casualties of Sickness, Decrepitude, and Mortality* (London: republished from the Apr., 1828, *Westminster Review* by Charles Knight, 1836), p. 12.

31. Michael J. MacCormack, *Medical Officer of Health's Report to the Vestry of the Parish of St. Mary, Lambeth,* Feb., 1872, pp. 2–3.

32. *Trans. Soc. M.O.H., 1883–1884,* p. 1.

33. *Brit. M.J.,* Aug. 16, 1873, p. 18. See also Dr. A. Carpenter, *Administrative Areas for Sanitary Purposes* (London: Spottiswood & Co., 1873), p. 15.

34. "Memorandum on the Advantages to be Derived From a Registration of Disease, and on the Mode which such a Record May be Obtained." Adopted at a Meeting of a Committee Representing the St. Andrew's Medical Graduates Association, the Medical Society of London, the Metropolitan Association of Medical Officers of Health, and the Poor Law Medical Officers Association.

35. *Trans. N.A.P.S.S., 1876,* p. 481ff. See also: *ibid., 1877,* p. 568; Soc. M.O.H., Minutes of Ordinary Meetings, May 20, 1881.

36. L.G.B. Misc. Corres., No. 81685/77, 27 Nov. 1877; Soc. M.O.H., Minutes of Annual Meetings, 1887.

37. Soc. M.O.H., Minutes of Ordinary Meetings, May 16, 1892; John F. J. Sykes, *Public Health Problems* (London: Walter Scott, 1892), pp. 347ff.

38. *Journal of the Royal Statistical Society,* LIX, Part I (Mar. 1896), 28.

39. L.G.B. Misc. Corres., No. 77189/78, Nov. 1878.

40. The deputation included representatives of the British Medical Association, the Social Science Association, and the National Health Society. Soc. M.O.H., Minutes of Council, May 17, 1881.

41. Beatrice and Sidney Webb, *The State and the Doctor,* pp. 46–47, 158–161. See also Soc. M.O.H., Minutes of Council, Dec. 11, 1884.

42. Edwin Chadwick, *The Evils of Disunity in Central and Local Administration* (London: Longmans, Green & Co., 1885), pp. 49–50. Actually, as Major Harry Barnes in *The Slum, Its Story* (London: P. S. King, 1931), points out, prior to 1870, legislation had given local authorities power to enter a house on the order of a Justice of the Peace (Nuisance Removal Act of 1855), while the Torrens Act of 1868 gave the medical officer of health power to investigate on his own initiative.

43. George Bernard Shaw, "Widower's Houses," in *The Collected Works of George Bernard Shaw,* Vol. VII (New York: William Wise & Co., 1930), p. 31.

44. John F. J. Sykes, M.D., *Public Health and Housing* (London: P. S. King, 1901), p. 141.

45. James M. Mackintosh, *Trends of Opinion About the Public Health, 1901–1951* (London: Geoffrey Cumberlege, Oxford University Press, 1953), p. 2.

46. James M. Mackintosh, *Housing and Family Life* (London: Cassell & Co., 1952), pp. 44–48.

47. T. S. Ashton, "The Treatment of Capitalism by Historians," in Fredrick A. von Hayek, ed., *Capitalism and the Historians* (Chicago: University of Chicago Press, 1954), pp. 50–51; Louis M. Hacker, "The Anti-Capitalist Bias of American Historians," in Hayek, *Capitalism and the Historians,* p. 68; Maurice Bruce, *The Coming of the Welfare State* (London: B. T. Batsford Ltd., 1961), pp. 117–121.

48. Cornelius Fox, M.D., "The Impairment of the Efficiency of the Medical Officer of Health. Produced by His Want of Independence as a Public Official," in *Dozen Papers Relating to Disease Prevention* (London: John Churchill, 1884), p. 5.

49. Alice Smith, *Memoirs of the Buchanan Family,* p. 20.

50. Barnes, *The Slum, Its Story,* p. 133.

51. The Home Office acknowledged the importance of the subject, but shelved any immediate action. Public Record Office File 058430/1: Letter from Medical Officers of Health of the Metropolis to the Home Office; P.R.O. Document O.S. 8430/2: Letter from Tom Taylor, Local Government Act Office, Feb. 22, 1870 to the Home Office. See also *Med. Press and Cir.,* Mar. 23, 1870, p. 233.

52. *Med. Times and Gaz.,* Oct. 20, 1870, p. 491.

53. Tatham, *Biennial Report on the Health of Salford for 1875 and 1876,* p. 8. See also D. M. Conan, *A History of the Public Health Department in Bermondsey* (Greenwich: Henry Richardson, 1935), pp. 134 and 153, for comments on Dr. James Vinen's views on housing.

54. In actuality, as Octavia Hill noted in 1875, all private housing improvement schemes in London during the previous thirty years had only rehoused 26,000, or about half the annual number of immigrants into London.

55. *Trans. N.A.P.S.S., 1878,* p. 501.

56. Soc. M.O.H. Minutes of Ordinary Meetings, Apr. 18, 1879.

57. See especially the testimony of John Dixon, M.D., Mr. Shirley F. Murphy, M.R.C.S., Mr. David Davids, M.R.C.S., Mr. Edward S. Angove, L.R.C.P. and Mr. W. H. J. Brown, M.B., Minutes of Evidence, *Report of the Royal Commission on the Housing of the Working Classes,* II, 1885.

58. *Public Health,* I (Sept., 1888), 146.

59. Minutes of Annual Provincial Meeting, Leeds, Oct. 3, 1891. See also the paper read to the Yorkshire Branch of the Society, *Public Health,* IV (Feb., 1892), 143–144.

60. James Niven, *Observations on the History of the Public Health Service in Manchester* (Manchester: John Heywood Ltd., 1923), p. 169.

61. See the following issues of *Public Health:* Sept., 1894, p. 393; May, 1885, pp. 288–289; Apr., 1899, p. 481; Dec., 1899, p. 137; Feb., 1900, p. 309; Oct., 1900, pp. 27–30.

62. *Public Health,* XII (Apr., 1900), 539.

63. See *Public Health,* IV (May, 1892), 232–235; (June, 1892), 285; and V (Apr., 1893), 206.

64. *Ibid.,* XII (Feb., 1900), 322.

65. Bernardino Ramazzini, *De morbis artificum diatriba.* Italian edition, Modena, 1670; English edition, 1705.

66. The detailed history of the factory acts is too long to include here. Useful summaries of this legislation appear in Ludwig Teleky, *History of Factory and Mine Hygiene* (New York: Columbia University Press, 1948); Thomas Oliver, ed., *Dangerous Trades* (New York: E. P. Dutton & Co., 1902), pp. 24–43; and T. K. Djang, *Factory Inspection in Great Britain* (London: Allen & Unwin Ltd., 1942), pp. 26–45.

67. The exception in the early years was Mr. Robert Baker, a Leeds surgeon, who joined the factory inspection staff in 1834, becoming an inspector in 1858. Djang, *Factory Inspection,* p. 32.

68. Henry A. Mess, *Factory Legislation and Its Administration, 1891–1924* (London: P. S. King & Sons, 1926), p. 184.

69. See, for example, *Annual Reports Upon the Health of Blackburn by James Wheatley, M.D., B.S., Medical Officer of Health and Police Surgeon, for the years 1891* (p. 26), *and 1893* (p. 60).

70. Oliver, *Dangerous Trades,* pp. 289–290.

71. *Annual Reports of the Medical Officer of Health for Durham, T. Eustace Hill, M.B., B.Sc., F.I.C., including a Summary of the Annual Reports of the District Medical Officers of Health, and other records, for the years 1891, 1896,* p. xliv, *and 1897,* p. xxxvii.

72. *Public Health,* IV (Mar., 1892), 169–170.

73. *Ibid.*, VIII (Jan., 1896), 124ff.

74. *Ibid.*, VIII (Apr., 1896), 228.

75. *Ibid.*, XII (Jan., 1900), 298–299.

76. George Goldie, L.R.C.P. (Edinburgh), M.R.C.S. (Edinburgh), *Report on the Sanitary Conditions of Leeds for the year 1876*, p. 79.

77. L.G.B. Misc. Corres., No. 8147/79, 29 Jan. 1879. (A bill to this effect was introduced into Parliament in the same Session, but was withdrawn because of the pressure of other business; see *ibid.*, No. 72521(R) (1) 15 Oct. 1879.)

78. Soc. M.O.H. Minutes of Council, Dec. 19, 1884 and June, 1885.

79. *Public Health*, X (Aug., 1898), 373.

80. *Ibid.*, VIII (July, 1896), 329; see also IX (Feb. ,1897), 174–175.

81. L.G.B. Misc. Corres., No. 63307/72, Nov. 18, 1872, Memorandum of the Association of Medical Officers of Health; See also Minutes of a Special Committee of the Metropolitan Members of the Association, Oct. 28, 1872.

82. *Public Health*, I (Jan., 1889), 269.

83. *Ibid.*, V (Sept., 1893), 354 ff.

84. *Ibid.*, IX (May, 1897), 269.

85. *Ibid.*, XI (May, 1899), 527 and 570. The Act, upon passage, was also reviewed extensively in the October, 1899, issue of *Public Health*, pp. 12ff.

86. L.G.B. Misc. Corres., May 19, 1876, No. 32822/76. Letter to President of the Local Government Board from J. Northcote Vinen, M.D.; also *Trans. Soc. M.O.H.*, *1876–1877*, pp. 16–17.

87. L.G.B. Misc. Corres., No. 4992/78, Petition from the Society of Medical Officers of Health. See also Petition of the Northwestern Association of Medical Officers of Health, L.G.B. Misc. Corres., No. 110.483/81, Nov. 28, 1881, and *Jubilee Issue of Public Health*, 1906, p. 103.

88. Soc. M.O.H. Minutes of Ordinary Meetings, Mar. 20, 1893; *Public Health*, IV (July, 1892), 290.

89. *Trans. Soc. M.O.H.* for 1886–1887, p. xxx; Minute Books of Annual Meetings for 1887; see also "Bacteriology in Relation to Public Health," Report of the Council of the Society of Medical Officers of Health, Session 1899–1900, also *Brit. M.J.*, Dec. 31, 1887, p. 1426.

90. Soc. M.O.H. Minutes of Ordinary Meetings, Dec. 19, 1892; *Public Health* Apr., 1897, p. 237; also Vol. 11 (1898–1899), pp. 225, 538, 618; Vol. 12 (1899–1900), pp. 232, 357, 639, etc.

91. *Public Health*, I (May, 1888), 27.

92. See, for example, Soc. M.O.H. Minutes of Ordinary Meetings, May 18, 1883.

93. Soc. M.O.H., Minutes of Council, May 21, 1894, May 20, 1896, Sept. 24, 1897, and Jan. 13, 1899.

94. *Public Health*, IX (May, 1897), 263–264.

Chapter VII. Auxiliary Central Government Medical Organization

1. Sir Henry Acland, *The Army Medical School* (London: Macmillan & Co., 1887), p. 9.

2. The Crimean medical and sanitary reforms are, of course, brilliantly described in Cecil Woodham-Smith's, *Florence Nightingale, 1802–1910* (London: Constable, 1950).

3. *Report of the Army Medical Department for 1898, Parl. Papers*, 1899, Vol. 53, p. 41.

4. "Memorandum by the Director-General Army Medical Service on the Physical

Unfitness of Men Offering Themselves for Enlistment in the Army," Apr. 2, 1903, *Parl. Papers*, 1903, Vol. 38, p. 4.

5. See Chapter IX, pp. 169–170 for a discussion of this report.

6. Walter Rivington, M.D., *The Medical Profession of the United Kingdom*, 2nd ed. (London: Longmans, Green & Co., 1888), pp. 420ff.

7. Peter Lovegrove, *Not Least in the Crusade, A Short History of the Royal Army Medical Corps* (Aldershot: Gale & Polden Ltd., 1952), p. 19.

8. "Letter from Sir Andrew Clark to the Secretary of State for War, Relative to the Status of Medical Officers of the Army, Jan. 17, 1891, and the Secretary of State's Reply, Feb. 2, 1891," *Parl. Papers*, 1890–1891, Vol. 50.

9. Lovegrove, *Not Least in the Crusade*, p. 25.

10. John Hay Beith, *One Hundred Years of Army Nursing, The Story of the British Army Nursing Services from the Time of Florence Nightingale to the Present Day* (London: Cassell & Co., 1953), pp. 40–53. See also Frederick Treves, *The Tale of a Field Hospital* (London: Cassell & Co., 1900).

11. "Report of the Royal Commission Appointed to Consider and Report Upon the Care and Treatment of the Sick and Wounded During the South African Campaign," 1901, *Parl. Papers*, 1901, Vol. 29, p. 4 and pp. 69–71.

12. "Report of Committee Appointed by the Secretary of State to Consider the Reorganization of the Army Medical Services," 1901.

13. *Medicine and the Navy, 1200–1900*, Vol. 4: *1815–1900*, by Christopher Lloyd and Jack L. S. Coulter (Edinburgh: E. & S. Livingstone Ltd., 1963), p. 241.

14. "Report to the Lords Commissioners of the Admiralty of the Committee Appointed to Inquire into the Organization and Training of Sick-Berth Staff of the Navy and the Nursing Staff of Royal Naval Hospitals, 1884," *Parl. Papers*, 1884, Vol. 170, p. vl.

15. "Report of the [War Office] Committee Appointed to Enquire into the Pay Status and Conditions of Service of Medical Officers of the Army and Navy, 1889, *Parl. Papers*, 1889, Vol. 17, p. 11.

16. "Statistical Report on the Health of the Navy for the Year 1898," *Parl. Papers*, 1889, Vol. 55, p. 6. See also Lloyd and Coulter, *Medicine and the Navy*, pp. 199–201.

17. See the "Correspondence or Extracts Therefrom Relating to the Repeal of the Contagious Disease Ordinances and Regulations in the Crown Colonies," *passim.*, in *Parl. Papers*, 1887, Vol. 57.

18. Julian Amery, *The Life of Joseph Chamberlain*, Vol. IV (1901–1903) (London: Macmillan & Co., 1951), pp. 222–233.

19. The following medical corporations were represented on the Council: the Royal College of Physicians of London; the Royal College of Surgeons of England; the Apothecaries' Society of London: the Universities of Oxford, Cambridge, Durham, and London; the Royal College of Physicians of Edinburgh; the Royal College of Surgeons of Edinburgh; the Faculty of Physicians and Surgeons of Glasgow; the University of Edinburgh in combination with the University of Aberdeen; the University of Glasgow in combination with the University of St. Andrews; the King and Queen's College of Physicians in Ireland; the Royal College of Surgeons in Ireland; the Apothecaries' Hall of Ireland; the University of Dublin; and the Queen's University; together with six Crown nominees and a president. See Rivington, *The Medical Profession* (1888 ed.), p. 187.

20. Ann Beck, "The British Medical Council and British Medical Education in the Nineteenth Century," *Bull. Hist. Med.* XXX (Mar.–Apr., 1956), 152.

21. The list of subjects suggested in 1869 by a committee of the General Medical Council, for example, for a diploma in State Medicine and for entry into the public medical services included: Forensic Medicine, Toxicology, Morbid Anatomy, Psychological Medicine, Laws of Evidence, Preventive Medicine, Vital and Sanitary Sta-

tistics, Medical Topography, and certain portions of Engineering Science and Practice. Many diplomas in State Medicine were granted, and many medical practitioners served in the public medical services without this training long after 1869. See *Brit. M.J.*, Oct. 2, 1869, p. 383.

22. Rivington, *The Medical Profession* (1888 ed.), p. 100: See also Chap. VIII of the present study, p. 148.

23. *Minutes Gen. Med. Council*, Feb. 29, 1872.

24. *Minutes Gen. Med. Council*, Nov. 1889, pp. 166–167; May 28, 1890, pp. 69–71.

25. Public Record Office, Home Office Papers, O.S. 6587, "Letter from Alexander Redgrave to Spencer Walpole," Dec. 14, 1858.

26. See Rivington *The Medical Profession* (1879 ed.), p. 240, and Djang, *Factory Inspection*, pp. 55–56.

27. "Report of the Inspector of Factories for the Half-year Ending 31 Oct. 1868," in *Parl. Papers*, 1868, Vol. 14, pp. 203–204. See also "Reports of Inspectors of Factories," Apr. 30, 1875 in *Parl. Papers*, 1875, Vol. 16, p. 84.

28. *The Lancet*, Jan. 9, 1869, p. 60.

29. In 1896, there were 1,897 certifying surgeons; in 1897, the number increased to 2,003. (*Ann. Rep. Chief Inspector of Factories and Workshops for 1897*, p. 241.)

30. *Ibid.* See also *Ann. Rep. Chief Inspector of Factories and Workshops for 1898*, p. 13.

31. See Whitelegge's obituary notice written by Sir George Newman in *The Lancet*, May 6, 1933, p. 990.

32. See Legge's obituary in the *Brit. M.J.*, May 14, 1932, pp. 913–914.

Chapter VIII. The Private Practitioner and the Role of the State, 1870–1900

1. *Brit. M.J.*, Sept. 11, 1869, p. 268. Dr. Charles Newman in his *Evolution of Medical Education in the Nineteenth Century* points out (pp. 200–201) that during the second half of the century the purely cultural aspects of medical education gradually disappeared.

2. "The Medical Profession and Its Morality" (anon.), reprinted with additions from *The Modern Review* of 1881 (London: Pewtress & Co., 1886), p. 11.

3. For a discussion of the roles of the physicians and apothecaries in the century previous, see Bernice Hamilton, "The Medical Profession in the Eighteenth Century," *The Economic History Review*, 2nd series, IV, 141–169.

4. By 1879, the Universities of Durham and Dublin still retained the right to confer licenses to practice medicine, although these had been given up by Oxford and Cambridge. Training in medical education, and the conferring of medical degrees (M.B., M.D., etc.) were, of course, part of the university function. See Rivington, *The Medical Profession* (1879 ed.), p. 46, and Edwin Wooton, *A Guide to the Medical Profession: A Comprehensive Manual Conveying the Means of Entering the Medical Profession in the Chief Countries of the World*, edited by L. Forbes Winslow, M.B. (London: L. Upcott Gill, 1882), Chaps. 1–6; and Charles Newman, *The Evolution of Medical Education in the Nineteenth Century*, Chap. II.

5. See also Chap. VII, pp. 142–143. A clear outline of the functions of the General Medical Council appears in A. M. Carr-Saunders and P. A. Wilson, *The Professions* (Oxford: Clarendon Press, 1933), pp. 83–89.

6. *Brit. M.J.*, Mar., 1868 and Dec. 19, 1874, p. 780.

7. As a result of this obstructive action, which was taken by the British Medical

Association's Direct Representation Committee, a number of well-known medical reformers resigned from the Association, including Drs. William Stokes, C. E. Paget, H. W. Acland, D. Embleton, and H. W. Rumsey. *The Lancet,* June 10, 1871, p. 789, and June 17, 1871, p. 838.

8. Sprigge, *Medicine and the Public,* pp. 26–27; also A. S. Comyns Carr, W. H. Stuart Garnett, and J. H. Taylor, *National Insurance,* 3rd ed. (London: Macmillan & Co., 1912), pp. 52ff.

9. *Med. Times and Gaz.,* Aug. 20, 1870, p. 215.

10. *The Lancet,* Sept. 3, 1870, p. 347. Prior to the passage of the Coroner's (Amendment) Act of 1926, no special qualifications were necessary for appointment as Coroner or Deputy Coroner. See Thomas Ottaway, *The Law and Practice Relating to Coroners* (London: Butterworth & Co., 1927), p. 1.

11. *Brit. M.J.,* Jan. 29, 1887, p. 192.

12. *Ibid.,* Aug. 4, 1894, p. 238.

13. Simon, *English Sanitary Institutions,* 1st ed., p. 463.

14. *Brit. M.J.,* June 10, 1871, pp. 606–607; *The Lancet,* June 10, 1871, pp. 771ff.

15. *The Lancet,* June 17, 1871, pp. 810–811. *The Doctor,* July 1, 1871, p. 127.

16. Sir George Newman, *The Place of Public Opinion in Preventive Medicine* (London: Ministry of Health, 1920), p. 26.

17. The Health Section of the Thirteenth Annual Congress of the National Association for the Promotion of Health Science, led by Dr. Symonds, Dr. Lankester, and Dr. William Budd, listed as its objects, "a consideration of various questions relating to the public health; it collects statistical evidence of the relative healthiness of different localities, of different industrial occupations and generally the influence of external circumstances in the production of health or disease; it discusses improvements in house construction, in drainage, warming, ventilation, public baths and wash-houses, adulteration of food and its effects . . . the function of Government in relation to public health; the legislative and administrative machinery expedient for its preservation, sanitary police, quarantine, poverty in relation to disease; and the effects of unhealthiness on the prosperity of places and nations." See note in *Scientific Opinion,* Sept. 29, 1869.

18. For example, see the paper by Dr. Richard Caton, "On the Teaching of Hygiene in Government Schools," *Reports, Brit Assoc. for the Advancement of Science,* 1874, p. 198; Dr. Henry Ashby's paper on "Infantile Mortality," *Trans. N.A.P.S.S.,* 1884, p. 497; Dr. G. B. Barron's paper, "The Constitutional Characteristics of Those Who Dwell in Large Towns," 1888, pp. 836–837; "The Degeneracy of the Race in Towns," a paper presented by Dr. H. W. Rumsey to the Annual Meeting of the N.A.P.S.S., 1871 (See *Brit. M.J.,* Oct. 21, 1871, pp. 482ff.)

19. *Brit. M.J.,* May 11, 1889, p. 1095.

20. J. L. Garvin, *The Life of Joseph Chamberlain,* Vol. I, 1836–1885 (London: Macmillan & Co., 1935), pp. 188ff.

21. Jeremy Bentham, *Constitutional Code* as cited by Sir Arthur MacNalty, *A Biography of Sir Benjamin Ward Richardson* (London: Harvey & Blythe, 1950), p. 57.

22. T. W. Grimshaw, "Sanitary Legislation and Organization," *Reports of the Brit. Assoc. for the Advancement of Science,* 1874, pp. 206–208.

23. Benjamin Ward Richardson, *Hygeia: A City of Health* (London, 1876); see the discussion of this in James Cassedy, "Hygeia: A Mid-Victorian Dream of a City of Health," *J. Hist. Med. and Allied Sciences,* XVII (Apr., 1962), 217–228; MacNalty, *A Biography of Sir Benjamin Ward Richardson,* p. 54; and Newsholme, *Fifty Years of Public Health,* pp. 103–104.

24. B. W. Richardson, *A Ministry of Health, and other addresses* (London: Chatto & Windus, 1879)

25. John Leyland, ed. *Contemporary Medical Men*, Vol. II (Leicester: *Provincial Medical Journal*, 1888), p. 99. Neither of Mackenzie's biographers, Hugh Haweis or R. Scott Stevenson, give any details on this plan.

26. *Brit. M.J.*, Aug. 31, 1889, p. 446.

27. L.G.B. Misc. Corres., No. 47603/95, dated Apr. 5, 1895.

28. Robert Reid Rentoul, *The Reform of Our Voluntary Medical Charities, Some Serious Considerations for the Philanthropic* (London: Balliere, Tindall and Cox, 1891). Earlier outlines of the plan were published in the medical journals in 1889, complete with details on projected fees for such services as "the washing out of the stomach—three shillings sixpence," and "leeching at two and six." *Brit. M.J.*, Sept. 28, 1889, pp. 742–743.

29. *Brit. M.J.*, June 29, 1889, p. 1495. Also see Chap. X ("Voluntary Effort in Medical Care at the Beginning of the Twentieth Century") for further detail on medical charities and the "club" system by the turn of the century.

30. *Brit. M.J.*, Nov. 28, 1889, p. 1194.

31. *Ibid.*, July 26, 1890, pp. 237ff. Three branches, numbering 426 members, approved of the plan; 2 branches, with 318 members, were neutral, and 16 branches, with a membership of 4,497 members opposed the Rentoul Plan, as did a majority of the Investigating Committee.

32. Sir Humphrey Rolleston in his "History of the *Practitioner*" states that the main object of the periodical was to act as a special medium for the intercommunication of information about remedies. (*Practitioner*, CL (June, 1943), 321–328). In a survey of the *Medical Press and Circular* by Robert Rowlette (London: *Medical Press and Circular*, 1939), little emerges to show that the journal took any major part in public health reform apart from supporting a single medical licensing system, reforms in the Army Medical Service, and calling attention to poor housing conditions in Dublin. Editorials of this journal, however, from time to time passed judgment on the ineffectiveness of such legislation as the Factory Acts (see issue of Oct. 13, 1875). The *Medical Times and Gazette* and *The Doctor* contain a number of liberal editorials urging investigation of a variety of sanitary evils. None of these periodicals, however, directly fostered investigating commissions or brought pressure to bear upon Parliament to the degree that the editors of the *British Medical Journal* and *The Lancet* did.

33. E. Muirhead Little, "Ernest Hart: A Study of Character," Nov. 1924, p. 6. (Photostat, in the Library of the Royal Society of Medicine, of a 14-page typed manuscript.) Hart resigned as editor in 1869, but was again appointed in 1870. See also Paul Vaughan, *Doctors' Commons, A Short History of the British Medical Association* (London: William Heinemann, 1959), pp. 136–139.

34. *Brit. M.J.*, Apr. 26, 1890, pp. 965–966.

35. *The Lancet*, Mar. 18, 1871, p. 386.

36. *Ibid.*, Sept. 21, 1872, p. 418.

37. *Ibid.*, Aug. 21, 1875, p. 285.

38. E. M. Brockbank, *A Centenary History of the Manchester Medical Society* (Manchester: Sherratt & Hughes, 1934), pp. 32ff.

39. L.G.B. Misc. Corres., No. 86397, Dec. 12, 1878; No. 97287/79, Dec. 30, 1879; No. 85718/79, Nov. 18, 1879; No. 58402/80, June 29, 1880.

40. L.G.B. Misc. Corres., No. 51953/88, "Kingston Memorial on Mr. G. Hastings' Bill."

41. *Brit. M.J.*, Mar. 23, 1895, p. 675; May 11, 1895, p. 1073.

42. Ernest Little, *A History of the British Medical Association, 1832–1932* (London: British Medical Association, 1932), pp. 79ff.

43. *Brit. M.J.*, Jan. 14, 1871, p. 40, and Aug. 12, 1871, p. 190. The *Medical Register* for 1900 lists a total of 35,836 registered practitioners in England, Scotland,

and Ireland (4,979 were in Ireland). This total, however, included many practitioners who served with the Army, Navy, and in the colonies.

44. Horatio N. Hardy, *The State of the Medical Profession in Great Britain and Ireland* (London: Bailliere, Tindall and Cox, 1901), p. 26.

45. *Med. Times and Gaz.*, Jan. 8, 1870, p. 37.

46. *The Doctor*, July 1, 1873, p. 117.

47. *Brit. M.J.*, Aug. 10, 1872, p. 153.

48. *Ibid.*, Dec. 20, 1873, p. 727.

49. Little, *History of the British Medical Association*, p. 138.

50. Robert Farquharson, *In and Out of Parliament* (London: Williams & Norgate, 1911), p. 118.

51. *Brit. M.J.*, Aug. 12, 1871, pp. 178–179.

52. *Ibid.*, Jan. 18, 1896, p. 162.

53. Little, *History of the British Medical Association*, p. 134. See also L.G.B. Misc. Corres., No. 4710/90E of 1890.

54. *Brit. M.J.*, Sept. 14, 1895, p. 651.

Chapter IX. New Patterns of State Medicine

1. George Howell, M.P., *Conflicts of Capital and Labour, Being a History and Review of the Trade Unions of Great Britain*, 2nd rev. ed. (London: Macmillan & Co., 1890), p. 484.

2. George D. H. Cole, *A Short History of the British Working Class Movement, 1789–1947*, new ed. (London: Allen & Unwin Ltd., 1948), Vol. 2, p. 161.

3. Elie Halevy, *A History of the English People in the Nineteenth Century*, Vol. V (1895–1905: *Imperialism and the Rise of Labor*) (London: E. Benn Ltd., 1951), p. 211. See also D. C. Summerville, *British Politics Since 1900* (London: Andrew Dakers Ltd., 1950), pp. 46–47.

4. Masterman described the Liberal Party at this time as a "gigantic straddle between the conservative middle class element on the one hand and on the other the radical factor of working class representatives and their sympathisers." C. F. G. Masterman, "Liberalism and Labour," *The Nineteenth Century and After*, 1906, p. 717.

5. Henry Broadhurst, *Henry Broadhurst, M.P., The Story of His Life From a Stonemason's Bench to the Treasury Bench* (London: Hutchinson & Co., 1901), p. 147.

6. *The Times*, June 21, 1901, p. 9.

7. Beatrice Webb, *My Apprenticeship*, p. 186.

8. Charles Booth, *Life and Labour of the People in London* (London: Macmillan & Co., 1892–1897), Vol. IX, p. 420.

9. *Ibid.*, 1903 ed., Vol. XVII, pp. 213 and 439.

10. This was Haldane's final estimate. *Richard Burdon Haldane, An Autobiography* (New York: Doubleday Doran & Co., 1929), p. 113.

11. Edward Pease, *The History of the Fabian Society* (New York: E. P. Dutton & Co., 1919), p. 37.

12. B. L. Hutchins, "What a Health Committee Can Do," Fabian Society Tract, London, 1908. F. Lawson Dodd, "A National Medical Service," Fabian Society Tract, London, 1911.

13. *The Times*, June 21, 1901, p. 9.

14. See especially *The Lancet* 1904 issues of Aug. 6 (pp. 390–392), Aug. 20 (pp. 557–558), and Sept. 10 (pp. 785–787).

15. *The Lancet*, Jan. 14, 1905, p. 93.

16. *Brit. M.J.*, Aug. 6, 1904, p. 297.

17. Beatrice Webb, *My Apprenticeship*, p. 215.

18. See, for example, Dr. George F. McCleary's volumes, *The Maternity and Child Welfare Movement* (London: P. S. King & Sons, 1935) and *The Early History of the Infant Welfare Movement* (London: H. K. Lewis, 1933), also A. H. Hogarth, *The Medical Inspection of Schools* (Oxford: Henry Frowde, Hodder & Stoughton, 1909).

19. A. Newsholme, "A Discussion of the Public Medical Services," *Brit. M.J.*, Sept. 14, 1907, pp. 656–657.

20. *Ibid.*, p. 659; also Newsholme, *The Last Thirty Years in Public Health*, p. 72.

21. Sir Robert Philip, *Collected Papers on Tuberculosis* (London: Oxford University Press, Humphrey Milford, 1937), p. 97; Rosen, *History of Public Health*, pp. 385ff.

22. *Ibid.* (Philip), pp. 35–36.

23. Norman Wilson, *Municipal Health Services* (London: Allen & Unwin Ltd., 1946), p. 10.

24. Newsholme, "Public Health in Relation to the Struggle Against Tuberculosis in England," *Journal of Hygiene*, 1903, pp. 446ff.

25. *The Times*, July 24, 1901, p. 9.

26. *Brit. M.J.*, June 7, 1902, p. 1394; *The Lancet*, July 27, 1901, p. 215.

27. "Second Interim Report of the Royal Commission Appointed to Inquire into the Relations of Human and Animal Tuberculosis, Part I, 1907, *Parl. Papers*, 1907, Vol. 38, pp. 36–37.

28. Frazer, *History of English Public Health*, p. 315. (The Society of Medical Officers of Health in its Metropolitan Branch as early as 1906 had petitioned the Local Government Board and the London County Council for compulsory notification of phthisis in London.) See *Brit. M.J.*, Apr. 14, 1906, p. 864.

29. See, for example, *Brit. M.J.*, issues of Dec. 16, 1905, pp. 1597–1598; Jan. 4, 1902; Mar. 14, 1908, p. 623; Oct. 21, 1905, p. 1059; Dec. 19, 1908, p. 1826; also *The Lancet*, Apr. 6, 1907, pp. 956–957.

30. *Ann. Rep. M.O.L.G.B. for 1908–1909*, App. A, p. 238.

31. *The Lancet*, Mar. 20, 1909, p. 848.

32. *Ibid.*, Feb. 1, 1908, p. 387. At this time only Sheffield and Bolton had instituted systems of compulsory notification for tuberculosis.

33. *Ann. Rep. M.O.L.G.B. for 1910–1911*, p. xli.

34. *Ibid.*, p. xxxvi.

35. *Brit. M.J.*, Sept. 17, 1910, p. 800.

36. *Ann. Rep. M.O.L.G.B. for 1910–1911*, p. xlii.

37. "Report on Infant and Child Mortality," Supp. to the *Ann. Rep. M.O.L.G.B. for 1909–1910, Parl. Papers*, 1910, Vol. 39, p. 15.

38. McCleary, *The Maternity and Child Welfare Movement*, pp. 84–95.

39. Rosen, *History of Public Health*, pp. 351ff.

40. Little, *History of the British Medical Association*, pp. 127–130.

41. One of the leaders of the opposition was Dr. Robert Rentoul who testified before a Select Committee on Midwives Registration that he was entirely opposed to legislation which he felt would form any new order of midwifery practitioners. "Report of the Select Committee on Midwives Registration, 1892, Minutes of Evidence," *passim.*, *Parl. Papers*, 1892, Vol. 14. See also *Brit. M.J.*, Feb. 15, 1902, p. 408.

42. Section 12 of the Midwives Act of 1902.

43. *British Medical Journal* reflections on the Bill through its successive stages may be traced in the following issues: Feb. 15, 1902, p. 408; Feb. 22, 1902, p. 468; Mar. 1, 1902, p. 537; May 10, 1903, p. 1163; June 7, 1902, p. 1427.

44. *Parl. Debates*, 4th Series, Vol. 103 (Feb. 26, 1902), pp. 1165–1166.

45. *The Lancet*, Feb. 22, 1902, p. 532.

46. "Report of the Departmental Committee Appointed by the Lord President of the Council to Consider the Working of the Midwives Act, 1902, Vol. 1, pp. 2–3. *Parl. Papers*, 1909, Vol. 33. The British Medical Association followed this Departmental Committee's work closely, and was especially concerned that the State should guarantee a fixed fee to medical men who answered emergency calls of midwives who were required under the Act to summon them in special cases. *Ibid.*, p. 12; *Brit. M.J.*, Aug. 28, 1909, p. 565.

47. *Brit. M.J.*, Apr. 2, 1910, p. 825.

48. *Parl. Debates*, Fourth Series, Vol. 136, June 14, 1904, p. 14, and July 11, 1904, p. 1193.

49. *The Times*, Nov. 10, 1904, p. 7.

50. *Brit. M.J.*, June 16, 1906, p. 1422.

51. McCleary, *The Early History of the Infant Welfare Movement*, p. 135.

52. *Brit. M.J.*, Aug. 31, 1907, p. 541. See also *ibid.*, Sept. 14, 1907, p. 696.

53. *The Lancet*, Sept. 7, 1907, pp. 717–718.

54. *Public Health*, XII (Dec., 1889); Dr. H. M. Richard, "The Factors which Determine the Local Incidence of Fatal Infantile Diarrhoea," *Journal of Hygiene*, III (July, 1903), 325ff.

55. "Supplement on Infant and Child Mortality," *Ann. Rep. M.O.L.G.B. for 1909–1910*, pp. 76–77.

56. *Ann. Rep. M.O.L.G.B. for 1909–1910*, p. xxviii.

57. The steps to a nation's personal health services have been well detailed in Dr. Walsh McDermott's October, 1963, lecture at the National Institutes of Health, "The Role of Biomedical Research in International Development."

58. Hermann Cohn's researches on the eyesight of over 10,000 children at Breslau in 1866 was one of the classic pillars of the movement. *Ann. Rep. Chief Medical Officer of the Board of Education for 1908*, p. 2, *Parl. Papers*, 1910, Vol. 23; Rosen, *History of Public Health*, pp. 365–366.

59. Clement Dukes, *Health at School Considered in its Mental, Moral and Physical Aspects*, 4th rev. ed. (London: Rivingtons, 1905).

60. Francis Warner, M.D., "A Method of Examining Children in Schools as to Their Development and Brain Condition," *Brit. M.J.*, Sept. 22, 1888, pp. 659–660.

61. Little, *History of the British Medical Association*, p. 134.

62. *Ibid.*, also *Brit. M.J.*, July 18, 1896, pp. 140ff. (The cities concerned were London, Birmingham, Bristol, Brighton, Bradford, and Lewes.)

63. *Report of the Inter-departmental Committee on Physical Deterioration*, 1904, p. 72; see also Frazer, *History of English Public Health*, p. 256.

64. *The Times*, Sept. 14, 1904, p. 7.

65. "Report of the Inter-departmental Committee on Medical Inspection and Feeding of Children Attending Public Elementary Schools," *Parl. Papers*, 1906, Vol. 47, p. 31.

66. *The Lancet*, Sept. 8, 1906, p. 661.

67. A Select Committee which considered the Provision of Meals Bill, heard the testimony of Dr. Osmond Airy, Divisional Chief Inspector of the London Elementary Schools, and Dr. James Keir, Medical Officer of the London School Board and London County Council. Dr. Airy testified to the value of a Birmingham program of feeding school children, but was guarded in recommending the use of public funds for the purpose; Dr. Keir stated that it was necessary to feed those children whose constitutional deficiencies and environmental limitations made the action essential. *Report from the Select Committee on the Education (Provision of Meals) Bill*, 1906, pp. 132–133; pp. 139–141.

68. *Brit. M.J.*, Jan. 14, 1905, p. 85; Feb. 17, 1906, p. 401. Little, *History of the British Medical Association*, p. 136.

69. *Brit. M.J.*, July 21, 1906, p. 156.

70. *Ann. Rep. Chief Med. Off. for Schools,* 1908, p. 11.

71. *Brit. M.J.,* Sept. 21, 1907, p. 761. See also Hogarth, *The Medical Inspection of Schools,* p. 34.

72. Hogarth, *The Medical Inspection of Schools,* p. 209.

73. *Brit. M.J.,* Dec. 26, 1908, p. 1869.

74. *Ibid.,* Jan. 9, 1909, p. 108.

75. *Ibid.,* June 12, 1909, p. 1446.

76. *Ibid.,* Apr. 2, 1910, pp. 831–832.

77. Webb, *The State and the Doctor,* pp. 168–169.

78. *Ann. Rep. Chief Med. Off. of the Board of Education for 1909,* p. 186.

79. *Brit. M.J.,* Dec. 3, 1910, p. 1868.

80. *The Lancet,* Dec. 3, 1910, p. 1629.

81. *Ann. Rep. Chief Med. Off. of the Board of Education for 1908,* p. 14.

Chapter X. Further Paths to State Curative Medicine

1. Shryock, *The Development of Modern Medicine,* pp. 249ff.

2. *Ibid.,* pp. 176ff. Anesthesia was not, of course, unknown by the eighteen-forties. Sir Humphrey Davy had carried out chemical experiments with the inhalation of nitrous oxide and other gases, suggesting in 1800 that nitrous oxide might be used in surgical operations.

3. Sir Rickman Godlee, *Lord Lister,* 3rd rev. ed. (Oxford: Clarendon Press, 1924), p. 129; Frazer, *History of English Public Health,* p. 157.

4. Shryock, *The Development of Modern Medicine,* pp. 280–281.

5. *Ibid.,* p. 310.

6. Dr. David Walsh, "Recent Progress in Radiography," *The Hospital,* XXVII (Oct. 7, 1899), 5.

7. St. Bartholomew's Hospital was, of course, founded in the twelfth century and St. Thomas' Hospital in the thirteenth. The other great London teaching hospitals —The London Hospital, Guy's, and St. George's Hospitals—were all founded in the eighteenth century.

8. The "Hospital Sunday" fund, for example, had operated in Birmingham since 1859. Conceived by a clergyman, the collections on Hospital Sunday were made in the churches and chapels throughout Birmingham, and the proceeds rotated among the various hospitals. See *The Lancet,* Nov. 16, 1869, p. 651.

9. Sprigge, *Medicine and the Public,* p. 58.

10. *The Lancet, Special Supplement in Support of the Metropolitan Hospital Sunday Fund,* June 17, 1905, p. 1697.

11. Misc. Papers of the Charity Organization Society, pp. 1870ff. (British Museum).

12. Charles S. Loch, *Cross Purposes in Medical Reform* (London: Society for Organizing Relief and Repressing Mendacity, n.d.).

13. *Brit. M.J.,* July 22, 1893, p. 198.

14. Sprigge, *Medicine and the Public,* pp. 61–62.

15. *The Lancet, Special Supplement in Support of the Metropolitan Hospital Sunday Fund,* June 17, 1905, p. 1692.

16. *Brit. M.J.,* May 21, 1870, p. 534.

17. *Ibid.,* Apr. 10, 1875, p. 1183. See the series of articles on provident dispensaries, Mar.–May, 1875, in the *Brit. M.J.*

18. *Ibid.,* Mar. 27, 1875, pp. 416–417.

19. Alfred Carpenter, *A Chapter in the History of Provident Medical Associations* (Croydon: Jesse W. Ward, 1881), p. 3.

20. Sprigge, *Medicine and the Public,* p. 47.

21. *Brit. M.J.,* May 9, 1891, p. 1029.

22. International Labor Office, Geneva, "Voluntary Sickness Insurance," *Studies and Reports,* Series M. No. 7, pp. 234–235.

23. Tom Seth Newman, *The Story of Friendly Societies and Social Security* (London: Hearts of Oak Benefit Society, 1945), p. 19.

24. H. W. Rumsey, *Medical Relief for the Labouring Classes on the Principle of Mutual Insurance* (London: J. W. Parker, 1837), p. 11.

25. Rumsey, *Essays on State Medicine,* p. 159.

26. Little, *History of the British Medical Association,* p. 202.

27. S. and B. Webb, *The State and the Doctor,* pp. 137–138.

28. *Ibid.,* p. 138.

29. *Report by the Medico-Political Committee of the British Medical Association, "An Investigation into the Economic Conditions of Contract Medical Practice in the United Kingdom,"* July 22, 1905, *Supplement to the Brit. M.J.,* 1905, p. 13. (Hereafter cited as B.M.A., *Report on Contract Practice,* 1905.)

30. *The Lancet,* Dec. 22, 1894, p. 1498; Dec. 29, 1894, p. 1574; March 18, 1905, p. 738 (résumé).

31. *Brit. M.J.,* July 22, 1905, p. 195; B.M.A., *Report on Contract Practice,* 1905, pp. 1–2.

32. *Ibid.,* p. 25.

33. *Ibid.,* p. 27.

34. See Chap. V and also the author's: "The Parish Doctor: England's Poor Law Medical Officers and Medical Reform, 1870–1900," *Bull. Hist. of Med.,* XXXV (Mar.–Apr., 1961), 97–122.

35. Charles L. Mowat, *The Charity Organization Society, 1869–1913; Its Ideas and Work* (London: Methuen & Co., 1961), pp. 128–129.

36. R. C. K. Ensor, *England 1870–1914* (Oxford: Clarendon Press, 1936), pp. 516–517.

37. *Ann. Rep. L.G.B. for 1899–1900,* p. lxvii.

38. Beatrice Webb, *Our Partnership* (London: Longmans, Green, & Co. 1948), p. 317.

39. *Ann. Rep. L.G.B. for 1909–1910,* pp. xi, xxxiv, and xxxviii.

40. B. and S. Webb, *English Poor Law Policy,* Vol. 2, p. 471.

41. *The Times,* Aug. 3, 1905, p. 7.

42. *Brit. M.J.,* Dec. 2, 1905, p. 1472; *Supp. to Brit. M.J.,* Nov. 4, 1905, p. 260. Representatives of neither the poor law medical officers or of private practitioners were included on the Commission; although this had been suggested to the Prime Minister by the Council of the British Medical Association.

43. *The Lancet,* Dec. 16, 1905, p. 1783.

44. *The Times,* Nov. 29, 1905, p. 9.

45. Webb. *Our Partnership,* p. 348.

46. *Report of the Royal Comm. on the Poor Laws, 1909, Minutes of Evidence With Appendix,* Vol. IX, p. 862.

47. *Ibid.,* Appendix, Vol. IV., p. 280, *Parl. Papers,* 1909, Vol. 41.

48. *Ibid.,* Vol. IV, p. 100.

49. *Ibid.,* Vol. IV, Minutes of Evidence, Jan. 29, 1907, pp. 148ff.

50. *Ibid.,* p. 149.

51. John McVail, M.D., "Report on the Methods and Results of the Present System of Administering Indoor and Outdoor Poor Law Medical Relief in Certain Unions of England and Wales," *Parl. Papers,* 1909, Vol. 42, pp. 157–159.

52. *Ibid.,* p. 148.

53. There was also a dissenting memorandum submitted by Dr. Arthur Downes.

the medical member of the Commission, who signed the Majority Report, but dissented in the proposal of both the Majority and Minority Reports, which would remove the administration of relief from ad hoc authorities to the hands of county and county borough administrators.

54. *Rep. of the Roy. Comm. on the Poor Laws,* Part V, p. 289.

55. *Ibid.,* Part V, pp. 294–295.

56. Dr. W. M. Frazer in his *History of English Public Health, 1834–1939,* pp. 281–283, has a useful discussion of the significance of the Minority Report. See also Ensor, *England 1870–1914,* pp. 516–517.

57. *Minority Report of the Royal Commission on the Poor Laws and Relief of Distress,* 1909, p. 889. (Hereafter cited as *Minority Report*).

58. In support of their unification demand, the Minority Commissioners pointed out that the heads of all the four public departments concerned had urged such action (the Medical Officer of the Local Government Board, of the Board of Education, the Medical Commissioner of the Local Government Board for Ireland, and Dr. Leslie Mackenzie, Medical Member of the Local Government Board for Scotland). See also B. and S. Webb, *The State and the Doctor,* p. 219.

59. *Minority Report,* p. 890.

60. B. and S. Webb, *English Poor Law Policy,* p. 318.

61. B. and S. Webb, *English Poor Law History,* Vol. II, pp. 529–531.

62. *Brit. M.J.,* June 13, 1908, p. 1444.

63. *Ibid.,* Jan. 9, 1909, p. 108.

64. *Ibid.,* July 3, 1909, p. 36.

65. *Report of the Special Poor Law Reform Committee, Presented to the Council of the British Medical Association, Supplement to the Brit. M.J.,* Nov. 13, 1909, p. 307.

66. *Brit. M.J.,* July 3, 1909, pp. 36–37.

67. *Special Supp. to the Brit. M.J.,* July 17, 1909, p. 89.

68. *Brit. M.J.,* Oct. 9, 1909, pp. 1085–1086.

69. *Ibid.,* Feb. 26, 1910, p. 521.

70. *Ibid.,* Apr. 1910, p. 945.

71. *The Lancet,* Feb. 20, 1909, pp. 553–554.

72. *Ibid.,* July 23, 1910, pp. 228–233.

73. Newsholme, *The Last Thirty Years of Public Health,* p. 97.

74. Appendix H 15 (Report of Mr. Philip H. Bagenal, Inspector for the District comprising the "Union Counties of East and West Ridings of Yorkshire," *Ann. Rep. L.G.B. for 1909–1910,* pp. 86–87.

75. Newsholme, *The Last Thirty Years in Public Health,* pp. 97–98.

Chapter XI. The Medical Profession and the National Insurance Act

1. Winston Churchill, *Liberalism and the Social Problem, Speeches, 1906–1909* (London: Hodder & Stoughton, 1909), p. 309.

2. C. F. G. Masterman, "Liberalism and Labour," *The Nineteenth Century and After,* 1906, p. 717.

3. The term "Indian summer" in this instance is that of Dr. James M. Mackintosh in *Trends of Opinion About the Public Health, 1901–1951* (Oxford: Oxford University Press, 1953), p. 53. See also Ensor, *England 1870–1914,* Chaps. XII and XIII, *passim.*

4. William W. Davies, *Lloyd George, 1863–1914* (London: Constable, & Co., 1939), *passim*. A vivid picture of Lloyd George's personality in relation to the development and passage of the National Health Insurance Act emerges from *Lloyd George's Ambulance Wagon, Being the Memoirs of William J. Braithwaite, 1911–1912*, edited by Sir Henry N. Bunbury (London: Methuen, 1957). (Hereafter cited as *Braithwaite Memoirs*.)

5. *Braithwaite Memoirs*, p. 72; Harold Spender, *The Prime Minister* (London: Hodder & Stoughton, 1920), p. 155.

6. Rosen, *History of Public Health*, p. 443.

7. R. C. Williams, *The United States Public Health Service 1798–1950* (Washington, D.C.: Commissioned Officers Association of the U.S. Public Health Service, 1951), pp. 23–32.

8. H. E. Sigerist, *Landmarks in the History of Hygiene* (London: Geoffrey Cumberlege–Oxford University Press, 1956), pp. 65–66; Shryock, *The Development of Modern Medicine*, pp. 385–387; Sigerist, "From Bismarck to Beveridge. Developments and Trends in Social Security Legislation," *Bull. Hist. Med.*, XIII (Apr., 1943), 366–88.

9. H. E. Sigerist, *Medicine and Health in the Soviet Union* (New York: Citadel Press, 1947), pp. 10–21.

10. *Braithwaite Memoirs*, p. 77.

11. Webb, *Our Partnership*, p. 417.

12. *Braithwaite Memoirs*, p. 115.

13. Lucy B. Masterman, *C. F. G. Masterman, A Biography* (London: Nicholson & Watson, 1939), pp. 225–226.

14. David Lloyd George, *The People's Insurance, Explained by the Chancellor of the Exchequer*, From the Speech in the House of Commons, May 4, 1911 (London: Hodder & Stoughton, 1911), pp. 3–5; *Parl. Debates*, House of Commons, 5th Series, Vol. 25, 1911, pp. 613–615.

15. "Bill to Provide for Insurance Against Loss of Health and for the Prevention and Cure of Sickness and for Insurance Against Unemployment, and for Purposes Incidental Thereto." 1 & 2 George V, *passim, Parl. Papers*, 1911, Vol. 4.

16. Hermann Levy, *National Health Insurance, A Critical Study* (Cambridge: Cambridge University Press, 1944), p. 7.

17. This feature was lost in the final Act, to the regret of the medical profession. The provisions of the Bill are discussed in detail, with the additional exceptions and safeguarding features in Lloyd George's, *The People's Insurance*, pp. 67–150. The second half of the measure, relating to unemployment insurance, will not be considered in the present study.

18. Newsholme, *International Studies on the Relation Between the Private and Official Practice of Medicine* (London: Allen & Unwin Ltd., 1931), Vol. III, p. 109.

19. Sir Leo G. Chiozza Money, *Insurance Versus Poverty* (London: Methuen & Co., 1912), p. 4.

20. *Braithwaite Memoirs*, Introduction, p. 24.

21. *Parl. Debates*, House of Commons, 5th Series, Vol. 25, 1911, p. 659.

22. *Ibid.*, p. 655.

23. *Ibid.*, pp. 656–657.

24. *The Times*, May 5, 1911.

25. Webb, *Our Partnership*, p. 473. Charles Loch was another who responded as did Mrs. Webb, and prophesied that a response to the government's measure would, "if we yield to it, bring in its wake an ever-increasing burden of pauperization and taxation." Charles Loch, *The National Insurance Bill, A Paper* (London: Society for Organizing 'Charitable Relief and Repressing Mendacity,' 1911), p. 48.

26. In 1903, Southampton had formed such a public medical service, under the

guidance of Dr. A. A. MacKeith, which was operated under the auspices of the medical profession of Southampton. Little, *History of the British Medical Association*, p. 325.

27. *Brit. M.J.*, Feb. 26, 1910, p. 522.

28. *Ibid.*, Apr. 2, 1910, p. 835.

29. *Ibid.*, Apr. 23, 1910, p. 1008.

30. *Ibid.*

31. *Brit. M.J., Supp.*, Dec. 10, 1910, pp. 438–439.

32. *Brit. M.J.*, June 14, 1910, pp. 1345ff.

33. *Supp. to the Brit. M.J.*, May 13, 1911, p. 236.

34. *Ibid.*, May 27, 1911, p. 297.

35. *Ibid.*, May 13, 1911, pp. 1134–1136.

36. *The Lancet*, June 3, 1911, p. 1518; also issue of May 13, 1911, p. 1289.

37. *Special Supp., Brit. M.J.*, June 3, 1911, pp. 340–341; p. 363.

38. J. H. Harley Williams, *A Century of Public Health* (London: A. & C. Black, 1932), p. 49.

39. *Special Supplement of the British Medical Journal on the Special Representative Meeting to Discuss National Insurance*, June 1, 1911, p. 338.

40. *Special Supp., Brit. M.J.*, June 3, 1911, p. 345.

41. *Ibid.*, June 10, 1911, p. 403; see also Little, *History of the British Medical Association*, pp. 326–327.

42. *Braithwaite Memoirs*, p. 175.

43. *Reports of Deputations to the Chancellor of the Exchequer*, p. 4, 1911, *Parl. Papers*, 1911, Vol. 73.

44. *Braithwaite Memoirs*, p. 175.

45. *The Lancet*, June 10, 1911, p. 1585.

46. Alfred Cox, *Among the Doctors* (London: Christopher Johnson, 1950), p. 86.

47. *Ibid.*, p. 87.

48. David Lloyd George, *The Insurance of the People, A Speech Delivered at Birmingham on June 10, 1911* (London: Liberal Publications Department, 1911), p. 9.

49. Cox, *Among the Doctors*, p. 91.

50. Sir Christopher Addison, *Politics From Within, 1911–1918* (London: Herbert Jenkins, 1924), Vol. I, p. 20.

51. *The Lancet*, July 1, 1911, p. 25.

52. Little, *History of the British Medical Association*, p. 328; Vaughan, *Doctors' Common*, p. 203.

53. *Brit. M.J.*, Aug. 5, 1911, p. 289.

54. *Parl. Debates, House of Commons*, 5th Series, Vol. 32, 1911, p. 1498.

55. *Ibid.*, p. 1518. The small size of the minority vote probably represented less actual satisfaction of the majority with the Bill than the necessity for keeping a weather eye on the electorate in home districts.

56. *Brit. M.J.*, 1911, p. 1608. The phrase was Benjamin Franklin's, not Washington's, and was uttered at the signing of the Declaration of Independence.

57. Stephen Paget, *Sir Victor Horsley, A Study of His Life and Work* (London: Constable, 1919), p. 226.

58. *The Lancet*, Dec. 9, 1911, p. 1642.

59. Cox, *Among the Doctors*, p. 94.

60. C. J. Bond, *Recollection of Student Life and Later Days* (London: H. K. Lewis, 1939), p. 41.

61. *Ibid.*, p. 46.

62. *Brit. M.J.*, Dec. 23, 1911, p. 1666.

63. *The Lancet*, June 8, 1912, pp. 1564–1565.

64. *The Times*, Jan. 13, 1912, p. 6.

65. *Ibid.,* Jan. 9, 1912, p. 5.

66. Morant's biographer described him as consenting reluctantly to Lloyd George's request, but accepting on the opportunity it offered of ultimately working towards a unification of the national health services. Bernard Allen, *Sir Robert Morant, A Great Public Servant* (London: Macmillan & Co., 1934), p. 277.

67. *Braithwaite Memoirs,* p. 264.

68. *The Lancet,* Feb. 24, 1912, p. 516.

69. Allen, *Sir Robert Morant,* p. 277.

70. *Report of Sir William Plender to the Chancellor of the Exchequer on the Result of His Investigation Into Existing Conditions in Respect of Medical Attendance and Remuneration in Certain Towns,* 1912, p. 3, *Parl. Papers,* 1912–13, Vol. 78.

71. *Brit. M.J.,* July 20, 1912, p. 133. See also Vaughan, *Doctors' Common,* pp. 206–207.

72. *The Lancet,* Dec. 21, 1912, p. 1759.

73. *Braithwaite Memoirs,* Introduction, p. 38. The *Medical Register* for 1912 listed 40,913 medical practitioners licensed to practice in England, Scotland and Ireland (p. xc.)

74. *Brit. M.J.,* Dec. 28, 1912, p. 1764.

75. Addison, *Politics From Within, 1911–1918,* Vol. I, p. 23.

76. *The Lancet,* Dec. 21, 1912, p. 1760. For further information on the "Socialist, Pacifist, Christian and Republican" Dr. Salter, see Archibald F. Brockway, *Bermondsey Story: the Life of Albert Salter* (London: Allen & Unwin Ltd., 1949).

77. "Letter from the Chancellor of the Exchequer to the National Insurance Practitioner's Association," *Parl. Papers,* 1912–1913, Vol. 78.

78. The vicious newspaper campaign invoked against the Act is described in some detail in Masterman, *Liberalism and Labour,* pp. 226, 249–50.

79. Dr. Roberts was to end up with a larger list of panel patients than any other physician in England. He added a dentist to his staff as well as a medical masseur. The practice got the reputation it deserved, and the Ministry of Health acquired the habit of sending visitors from abroad who wished to see the panel system to Robert's flourishing establishment. Winefred Stamp, *Doctor Himself* (London: H. Hamilton, 1949), p. 75.

80. Webb, *Our Partnership,* p. 472; *Braithwaite Memoirs,* pp. 122–123.

81. Lloyd George, "Statements as to the Administration of Medical Benefit," etc., p. 7, in *Parl. Papers,* 1912–13, Vol. 78; *Braithwaite Memoirs,* pp. 141–142.

82. Sir Arthur Newsholme, *Health Problems in Organized Society* (London: P. S. King & Sons, 1927), p. 23; A. N. Simons and Nathan Sinai, *The Way of Health Insurance* (Chicago: University of Chicago Press, 1932), p. 59.

83. For a good comparison of the 1911 and 1946 Acts, see the excellent "Commentary" by Professor Richard Titmuss in the *Braithwaite Memoirs,* pp. 43–59.

84. *Brit. M.J.,* Dec. 7, 1912, p. 1635ff.

85. Cox, *Among the Doctors,* p. 99; Vaughan, *Doctors' Common,* p. 209.

86. *Supplement to the Brit. M.J.,* June 23, 1917, pp. 143–144.

Chapter XII. The Medical Profession and Government Action in Public Health by 1912—A Perspective

1. *Ann. Rep. M.O.L.G.B. for 1917–18,* pp. vi–vii.

2. Newsholme, *The Last Thirty Years in Public Health,* p. 60.

3. C. J. Bond, "Health and Healing in the Great State," in H. G. Wells, *The Great State* (London: Harper Bros., 1912), p. 145.

4. *Ann. Rep. M.O.L.G.B. for 1917–1918*, p. xv.

5. These figures refer to the continental United States. *Historical Statistics of the United States, Colonial Times to 1957*, prepared by the Bureau of the Census with the co-operation of the Social Science Research Council (Washington, D.C.: U.S. Government Printing Office, 1960), p. 8.

6. M. P. Ravenel, ed., *A Half Century of Public Health* (New York: American Public Health Association, 1921), p. 14.

7. R. C. Williams, *U.S. Public Health Service*, p. 76; H. Kramer, "Agitation for Public Health Reform in the 1870's," *loc. cit.*, pp. 84–86; Smillie, *Public Health*, p. 338.

8. Rosen, *History of Public Health*, p. 250.

9. R. C. Williams, *U.S. Public Health Service*, pp. 156–159.

10. James G. Burrow, *A.M.A., Voice of American Medicine* (Baltimore: The Johns Hopkins Press, 1963), pp. 21–23; p. 395.

11. Bernhard J. Stern, *Medical Services by Government, Local, and State and Federal* (New York: The Commonwealth Fund, 1946), pp. 6–14.

12. R. C. Williams, *U.S. Public Health Service*, pp. 41–47; 159.

13. The laws passed before 1910 for workmen's compensation which were not declared unconstitutional by state legislatures were only optional. In May, 1908, Theodore Roosevelt's administration passed a limited compensation act for the protection of some federal government employees. A useful chart of workmen's compensation legislation from 1902 to 1913 appears in I. M. Rubinow, *Social Insurance with Special Reference to American Conditions* (New York: Henry Holt & Co., 1912), pp. 169–170.

14. Odin Anderson, "Health Insurance in the United States, 1910–1920," *J. Hist. of Med. and Allied Sciences*, V (1950), 363.

15. *Journal of the American Medical Association*, May 1, 1920, p. 1319; Burrow, *A.M.A.*, p. 150.

16. *Journal of the American Medical Association*, Nov. 23, 1912, p. 1890.

17. *Ibid.*, p. 1891.

18. Anderson, *Health Insurance in the U.S.*, p. 392.

19. Irving Fisher, *A Report on National Vitality: Its Waste and Conservation* (Washington, D.C.: U.S. Government Printing Office, 1909), p. 126.

Selected Bibliography

I. PRIMARY SOURCES

A. MANUSCRIPT MATERIALS

Home Office Papers, 1864–1874.

Local Government Board: Government Office Correspondence Files and Miscellaneous Correspondence Files, 1871–1900.

Privy Council: Minutes, 1870–1874; Miscellaneous Memoranda on Public Health and Quarantine, 1862–1873.

Society of Medical Officers of Health: Minutes of Council, 1874–1900; Minutes of Ordinary Meetings, 1870–1900; Minutes of Annual Meetings, 1879–1891.

B. PRINTED CONTEMPORARY MATERIALS

1. Autobiographies and Personal Memoirs

ADDISON, CHRISTOPHER. *Politics From Within, 1911–1918.* 2 vols. London: Herbert Jenkins Ltd., 1924.

BOND, C. J. *Recollections of Student Life and Later Days.* London: H. K. Lewis, 1939.

BRAITHWAITE, WILLIAM J. *Lloyd George's Ambulance Wagon; Being the Memoirs of William J. Braithwaite, 1911–1912.* Edited by Sir Henry N. Bunbury, and with a commentary by Richard Titmuss. London: Methuen & Co., 1957.

BROADHURST H. *Henry Broadhurst, M.P., The Story of His Life From a Stonemason's Bench to the Treasury Bench.* London: Hutchinson & Co., 1901.

CHRISTISON, R. *The Life of Sir Robert Christison, Bart.* Edited by his sons. 2 vols. London: Blackwood & Sons, 1887.

COX, ALFRED. *Among the Doctors.* London: Christopher Johnson, 1949.

FARQUHARSON, ROBERT. _In and Out of Parliament._ London: Williams & Norgate, 1911.

HALDANE, R. B. _Richard Burdon Haldane, An Autobiography._ New York: Doubleday Doran & Co., 1929.

PRESTON-THOMAS, HERBERT. _The Work and Play of a Government Inspector._ London: William Blackwood & Sons, 1909.

ROGERS, JOSEPH. _Joseph Rogers, M.D., Reminiscences of a Workhouse Medical Officer._ Edited with a preface by Thorold Rogers. London: T. Fisher Unwin, 1889.

SIMON, JOHN. _Personal Recollections._ London: Privately Printed by the Wiltons Ltd., 1894.

WEBB, BEATRICE. _My Apprenticeship._ London: Longmans, Green & Co., 1950.

WEBB, BEATRICE. _Our Partnership._ Edited by Barbara Drake, Margaret Cole. London: Longmans, Green & Co., 1948.

2. Contemporary Authorities, General

ABBOTT, S. W. _Past and Present Condition of Public Health and Medicine in the United States._ Boston: Wright & Potter, 1900.

ACLAND, HENRY. _The Army Medical School, An Address Delivered at Netley Hospital, July 29, 1887._ London: Macmillan & Co., 1887.

———. _Memoir on the Cholera at Oxford in the Year 1854._ London, Oxford: John Churchill & J. Parker, 1856.

———. and Stokes, William, _et al. Medicine in Modern Times, Discourses Delivered at a Meeting of the British Medical Association at Oxford._ London: Macmillan & Co., 1869.

ASSOCIATION FOR EXTENDING THE CONTAGIOUS DISEASE ACTS. _The Effects of the Contagious Disease Acts._ Pamphlet, n.d.

BEVERIDGE, WILLIAM. _Unemployment; A Problem of Industry._ London, New York: Longmans, Green & Co., 1909.

BOOTH, CHARLES. _The Life and Labour of the People in London._ 9 vols. London: Macmillan & Co., 1892–1897; also 17 vols., 1902.

———. _The Aged Poor in England and Wales._ London: Macmillan & Co., 1894.

BRISTOWE, JOHN SYER. _A Treatise on the Theory and Practice of Medicine._ 1st ed. London: Smith, Elder & Co., 1876.

BUDD, WILLIAM. _Typhoid Fever, Its Nature, Mode of Spreading, and Prevention._ London, Longmans, Green & Co., 1873.

CARPENTER, ALFRED. _A Chapter in the History of Provident Medical Associations._ Croyden: Jesse W. Ward, 1881.

———. _Administrative Areas for Sanitary Purposes._ Read in the Health Section of the Social Science Association, Norwich Congress. London: Spottiswoode & Co., 1873.

CHADWICK, EDWIN. _The Evils of Disunity in Central and Local Administra-_

tion, Especially with Relation to the Metropolis. London: Longmans, Green & Co., 1885.

CHURCHILL, WINSTON. *Liberalism and the Social Problem, Speeches 1906–1909.* London: Hodder & Stoughton, 1909.

DE CHAUMONT, FRANÇOIS S.B. *Lectures on State Medicine, Delivered before the Society of Apothecaries.* London: Smith, Elder & Co., 1875.

DODD, F. L. "A National Medical Service," *Fabian Tracts, No. 160.* London: Fabian Society, 1911

FISHER, IRVING. *A Report on National Vitality: Its Waste and Conservation.* (Prepared for the National Conservation Commission by the Committee of One Hundred on National Health.) Washington, D.C.: U.S. Government Printing Office, 1909.

FOX, CORNELIUS. *Dozen Papers Relating to Disease Prevention.* London: Churchill, 1884.

GIFFEN, ROBERT. "Essay on the Progress of the Working Classes," *Journal of the Royal Statistical Society*, vol. 46 (Dec., 1883), p. 593.

GUY, WILLIAM. "Two Hundred and Fifty Years of Smallpox in London," *Journal of the Royal Statistical Society*, vol. 45 (Dec., 1882), pp. 399–443.

HARDY, H. NELSON. *The State of the Medical Profession in Great Britain and Ireland in 1900*, Carmichael Prize Essay. London: Bailliere, Tindall & Cox, 1901.

HART, ERNEST. *Essays on State Medicine.* Reprinted from the *British Medical Journal.* London: British Medical Association, 1894.

———. *Local Government as It Is and As It Ought To Be, Being the Address to the Sanitary Congress at Leicester, September 24, 1885.* London: Smith, Elder & Co., 1885.

———. *The Registration of Infectious Disease, A Report to the Parliamentary Bills Committee of the British Medical Association.* London: British Medical Association, 1879.

———. *The Sick Poor in Workhouses.* London: Smith, Elder & Co., 1895.

———. *The State and Its Servants, Being a Reprinted Series of Editorial Articles Published in the British Medical Journal on Medical and Sanitary Questions in Current Policies.* London: Smith, Elder & Co., 1893.

HAWKSLEY, THOMAS. *The Charities of London and Some Errors of their Administration.* London: John Churchill & Sons, 1869.

HOWELL, GEORGE. *The Conflicts of Capital and Labour.* London: Macmillan & Co., 1890.

LEGGE, THOMAS. *Industrial Maladies.* Edited by S. A. Henry. London: Humphrey Milford, 1934

LLOYD GEORGE, DAVID. *The Insurance of the People, A Speech Delivered at Birmingham on June 10, 1911.* London: Liberal Publications Department, 1911.

———. *The People's Insurance.* London: Hodder & Stoughton, 1911.

———. *The State and the People, Speeches Delivered at Aberdeen.* London: Liberal Publications Department, 1913.

LOCH, CHARLES S. *Cross Purposes in Medical Reform.* London: Society for Organizing Charitable Relief and Repressing Mendacity, n.d.

———. *The National Insurance Bill, A Paper.* London: Society for Organizing Charitable Relief and Repressing Mendacity, 1911.

LONSDALE, SOPHIE. *The English Poor Laws, Their History, Principles, and Administration.* London: P. S. King & Sons, 1897.

MACKAY, THOMAS. *On the Cooperation of Charitable Agencies With the Poor Law, A Paper Read At the Fourth Meeting of the Charity Organization Conference.* London: Spottiswood & Co., 1893.

———. *Public Relief of the Poor, Six Lectures.* London: John Murray, 1901.

MASTERMAN, C. F. G. "Liberalism and Labour." *The Nineteenth Century and After,* 1906.

McCULLOCH, J. R. *A Descriptive and Statistical Account of the British Empire.* London: Longmans, Green & Co., 1854.

McKAIL, DAVID, AND WILLIAM JONES. *A Public Medical Service.* London: Fabian Society, 1919.

"The Medical Profession and Its Morality" (Anon.). Reprinted with additions from *The Modern Review* of April, 1881. London: Pewtress & Co., 1886.

"Memorandum on the Advantage to be Derived From a Registration of Disease, and on the Mode Which Such a Record May be Obtained." Adopted at a Meeting of a Committee Representing the St. Andrew's Medical Graduates Association, the Medical Society of London, etc., n.d.

MILNES, ALFRED. *Speech of Alfred Milnes, M.A. at the Leicester Demonstration Against Compulsory Vaccination, March 23, 1885.* London: E. W. Allen, 1885.

MONEY, LEO G. CHIOZZA. *Insurance Versus Poverty.* London: Methuen & Co., 1912.

MORRIS, MALCOLM. *The Nation's Health.* London, New York: Cassell & Co., 1917.

———. *The Story of English Public Health.* London: Cassell & Co., 1919.

NATIONAL COMMITTEE TO PROMOTE THE BREAK-UP OF THE POOR LAW. *The Failure of the Poor Law.* London, 1909.

NEWMAN, GEORGE. *The Building of a Nation's Health.* London: Macmillan & Co., 1939.

———. *Health and Social Evolution.* London: G. Allen & Unwin Ltd., 1930.

———. *Infant Mortality, A Social Problem.* London: Methuen & Co., 1906.

———. *The Place of Public Opinion in Preventive Medicine.* Delivered before the National Health Society, April 22, 1920. London: The Ministry of Health, 1920.

———. *The Rise of Preventive Medicine.* London: Oxford University Press, 1932.

NEWSHOLME, ARTHUR. "The Coordination of the Public Medical Services," *British Medical Journal,* September 14, 1907.

———. *Evolution of Preventive Medicine.* Baltimore: Williams and Wilkins, 1927.

————. *Fifty Years in Public Health, A Personal Narrative With Comments.* London: G. Allen & Unwin, 1935.

————. *Health Problems in Organized Society, Studies in the Social Aspects of Public Health.* London: P. S. King & Son, 1927.

————. *International Studies on the Relation Between the Private and Official Practice of Medicine, With Special References to the Prevention of Disease,* III. London: Milbank Memorial Fund, 1931.

————. *The Last Thirty Years in Public Health, Recollections and Reflections on My Official Life and Post-Official Life.* London: G. Allen & Unwin Ltd., 1936.

————. *Medicine and the State, the Relation Between the Private and Official Practice of Medicine.* London: G. Allen & Unwin Ltd., 1932.

————. *Public Health and Insurance, American Addresses.* Baltimore: The Johns Hopkins Press, 1920.

————. "Public Health in Relation to the Struggle Against Tuberculosis," *Journal of Hygiene,* III (1903), 446ff.

NIVEN, JAMES. *"The Economics of Health,"* An Address Delivered at the Jubilee Conference of the Manchester and Salford Sanitary Association on April 25, 1902. Manchester: by the Society, 1902.

————. *Observations on the History of the Public Health Effort in Manchester.* Manchester and London: John Heywood Ltd., 1923.

OLIVER, THOMAS (ed.). *Dangerous Trades, The Historical, Social and Legal Aspects of Industrial Occupations as Affecting Health, by a Number of Experts.* New York: E. P. Dutton & Co.; London: John Murray, 1902.

PALMBERG, ALBERT J. *A Treatise on Public Health and Its Application in Different Countries.* Translated from the French edition and the section on England edited by Arthur Newsholme. 2nd ed. London: Sonnenschein, 1895.

PEASE, EDWARD R. *The History of the Fabian Society.* New York: E. P. Dutton & Co., 1919.

PHILIP, ROBERT. *Collected Papers on Tuberculosis.* London: Oxford University Press, 1937.

RANSOME, ARTHUR. *Some Causes of Preventable Disease.* London: John Heywood for the Manchester and Salford Sanitary Association, 1886.

RENTOUL, ROBERT RIED. *The Reform of Our Voluntary Medical Charities, Some Serious Considerations for the Philanthropic.* London: Bailliere, Tindall & Cox, 1891.

RICHARDSON, BENJAMIN W. *The Health of Nations, A Review of the Works of Edwin Chadwick.* 2 vols. London: Longmans, Green & Co., 1887.

————. *Hygeia, A City of Health.* London: Macmillan & Co., 1876.

————. *A Ministry of Health, and Other Addresses.* London: Chatto & Windus, 1879.

RICKETTS, THOMAS FRANK. *The Diagnosis of Small-Pox.* London: Cassell & Co., 1908.

RIVINGTON, WALTER. *The Medical Profession: Being the Essay to which was*

Awarded the First Carmichael Prize. London: Longmans, Green Co., 1879; also republished in expanded form in 1888 by the same publishers under the title, *The Medical Profession of the United Kingdom.*

ROWNTREE, B. SEEBOHM. *Poverty: A Study of Town Life.* London: Macmillan & Co., Ltd., 1901.

RUMSEY, HENRY WYLDBORE. *Essays on State Medicine.* London: John Churchill, 1856.

———. *Medical Relief for the Labouring Classes on the Principle of Mutual Insurance.* London: J. W. Parker, 1837.

SEATON, EDWARD CATOR. *A Handbook of Vaccination.* London: Macmillan, 1868.

SHAW, GEORGE B. "Widower's Houses," in *The Collected Works of George Bernard Shaw.* Vol. VII. New York: William H. Wise & Co., 1930.

SIMON, JOHN. *Public Health Reports.* 2 Vols. Edited for the Sanitary Institute of Great Britain by Edward Seaton. London: Offices of the Sanitary Institute, 1887.

———. *English Sanitary Institutions.* London, Paris, New York: Cassell & Co. Ltd, 1890; also, 2nd ed. London: John Murray, 1897.

———. *Reports Relating to the Sanitary Condition of the City of London.* London: John Parker & Son for Private Circulation, 1854.

———. *Report to the Local Board of Health, Croyden.* Croyden: J. L. Wright, 1853.

SNOW, JOHN. *On the Mode of Communication of Cholera.* 2nd ed. London: John Churchill, 1855.

———. *Snow on Cholera, Being a Reprint of Two Papers of John Snow, Together With a Biographical Memoir by B. W. Richardson.* New York: The Commonwealth Fund, 1936.

SYKES, JOHN F. *Public Health and Housing, Milroy Lectures, Delivered Before the Royal College of Physicians.* London: P. S. King & Sons, 1901.

———. *Public Health Problems.* London: Walter Scott, 1892.

SMITH, EDWARD. *Manual for Medical Officers of Health.* London: Knight & Co., 1873.

SMITH, STEPHEN. *The City That Was.* New York: F. Allaben, 1911.

TAYLOR, P. A. *Vaccination, A Letter to Dr. W. B. Carpenter.* London: E. W. Allen for the London Society for the Abolition of Compulsory Vaccination, 1881.

THORNE THORNE, RICHARD. *The Administrative Control of Tuberculosis, Being the Harben Lectures Delivered in 1898 before the Royal Institute of Public Health.* London: Bailliere, Tindall and Cox, 1899.

———. *Diphtheria, Its Natural History and Prevention, Milroy Lectures Delivered Before the Royal College of Physicians of London.* London: Macmillan & Co., 1891.

———. *On the Progress of Preventive Medicine During the Victorian Era, Being the Inaugural Addresses Delivered Before the Epidemiological Society of London.* London: Shaw & Sons, 1888.

THUDICHUM, J. L. W. *A Treatise on the Chemical Composition of the Brain, based throughout upon original researches.* London: Bailliere, Tindall and Cox, 1884.

TWINING, LOUISA. *Out-Relief and Charity, Notes by a Lady Guardian, Reprinted from A Threefold Cord.* London, 1892.

TREVES, FREDERICK. *The Tale of a Field Hospital.* London: Cassell & Co., 1900.

WEBB, BEATRICE. *The Poor Law Medical Officer and His Future* (Papers used at the Conference of the Association of Poor Law Medical Officers, July 6, 1909). London: National Committee for the Break-up of the Poor Law, 1909.

WEBB, BEATRICE AND SIDNEY. *English Poor Law History,* Part II: *The Last Hundred Years.* 2 vols. London: printed by the authors, 1929.

————. *English Poor Law Policy.* London: Longmans, Green & Co., 1910.

————. *The State and the Doctor.* London: Longmans, Green & Co., 1910.

WELLINGTON, R. HENSLOW. *The King's Coroner.* London: Wm. Clowes & Sons Ltd., 1904.

WELLS, H. G. *The Great State.* London: Harper Bros., 1912.

WOOTON, EDWIN AND L. FORBES WINSTON. *A Guide to the Medical Profession: A Comprehensive Manual Conveying the Means of Entering the Medical Profession in the Chief Countries of the World.* London: L. Upcott Gill, 1882.

3. Official Publications (General)

Reports of rural and urban local medical officers of health, annual and special, during the years 1870–1900 have been used on a sampling basis from those available in London libraries and from the excellent collection available at the National Library of Medicine, Bethesda, Md.

The Medical Register, published by the General Council of Medical Education and Registration.

Metropolitan Asylum Board, Annual Reports, 1898–1900.

Minutes of the General Council of Medical Education and Registration of the United Kingdom, and of the Branch Councils.

Resolutions of the General Medical Council, Adopted July 9 and July 12, 1869, with Report of the Committee on State Medicine. London: W. J. Golborn, 1869.

4. Official Publications, Parliamentary Papers

a) *Hansard, Parliamentary Debates.*

b) *Annual Reports of Government Departments:*
Army Medical Department, 1870–1900.
Chief Inspector of Factories and Workshops, Reports of the Medical Inspector, 1898–1900.

Chief Medical Officer for the Board of Education, 1908–1910.
Local Government Board, 1871–1918.
Medical Officer of the Local Government Board, 1873–1918.
Medical Officer of the Privy Council, 1865–1870.
Poor Law Board.
Registrar-General, Annual Reports and Decennial Supplements.

c. Topical Reports:

Army Medical Service. Letter Dated 17 January 1891 from Sir Andrew Clark, Bart., M.D., to Secretary of State for War, Relative to the Status of Medical Officers of the Army. (*Parl. Papers,* 1890–91, Vol. 50.)

Memorandum by the Director General Army Medical Service on the Physical Unfitness of Men Offering Themselves for Enlistment in the Army. 1903. (*Parl. Papers,* 1903, Vol. 38.)

Report of Committee Appointed by the Secretary of State to Consider the Reorganization of the Army Medical Service, 1901. (*Parl. Papers,* 1902, Vol. 10.)

Cholera. Report of the General Board of Health on the Cholera Epidemics of 1846–50, and 1852–53. (*Parl. Papers,* 1852–53, Vol. 41.)

Contagious Disease. Correspondence or Extracts Therefrom Relating to the Repeal of the Contagious Disease Acts and Regulations in the Crown Colonies. (*Parl. Papers,* 1887, Vol. 57.)

Dangerous Trades. Final Report of the Departmental Committee Appointed to Inquire Into and Report Upon Certain Miscellaneous Dangerous Trades, 1899. (*Parl. Papers,* 1899, Vol. 12.)

Hospitals. Report and Papers on the Use and Influence of Hospitals for Infectious Diseases. (*Parl. Papers,* 1882. Vol. 30, Part II.)

Housing. First Report of the Royal Commission on the Housing of the Working Classes, 1885. (*Parl. Papers,* 1884–1885, Vol. 31.)

Infant Mortality. Report on Infant Mortality, Supplement to the Annual Report, Medical Officer of the Local Government Board for 1909–1910. (*Parl. Papers,* 1910.)

Influenza. Further Report and Papers on the Influenza Epidemic 1889–1892. (*Parl. Papers,* 1893–94, Vol. 42.)
Memoranda on Epidemic Influenza, March, 1895. (*Parl. Papers,* 1895, Vol. 51.)
Report by Dr. Parsons on the Influenza Epidemic of 1889–1890. (*Parl. Papers,* 1890–1891, Vol. 34.)

Labor. Reports of the Royal Commission on Labour. (*Parl. Papers,* 1892–1894.)
Report to the Local Government Board on Proposed Changes in Hours and Ages of Employment in Textile Factories, by Dr. J. H. Bridges and Mr. T. Holmes. (*Parl. Papers,* 1873, Vol. 55.)

Midwives. Report of the Select Committee on the Midwives Registration Act. (*Parl. Papers,* 1892, Vol. 14.)

National Insurance. "A Bill to Provide for Insurance Against the Loss of Health, etc. 1 & 2 Geo 5." (*Parl. Papers,* 1911, Vol. 4.)

Reports of Deputations to the Chancellor of the Exchequer, 1911. (*Parl. Papers,* 1911, Vol. 73.)

Medical Benefit Under the German Insurance Legislation. (*Parl. Papers,* 1912–1913. Vol. 78.)

Report of Sir William Plender to the Chancellor of the Exchequer on the Result of His Investigation Into Existing Conditions in Respect of Medical Attendance and Remuneration in Certain Towns. (*Parl. Papers,* 1912–13, Vol. 78.)

National Insurance. Statements as to the Administration of Medical Benefit and Correspondence Thereon Between the Chancellor of the Exchequer and the British Medical Association. (*Parl. Papers,* 1912–13, Vol. 78.)

Naval & Military Departments. Preliminary and Further Reports of the Royal Commissions Appointed to Inquire Into Civil and Professional Administration of Naval and Military Departments. (*Parl. Papers,* 1890, Vol. 19.)

Report of the Committee Appointed to Enquire Into the Pay, Status and Conditions of Service of Medical Officers of the Army and Navy, 1889. (*Parl. Papers,* 1889, Vol. 17.)

Report to the Lords Commissioners Appointed to Inquire Into the Organization and Training of Sick Berth Staff of the Navy and the Nursing Staff of the Royal Naval Hospitals, 1884. (*Parl. Papers,* 1884, Vol. 17.)

Statistical Report on the Health of the Navy for the Years 1898, and 1899. (*Parl. Papers,* 1899, Vol. 55.)

Physical Deterioration. Report of the Inter-Departmental Committee on Physical Deterioration. (*Parl. Papers,* 1904, Vol. 32.)

Poor Laws. Report of the Royal Commission on the Aged Poor, 1895. (*Parl. Papers,* 1895, Vols. 14, 15.)

Report of a Committee Appointed by the President of the Local Government Board to Inquire Into the Question of Workhouse Dietaries, 17 June 1898. (*Parl. Papers,* 1898, Vol. 51.)

Report of the Royal Commission on the Poor Laws and the Relief of Distress, 1909. (*Parl. Papers,* 1909–10.)

Report of the Select Committee on the Aged Deserving Poor. (*Parl. Papers,* 1899, Vol. 8.)

Report of the Select Committee of the House of Lords on Poor Law Relief, 1888. (*Parl. Papers,* 1888, Vol. 15.)

Public Health Acts. Report of Select Committee on the Public Health Act (1875) Amendment Bill, 1878. (*Parl. Papers,* 1878, Vol. 18.)

Reports of the Local Government Board Inspectors on the Working of the Public Health Act, 1872. (*Parl. Papers,* 1875, Vol. 40.)

Sanitary Conditions. Particular of All Local Visitations Made by Medical Inspectors Under the Direction of the Local Government Board from the Establishment of the Board to 1 January 1880, with regard to the prevalence of disease in particular places and defects in sanitary administration, 1880. (*Parl. Papers,* Vol. 61, 1880.)

Report on the Sanitary Conditions of the Labouring Population of Great Britain. (*Parl. Papers,* 1842.)

Report on the Inland Sanitary Survey, 1893–1895. (*Parl. Papers,* 1896, Vol. 37.)

Reports of the Commission on the Operation of the Sanitary Laws; Evidence and Appendix (Royal Commission). (*Parl. Papers,* 1869–1871.)

School Children. Proceedings of the Select Committee on Education (Provision of Meals) Bill, 1906. (*Parl. Papers,* 1906, Vol. 7.)

Report of the Inter-Departmental Committee on Medical Inspection and Feeding of Children Attending Public Elementary Schools, 1906. (*Parl. Papers,* 1906, Vol. 47.)

Small Pox. Hutchinson, J. R., "An Historical Note on the Prevention of Small Pox in England and the Foundation of the Government Lymph Establishment, *Annual Report, Ministry of Health,* 1946

Report of the Commission on Small Pox and Fever Hospitals, 1882. (*Parl. Papers,* 1882, Vol. 29.)

South African Campaign. Report of the Royal Commission Appointed to Consider and Report Upon the Care and Treatment of the Sick and Wounded During the South African Campaign, 1901. (*Parl. Papers,* 1901, Vols. 29 and 30.)

Taxation. Final Report of His Majesty's Commissioners Appointed to Inquire Into the Subject of Local Taxation, 1901. (*Parl. Papers,* 1901, Vol. 24.)

Tuberculosis. Reports of the Royal Commission to Inquire Into the Relations of Human and Animal Tuberculosis. (*Parl. Papers,* 1904–1909.)

Typhus. Low, Bruce. The Epidemiology of Typhus Exanthematous in Recent Years. (*Parl. Papers,* 1914–16, Vol. 25.)

Vaccination. Reports of the Royal Commission on the Subject of Vaccination (*Parl. Papers,* 1889–1896.)

Reports of the Select Committee on the Operation of the Vaccination Act, 1867. (*Parl. Papers,* 1871, Vol. 13.)

5. Contemporary Periodical Publications*

The British Medical Journal. The Journal of the British Medical Association. 1865–1912.

The Doctor. A Monthly Review of the British and Foreign Medical Practice and Literature. 1871–1878.

The Hospital. Journal of the Hospitals Association (London).

Journal of the American Medical Association.

The Journal of Hygiene. 1901–1911.

The Journal of the Royal Sanitary Institute of Great Britain.

The Journal of the Royal Statistical Society.

The Journal of the Social Sciences.

The Journal of State Medicine. The Official Organ of the British Institute of Public Health.

The Lancet. A Journal of British and Foreign Medicine, Surgery, Obstetrics, Physiology, Chemistry, Pharmacology, Public Health, and News. 1865–1912.

The Medical Press and Circular. 1868–1875.

The Medical Times and Gazette. A Journal of Medical Science, Literature, Criticism, and News. 1869–1875.

The Practitioner. A Monthly Journal of Therapeutics, 1868–1871.

Public Health. The Journal of the Medical Officers of Health. 1888–1911.

Macmillan's Magazine.

Punch.

Scientific Opinion. A Weekly Record of Scientific Progress at Home and Abroad. 1869–1870.

The Times (London).

6. Contemporary Reports, Records, and Transactions of Societies and Organizations and Special Conferences

BRITISH ASSOCIATIONS FOR THE ADVANCEMENT OF SCIENCE. *Transactions,* 1870–1890.

BRITISH MEDICAL ASSOCIATION. Reports of annual meetings and other topical reports of the Association have been used as they appear in the *British Medical Journal,* 1865–1911, and special supplementary issues.

————. *Interim Report of the Insurance Acts Committee on the Future of the Insurance Acts.* Supplement to the *British Medical Journal,* June 23, 1917.

————. *Report of the Special Poor Law Reform Committee.* Supplement to the *British Medical Journal,* November 13, 1909.

————. *Investigation Into the Economic Conditions of Contract Practice in the United Kingdom.* Supplement to the *British Medical Journal,* July 22, 1905.

CHARITY ORGANIZATION SOCIETY. *Miscellaneous Papers.* 1870ff. (Pamphlet File in the British Museum.)

* Where the years of issue are not specified, only occasional references in these periodicals have been used in topical reference.

INTERNATIONAL HEALTH EXHIBITION, 1884. *Records.* 19 vols. London: William Clowes & Son, 1884. A single volume edition of *Papers and Discussion Records* has also been used.

LOCAL MEDICAL SOCIETIES. (Reports of meetings as they appear in the *British Medical Journal* and *The Lancet*).

MANCHESTER AND SALFORD SANITARY ASSOCIATION. *Committee Reports.* 1853–1863. (File at the London School of Economics and Political Science Library.)

MEDICAL OFFICERS OF HEALTH, SOCIETY OF. *Transactions* and *Annual Reports,* 1874–1887.

MEDICAL SOCIETY OF LONDON. *Proceedings and Transactions.* 1872–1900. London: John Langton, 1911.

NATIONAL ASSOCIATION FOR THE PROMOTION OF SOCIAL SCIENCE. *Transactions.* 1871–1884. London: Longmans, Green & Co.

TOWN PLANNING CONFERENCE, OCTOBER 1910. *Transactions.* Royal Institute of British Architects.

II. SECONDARY SOURCES

A. BIOGRAPHIES, OBITUARIES, MEMOIRS.

ALLEN, BERNARD M. *Sir Robert Morant. A Great Public Servant.* London: Macmillan & Co., 1934.

AMERY, JULIAN. *The Life of Joseph Chamberlain.* Vol. IV (1901–1903), London: Macmillan & Co., 1951.

ASHWORTH UNDERWOOD, E. "Charles Crieghton, M.A. M.D. (1847–1927): Scholar, Historian and Epidemiologist," *Proceedings of the Royal Society of Medicine,* XLI (1948), 869–876.

ATLAY, JAMES B. *Sir Henry Wentworth Acland, Bart., K.C.B., F.R.S., A Memoir.* London: Smith, Elder Co., 1903.

BROCKWAY, ARCHIBALD FENNER. *Bermondsey Story: The Life of Alfred Salter.* London: Allen & Unwin, Ltd. 1949.

BROOK, CHARLES. *Battling Surgeon.* Glasgow: The Strickland Press, 1945.
———. *Thomas Wakley.* London: Socialist Medical Association, 1962.

CHARLES, JOHN. "Presidential Address on John Simon and Some Contemporaries—A Brief Retrospect," *Journal of the Royal Sanitary Institute,* LXXI (July 1951), 286–295.

CHURCHILL, EDWARD D. *To Work in the Vineyard of Surgery, The Reminiscences of J. Collins Warner, 1842–1927.* Cambridge: Harvard University Press, 1958.

COLLINS, SIR WILLIAM. *The Life and Doctrine of Sir Edwin Chadwick.* Surrey: The Chadwick Trust, 1924.

COPE, ZACHARY. *Florence Nightingale and the Doctors.* London: Museum Press, 1958.

DAVIES, WILLIAM W. *Lloyd George, 1863–1914.* London: Constable & Co. Ltd., 1939.

Dictionary of National Biography. Edited by Leslie Stephen. London: Smith, Elder & Co., 1885–.

FINER, S. E. *The Life and Times of Edwin Chadwick.* London: Metheun & Co., 1952.

FLEXNER, SIMON AND JAMES T. FLEXNER. *William Henry Welch and the Heroic Age of American Medicine.* New York: The Viking Press, 1941.

FRAZER, WILLIAM M. *Duncan of Liverpool, Being an Account of the Work of Dr. W. H. Duncan, Medical Officer of Health of Liverpool, 1847–1863.* London: Hamish Hamilton Medical Books, 1947.

GARVIN, J. L. *The Life of Joseph Chamberlain.* 3 vols. London: Macmillan & Co., 1935–. (Continued in Amery, J. with Vol. 4.)

GODLEE, RICKMAN J. *Lord Lister.* 3rd rev. ed. Oxford: Clarendon Press, 1924.

GOODALL, EDWARD W. *William Budd.* Bristol: Arrowsmith, 1936.

GREENWOOD, MAJOR. *Some British Pioneers of Social Medicine.* University of London, Heath Clark Lectures, 1946. London: Oxford University Press, 1948.

GWYNN, STEPHEN AND GERTRUDE TUCKWELL. *The Life of the Right Honourable Sir Charles W. Dilke, Bart., M.P.* 2 vols. London: John Murray, 1917.

HALE-WHITE, WILLIAM. *Great Doctors of the Nineteenth Century.* London: E. Arnold & Co., 1935.

HAMMOND, J. L. AND BARBARA. *James Stansfeld. A Victorian Champion of Sex Equality.* London: Longmans, Green & Co., 1932.

HAWEIS, H. R. *Sir Morell Mackenzie, Physician and Operator, A Memoir.* London: W. H. Allen & Co., 1893.

LEWES, GERTRUDE. *Doctor Southwood Smith, A Retrospect.* Edinburgh: Blackwood, 1898.

LEWIS, RICHARD, A. *Edwin Chadwick and the Public Health Movement, 1832–1854.* London: Longmans, Green & Co., 1952.

LEYLAND, JOHN. *Contemporary Medical Men and Their Professional Work.* 2 vols. Leicester: Offices of the *Provincial Medical Journal,* 1888.

LITTLE, E. M. "Ernest Hart: A Study of Character," November 1924. (Photostat of a 14-page typed manuscript in the Library of the Royal Society of Medicine.)

Lives of the Fellows of the Royal College of Physicians of London, Munk's Roll.

MACNALTY, ARTHUR. *A Biography of Sir Benjamin Ward Richardson, 1828–1896.* London: Harvey & Blythe Ltd., 1950.

———. "Sir John Burdon Sanderson," *Proceedings of the Royal Society of Medicine,* XLVII (1954), 754–758.

MARKHAM, VIOLET. *May Tenant. A Portrait.* London: Falcon Press, 1949.

McCRACKEN, IAN E. "How Sir John Simon Entered the Public Health Service," *Medical Officer,* LXXX (1948), 157–158.

McIlwain, Henry. "Thudichum and the Medical Chemistry of the 1860's to 1880's," *Proceedings of the Royal Society of Medicine,* vol. 51, pp. 5–10.

Masterman, Lucy. *C F. G. Masterman, A Biography.* London: Nicholson & Watson, 1939.

Newman, George. Obituary of, in the *British Medical Journal,* June 5, 1948, pp. 1112–1113.

Newsholme, Arthur. Obituary: "The Life Work of Sir John Simon," *Journal of Hygiene,* V (Jan., 1905), 1–6.

Oliver, Wade Wright. *The Man Who Lived for Tomorrow, A Biography of William Hallock Park, M. D.* New York: E. P. Dutton & Co., 1941.

Paget, Stephen. *Sir Victor Horsley. A Study of His Life and Work.* London: Constable & Co., 1919.

Plarr, Victor G. "The Late Sir John Simon" (Letter to the Editors), *The Lancet,* August 13, 1904, pp. 488–489.

Raine, G. E. *The Real Lloyd George.* London: George Allen & Co., 1913.

Reid, Wemyss. *Memoirs and Correspondence of Lyon Playfair.* London: Cassell & Co., 1899.

Sanderson, John Burdon. "[Obituary of] Sir John Simon, 1816–1904," *Proceedings of the Royal Society of London,* LXXV (1905), 336–346.

Simon, John. Anonymous Obituary of Simon. *Transactions of the Epidemiological Society of London,* New Series, XXIII (1903–1904), 253–258.

Smith, Alice L. *A Memoir of the Buchanan Family, and in Particular of George Buchanan.* Aberdeen: printed privately at the Aberdeen University Press, 1941.

Smith, Frank. *The Life and Work of Sir James Kay-Shuttleworth.* London: John Murray, 1923.

Spender, Harold. *The Prime Minister.* New York: George Doran & Co., 1920.

Sprigge, Samuel Squire. *The Life and Times of Thomas Wakley, Founder and First Editor of the Lancet.* London: Longmans, Green & Co., 1897.

Stamp, Winifred. *Doctor Himself, An Unorthodox Biography of Harry Roberts, 1871–1946.* London: Hamish Hamilton, 1949.

Stokes, William. *His Life and Work, by his Son, William Stokes.* London: T. Fisher Unwin, 1898.

Thudichum, J. L. W. "Obituary, J. L. W. Thudichum, M.D., F.R.C.P., *British Medical Journal,* II (Sept. 14, 1901), 726.

West, Algernon. *Contemporary Portraits.* London: Thomas Nelson & Sons, 1920.

Woodham Smith, Cecil. *Florence Nightingale, 1820–1910.* London: Constable, 1950.

B. GENERAL HISTORICAL AND TOPICAL STUDIES

Anderson, Odin. "Health Insurance in the United States, 1910–1920," *J. Hist. Med. and Allied Sciences,* V (1950), 363–396.

ASCHROTT, PAUL F. *The English Poor Law System, Past and Present.* London: Knight & Co., 1888.

ASHWORTH UNDERWOOD, E. "The Fieldworkers in the English Public Health Movement, 1847–75," *Bull. Soc. of the Hist. of Med. of Chicago,* VI (1948), 31–48.

BARNES, HARRY. *The Slum, Its Story and Solution.* London: P. S. King, 1931.

BEALES, H. L. *The Making of Social Policy.* Hobhouse Memorial Trust Lecture No. 15, delivered on 23 May 1945. London: Oxford University Press, 1946.

BECK, ANN. "The British Medical Council and British Medical Education in the Nineteenth Century," *Bull. Hist. Med.,* XXX (Mar.–Apr., 1956), 150–162.

BICKERTON, THOMAS H. *A Medical History of Liverpool From the Earliest Days to the Year 1920.* London: John Murray, 1936.

BLAKE, JOHN B. "Scientific Institutions Since the Renaissance, Their Role in Medical Research," *Proceedings of the American Philosophical Society,* Vol. 101 (1957), pp. 31–62.

BRAND, JEANNE L. "The British Medical Profession and State Intervention in Public Health, 1870–1911." Ph.D. dissertation, University of London, 1953.

———. "The Parish Doctor: England's Poor Law Medical Officers and Medical Reform, 1870–1900," *Bull. Hist. Med.,* XXXV (Mar.–Apr., 1961), 97–122.

———. "John Simon and the Local Government Board Bureaucrats: 1871–1876," *Bull. Hist. Med., XXXVII* (Mar.–Apr., 1963), 184–194.

BREND, WILLIAM A. *Health and the State.* London: Constable & Co., 1917.

BRIGGS, ASA. *The Age of Improvement.* London: Longmans, Green & Co., 1959.

———. *A Study of the Work of Seebohm Rowntree, 1871–1954.* London: Longmans, Green & Co., 1961.

———. *Victorian People, Some Reassessments of People, Institutions, Ideas and Events, 1851–1867.* London: Oldhams Press Ltd., 1954.

BRINTON, CLARENCE CRANE. *English Political Thought in the Nineteenth Century.* London: E. Benn Ltd., 1933.

BROCKBANK, EDWARD. *A Centenary History of the Manchester Medical Society.* Manchester: Sherratt & Hughes, 1934.

BROCKINGTON, COLIN FRASER. *Medical Officers of Health, 1848 to 1855, An Essay in Local History.* London: Hodgetts Ltd., 1957.

———. "Public Health at the Privy Council, 1858–1871," a series of articles published in *The Medical Officer,* Mar.–May, 1959.

———. *A Short History of Public Health.* London: J & A Churchill Ltd., 1956.

BRUCE, MAURICE. *The Coming of the Welfare State.* London: B. T. Batsford Ltd., 1961.

BUER, M. C. *Health, Wealth and Population in the Early Days of the Industrial Revolution.* London: G. Routledge & Sons, 1926.

BULLOCH, WILLIAM. *The History of Bacteriology*. London: Oxford University Press, 1938.

BURROW, JAMES G. *A.M.A., Voice of American Medicine*, Baltimore: The Johns Hopkins Press, 1963.

CARR (A. S. COMYNS), GARNETT (W. H. STUART), AND J. H. TAYLOR. *National Insurance*. 3rd ed. London: Macmillan & Co., 1912.

CARR-SAUNDERS, A. M. AND P. A. WILSON. *The Professions*. Oxford: Clarendon Press, 1933.

CASSEDY, JAMES H. "Hygeia: A Mid-Victorian Dream of a City of Health," *Journal of the History of Medicine and Allied Sciences*, XVII (Apr. 1962), 217–228.

CHARLES, JOHN. *Research and Public Health*. The Heath Clark Lectures, 1959. London: Oxford University Press, 1961.

CLAPHAM, J. H. *The Economic History of Modern Britain: Free Trade and Steel, 1850–1886*. Cambridge: University Press, 1952.

COLE, G. D. H. *A Short History of the British Working Class Movement, 1789–1947*. Rev. ed. London: Allen & Unwin Ltd., 1948.

CONNAN, D. M. *A History of the Public Health Department in Bermondsey*. Greenwich: Henry Richardson, 1935.

CREIGHTON, CHARLES. *A History of Epidemics in Britain, 1668–1893*. 2 vols. Cambridge: Cambridge University Press, 1891–94.

CRICHTON-BROWNE, JAMES. *Physical Efficiency in Children*. London: King, 1902.

DELMEGE, J. ANTHONY. *Towards National Health*. London: William Heinemann, 1931.

DICEY, A. V. *Lectures on the Relation Between Law and Public Opinion in England During the Nineteenth Century*. London: Macmillan & Co., 1948.

DJANG, TIEN KAI. *Factory Inspection in Great Britain*. London: Allen & Unwin, 1942.

DUDFIELD, REGINALD. "History of the Society of Medical Officers of Health," Jubilee Number of *Public Health,* 1906.

DUKES, CLEMENT. *Health At School, Considered in Its Mental, Moral and Physical Aspects*. 4th rev. ed. London: Rivington, 1905.

ECKSTEIN, HARRY H. "The Politics of the British Medical Association," *Political Quarterly*, XXVI (Oct.–Dec., 1955), 345–359.

ENSOR, R. C. K. *England 1870–1914*. Oxford: Clarendon Press, 1936.

FERGUSON, THOMAS. *The Dawn of Scottish Social Welfare*. London, New York: Thomas Nelson & Sons, 1948.

FISHBEIN, MORRIS. *A History of the American Medical Association 1847 to 1947*. Philadelphia & London: W. B. Saunders Co., 1947.

FRAZER, WILLIAM M. *A History of English Public Health, 1834–1939*. London: Bailliere, Tindall and Cox, 1950.

GALDSTON, IAGO. *The Meaning of Social Medicine*. Cambridge, Mass.: Published for the Commonwealth Fund by Harvard University Press, 1954.

GALE, ARTHUR HAROLD. *Epidemic Diseases.* London: Penguin Books, 1959.

GREENWOOD, MAJOR. *The Law Relating to Poor Law Medical Service and Vaccination.* London: Bailliere, Tindall & Cox, 1901.

HALEVY, ELIE. *A History of the English People, 1895–1905 (Imperialism and the Rise of Labour).* London: E. Benn Ltd., 1951.

HAMILTON, BERNICE. "The Medical Professions in the Eighteenth Century," *Economic History Review,* IV, No. 2 (1951), 141–169.

HARRIS, R. W. *National Health Insurance in Great Britain, 1911–1946.* London: Allen & Unwin Ltd., 1946.

HASSALL, A. H. *Food and Its Adulteration.* London: Longmans Brown, Green & Longmans, 1855.

HAYEK, FREDRICK A. VON (ed.). *Capitalism and the Historians.* Chicago: University of Chicago Press, 1954.

HODGKINSON, RUTH G. "The Medical Services of the New Poor Law, 1834–1871." 2 vols. Ph. D. dissertation, University of London, 1950.

———. "Poor Law Medical Officers of England, 1834–1871," *J. Hist. Med. and Allied Sciences,* II (1956), 299–338.

HOGARTH, A. H. *Medical Inspection of Schools.* Oxford, London: Henry Frowde, Hodder & Stoughton, 1909.

HOHMAN, H. F. *The Development of Social Insurance and Minimum Wage Legislation in Great Britain.* Boston: Houghton Mifflin Co., 1933.

HORNER, NORMAN G. *The Growth of the General Practitioner of Medicine in England.* London: Bridge & Co. for the Author, 1922.

HOWELL, GEORGE M. P. *Conflicts of Capital and Labour, Being A History and Review of the Trade Unions of Great Britain.* 2nd rev. ed. London: Macmillan & Co., 1890.

HUNTER, DONALD. *Health in Industry.* Harmondsworth: Penguin Books, 1959.

HURWITZ, SAMUEL J. *State Intervention in Great Britain. A Study of Economic Control and Social Response, 1914–1919.* New York: Columbia University press, 1949.

HUTCHINS, B. L. *The Public Health Agitation, 1833–1848.* London: A. C. Fifield, 1909.

———. "What a Health Committee Can Do," *Fabian Tracts,* No. 148, 1910.

HUTCHINS, B. L. AND A. HARRISON. *A History of Factory Legislation.* 2nd rev. ed. London: The London School of Economics and Political Science Studies, No. 10, 1911.

HUTCHINSON, J. R. "An Historical Note on the Prevention of Smallpox in England and the Foundation of the Government Lymph Establishment," in *Annual Report, Ministry of Health for the Year Ending 31 Mar. 1946,* Appendix A.

INTERNATIONAL LABOUR OFFICE. "Voluntary Sickness Insurance," in *Studies and Reports, Series M (Social Insurance),* No. 7. Geneva, 1925–40.

JEWKES, JOHN AND SYLVIA. *The Genesis of the British National Health Service.* 2nd ed. Oxford: Basil Blackwell, 1961.

JONES, DORSEY P. *Edwin Chadwick and the Early Public Health Movement in England.* Iowa City: Iowa University Press, 1929.

KEEVIL, JOHN JOYCE. *Medicine and the Navy, 1200–1900.* Vol. 4: *1815–1900* by Christopher Lloyd and Jack L. S. Coulter. Edinburgh: E & S Livingstone, 1963.

KEITH-LUCAS, B. "Some influences Affecting the Development of Sanitary Legislation in England," *Economic History Review,* IV (Apr., 1954). 290–296.

KELYNACK, T. N. (ed.). *Medical Examination of Schools and Scholars.* London: P. S. King & Son, 1910.

KRAMER, HOWARD D. "Agitation for Public Health Reform in the 1870's," *J. Hist. Med.,* Vol. 3 (1948), pp. 473–488; Vol. 4 (1949), pp. 75–89.

————. "The Beginnings of the Public Health Movement in the United States." *Bull. Hist. Med.* XXI (1947), 352–76.

————. "The Germ Theory and the Early Public Health Program in the United States," *Bull. Hist. Med.,* XXII (May–June, 1948), 233–247.

LAMBERT, ROYSTON J. "Central and Local Relations in Mid-Victorian England: The Local Government Act Office, 1853–71," *Victorian Studies,* IV (December, 1962), 121–150.

————. *Sir John Simon, 1816–1904, and English Social Administration.* London: Macgibbon & Kee Ltd., 1963.

————. "A Victorian National Health Service: State Vaccination," *The Historical Journal,* V, No. 1 (1962), 1–18.

LEIPER, R. T. *Periodicals of Medicine and the Allied Sciences in British Libraries.* London: British Medical Association, 1923.

LEVY, HERMAN. *National Health Insurance, A Critical Study.* Cambridge: Cambridge University Press, 1944.

LINDSEY, ALMONT. *Socialized Medicine in England and Wales, The National Health Service, 1948–1961.* Chapel Hill: University of North Carolina Press, 1962.

LITTLE, ERNEST M. *A History of the British Medical Association, 1832–1932.* London: British Medical Association, 1932.

LOVEGROVE, PETER. *Not Least in the Crusade, A Short History of the Royal Army Medical Corps.* Aldershot: Gale and Polden Ltd., 1952.

LYNCH, MATHEW J. AND STANLEY S. RAPHAEL. *Medicine and the State.* Springfield, Ill.: Thomas, 1963.

MACKAY, THOMAS. *A History of the English Poor Law,* Vol. III (Supplementary Volume to G. Nicholls, *A History of the English Poor Law*). London: P. S. King & Sons, 1898.

————. *Public Relief of the Poor, Six Lectures.* London: John Murray, 1901.

MACKINTOSH, JAMES M. *Housing and Family Life.* London: Cassell & Co., 1952.

————. *Trends of Opinion About the Public Health, 1901–1951.* London: Oxford University Press, 1953.

MACNALTY, ARTHUR S. *The History of State Medicine in England, Being the*

Fitzpatrick Lectures of the Royal College of Physicians of London for 1946 and 1947. London: Royal Institute of Public Health and Hygiene, 1948.

McLEARY, GEORGE F. *The Early History of the Infant Welfare Movement.* London: H. K. Lewis, 1933.

————. *The Maternity and Child Welfare Movement.* London: P. S. King & Sons, 1935.

————. *National Health Insurance.* London: H. K. Lewis, 1932.

McDONALD, J. C. "The History of Quarantine in Britain During the Nineteenth Century," *Bull. Hist. Med.* XXV (1951), 22–44.

MEACHEN, G. NORMAN. *A Short History of Tuberculosis.* London: John Bale, Sons & Danielsson Ltd., 1936.

MESS, H. A. *Factory Legislation and Its Administration, 1891–1924.* (London School of Economics Studies in Economics and Political Science No. 84). P. S. King Ltd., 1926.

MOORE, NORMAN AND PAGET. *The Royal Medical and Chirurgical Society, 1805–1905.* London: Royal Medical and Chirurgical Society, 1905.

MOWAT, CHARLES LOCH. *The Charity Organization Society, 1869–1913; Its Ideas and Work.* London: Methuen, 1961.

NEWMAN, CHARLES. *The Evolution of Medical Education in the Nineteenth Century.* London, New York: Oxford University Press, 1957.

NEWMAN, TOM SETH. *The Story of Friendly Societies and Social Security, Past, Present and Future.* London: Hearts of Oak Benefit Society, 1945.

NICHOLLS, GEORGE. *A History of the English Poor Law.* 2 vols., new ed. London: P. S. King, 1900.

OAKESHOTT, JOSEPH, P. *The Humanizing of the Poor Law.* London: The Fabian Society, 1897.

OTTAWAY, THOMAS. *The Law and Practice Relating to Coroners.* London: Butterworth & Co., 1927.

"Our Medical Officers of Health," A Study of the Medical Officer of Health of the Larger Towns in the 'Seventies' by the Students of the History Seminar, London School of Hygiene and Tropical Medicine, 1947–1948, *Public Health,* LXI (Aug. 1948), pp. 210–213.

PATRICK, ADAMS. *The Enteric Fevers, 1800–1920* [Being the Sydney Watson Smith Lecture for 1954, Royal College of Physicians of Edinburgh.] Edinburgh: Royal College of Physicians, 1955.

POWER, D'ARCY (ed.). *British Medical Societies.* London Medical Press and Circular, 1939.

PYKE-LEES, WALTER. *Centenary of the General Medical Council, 1858–1958: The History and Present Work of the Council.* London: Spottiswoode, Ballantyne & Co., 1958.

RAVENEL, M. P. (ed.). *A Half Century of Public Health,* Jubilee Historical Volume of the American Public Health Association. New York: American Public Health Association, 1921.

ROBSON, WILLIAM A. *The Development of Local Government.* London: Allen & Unwin Ltd., 1931.

————. *From Patronage to Proficiency in the Public Service*. London: Fabian Society, 1922.

ROLLESTON, HUMPHREY. "The History of *The Practitioner*," *The Practitioner*, CL (June, 1943), 321–328.

ROSEN, GEORGE. *A History of Public Health*. New York: M.D. Publications, Inc., 1958.

————. "Carl Ludwig and his American Students," *Bulletin of the Institute for the History of Medicine*, Vol. 4 (1936), pp. 609–650.

ROSS, JAMES STIRLING. *The National Health Service in Great Britain, An Historical and Descriptive Study*. London: Oxford University Press, 1952.

ROWLETTE, ROBERT J. *The Medical Press and Circular, 1839–1939, A Hundred Years in the Life of a Medical Journal*. London: Medical Press and Circular, 1939.

RUBINOW, I. M. *Social Insurance with Special Reference to American Conditions*. New York: Henry Holt & Co., 1913.

SAVAGE, WILLIAM C. *Rural Housing*. London: T. Fisher Unwin, 1915.

SHRYOCK, RICHARD H. *American Medical Research, Past & Present*, New York: Commonwealth Fund, 1947.

————. *The Development of Modern Medicine: An interpretation of the Social and Scientific Factors Involved*. 2nd ed. New York: Alfred Knopf, 1947.

SIGERIST, HENRY E. *American Medicine*. New York: W. W. Norton & Co., 1934.

————. *Civilization and Disease*. Ithaca: Cornell University Press, 1944.

————. "From Bismarck to Beveridge, Developments and Trends in Social Security Legislation," *Bull. Hist. Med.*, XIII (Apr., 1943), 365–388.

————. *Great Doctors, A Biographical History of Medicine*. London: Allen & Unwin Ltd., 1933.

————. *Landmarks in the History of Hygiene*, Heath Clark Lectures, University of London 1952. London: Geoffrey Cumberlege–Oxford University Press, 1956.

————. *Man and Medicine. An Introduction to Medical Knowledge*. Translated by M. G. Boise. New York: W. W. Norton & Co., Inc., 1932.

————. *Medicine and Health in the Soviet Union*. New York: Citadel Press, 1947.

SIMONS, ALGIE AND NATHAN SINAI. *The Way of Health Insurance*. Chicago: University of Chicago Press, 1932.

SMELLIE, K. B. *A History of Local Government*, Rev. ed., London: Allen & Unwin Ltd., 1949.

————. *A Hundred Years of English Government*. London: Duckworth, 1937.

SMILLIE, WILSON G. *Public Health, its Promise for the Future; a chronicle of the development of public health in the U.S., 1607–1914*. New York: Macmillan, 1955.

SPRIGGE, SAMUEL. *Medicine and the Public*. London: William Heinemann, 1905.

STERN, BERNHARD J. *Medical Services by Government, Local, State and Federal.* New York: The Commonwealth Fund, 1946.

SUMMERVILLE, D. C. *British Politics Since 1900.* London: Andrew Dakers Ltd., 1950.

TELEKY, LUDWIG. *History of Factory and Mine Hygiene.* New York: Columbia University Press, 1948.

VAUGHAN, PAUL. *Doctors' Commons, A Short History of the British Medical Association.* London: William Heinemann, 1959.

WALTON, W. S. "The History of the Society of Medical Officers of Health, 1856–1956," *Public Health,* Vol. 69 (May, 1956), pp. 160–226.

WEBB, SIDNEY AND BEATRICE. *English Poor Law History: The Last Hundred Years.* 2 Vols. London: Longmans, Green Co., 1931.

WHITE, BRIAN D. *A History of the Corporation of Liverpool, 1835–1914.* Liverpool: University Press, 1951.

WILLIAMS, HARLEY. *A Century of Public Health in Britain, 1832–1929.* London: A & C. Black, 1932.

WILLIAMS, HUNTINGTON. "The Influence of Edwin Chadwick on American Public Health," *Medical Officer,* Vol. 95 (1956), pp. 273–279.

WILLIAMS, RALPH CHESTER. *The United States Public Health Service, 1798–1950.* Washington, D.C.: Commissioned Officers Association of the U.S. Public Health Service, 1951.

WILLIS, W. ADDINGTON. *National Health Insurance Through Approved Societies: Being A Practical Legal Treatise Incorporating the Operative Orders and Regulations.* London: University of London Press by Hodder & Stoughton, 1914.

WILSON, NORMAN. *Municipal Health Services.* London: Allen & Unwin Ltd., 1946.

———. *Public Health Services.* London: William Hodge & Co., 1938.

WINSLOW, C. E. A. *The Evolution and Significance of the Modern Public Health Campaign.* New Haven: Yale University Press, 1923.

"Workhouse Infirmaries." *MacMillan's Magazine,* July, 1881.

Index

Aberdeen, 62

Acland, Sir Henry W. D.: Royal Sanitary Commission, 11; and Public Health Act (1872), 18; on cholera, 41; on central versus local government, 81; on Army medicine, 137; on national health, 150

Acts of Parliament: Adulteration (1860, 1872), 4, 69, 131, 132. Alkali (1863, 1874), 4, 130. Artizans and Labourers' Dwellings (1868), 16. Artizans and Labourers' Dwellings Improvement (1875), 128. Bakehouse Regulation (1822, 1836), 16. Burials (1852), 4. Children (1908), 178. Common Lodging Houses (1848–52), 16. Contagious Diseases (1864, 1866), 16, 64, 134, 135, 141. Cross' (Housing) (1875, 1879), 122. Diseases Prevention (1883), 45, 119, 254 n29. Education (1870), 183; (1902), 166. Education (Administrative Provisions) (1907), 171, 186, 189. Education (Provision of Meals) (1906), 185, 189. Factory, 4, 166; (1844), 143; (1878, 1889), 128. Factories and Workshops (1867), 126; (1891, 1895), 128. Franchise (1867), 7. Health and Morals of Apprentices (1802), 126. Housing and Town Planning (1909), 167. Housing of the Working Classes (1885), 35, 124; (1890), 124, 125. Infant Life Protection (1872, 1897), 178. Infectious Diseases Notification (1889), 62–63, 117; (1899), 62, 118. Infectious Diseases Prevention (1890), 112. Isolation Hospitals (1893), 52. Labouring Classes Lodging Houses (1851, 1853), 4, 124. Local Government (Board) (1871), 14, 15, 18, 19, 109, 162. Medical (1858), 88, 142, 148, 163; (1886), 142, 143, 148, 162, 163. Medical Relief Disqualification Removal, (1885), 119. Metropolis Management (1855), 102. Metropolitan Poor (1867), 87, 95, 100. Midwives (1902), 179, 183. National Health Service (1946), 241. National Insurance (1911), 171, 174, 176, 209–32, 271 n17. Notification of Births (1907), 181, 183. Nuisances Removal (1855, 1860, 1863), 4, 16, 19, 68, 130. Old Age Pensions (1908), 210, 211, 216. Parliament (1911), 210. Pharmacy (1868), 4. Poor Law (1889), 95. Poor Law Amendment (1834), 5, 85, 103. Public Health (1848), 3, 19; (1859), 19; (1872), 15, 18, 19, 69, 71, 108, 110; (1875), 18, 19, 20, 51, 113, 122, 130, 135, 175; (1896), 4. Public Health (London) (1891), 95, 119, 133. Sale of Food and Drugs (1899), 132, 133. Lord Salisbury's (school fees) (1891), 183. Sanitary (1866), 5, 6, 9, 19; (1868), 19; (1870), 19. Sewage Utilization (1865), 19. Smoke Abatement, 130. Torrens (housing) (1868), 122, 124. Unemployed Workmen (1905), 209. Workmen's Compensation (1897), 166

Adderley, Sir Charles, First Baron Norton, 10, 14

Addison, Dr. Christopher, 221–30 *passim*

Admiralty, 24

Adulteration of food and drugs, 131–32, 135, 156, 162

Afghan Wars, 139

Air Pollution, 12, 54, 131. *See also* Alkali Acts; Smoke Abatement Acts

Albert, Prince Consort of England, 14n

Albutt, Sir T. Clifford, 225

Aldershot, 140

Alexander II, Czar of Russia, 212

Alison, Dr. William Pulteney, 110

Allan, Dr. Francis J., 129

American Association for Labor Legislation, 239, 240

American Medical Association, 238–40

American Public Health Association, 5

Anesthetics: and Snow, 40; in poor law care, 105; in Army medicine, 139; chloroform inhaler, 153; in surgery, 190–91

Anthrax, 78, 79, 128, 145

Antiseptic procedures, 191